Recent Advances in
Otolaryngology
Head and Neck Surgery

Recent Advances in
Otolaryngology
Head and Neck Surgery

Anil K Lalwani MD
Professor of Otolaryngology and
Vice-Chair for Research,
Director of Division of Otology
Director of the Columbia Cochlear Implant Program,
Columbia University
College of Physicians and Surgeons
New York, USA

Markus HF Pfister MD
Otolaryngologist
Sarnen, Switzerland

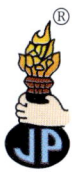

JAYPEE BROTHERS MEDICAL PUBLISHERS (P) LTD

New Delhi • Panama City • London

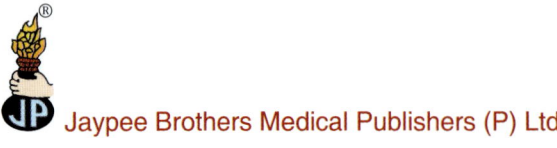

Jaypee Brothers Medical Publishers (P) Ltd.

Headquarter

Jaypee Brothers Medical Publishers (P) Ltd
4838/24, Ansari Road, Daryaganj
New Delhi 110 002, India
Phone: +91-11-43574357
Fax: +91-11-43574314
Email: jaypee@jaypeebrothers.com

Overseas Offices

J.P. Medical Ltd.,
83 Victoria Street London
SW1H 0HW (UK)
Phone: +44-2031708910
Fax: +02-03-0086180
Email: info@jpmedpub.com

Jaypee-Highlights Medical Publishers Inc.
City of Knowledge, Bld. 237, Clayton
Panama City, Panama
Phone: +50-73-010496
Fax: +50-73-010499
Email: cservice@jphmedical.com

Website: www.jaypeebrothers.com
Website: www.jaypeedigital.com

Recent Advances in Otolaryngology – Head and Neck Surgery
First Edition: 2012

ISBN 978-93-5025-790-6

Printed at Ajanta Offset & Packagings Ltd., New Delhi

Dedicated to

This book is dedicated to my parents, Madan and Gulab Lalwani; my in-laws, Rikhab and Ratan Bhansali; my children, Nikita and Sahil and most specially to my wife, Renu Bhansali Lalwani, a wonderful partner, friend, mother, community activist and the smartest internist I know!

Anil K Lalwani

To my parents, Ingeborg and Hermann Pfister; my uncle and aunt, Alfred and Isolde Demmler, and most specially to my beloved Doris, a wonderful partner and my center of inspiration.

Markus HF Pfister

International Editorial Board

Contributors

Abbas A Anwar
Medical student
New York University School of Medicine

Amin R Javer MD, FRCSC FARS
Director, St. Paul's Sinus Centre
Assistant Clinical Professor, UBC
ENT Clinic, 1081 Burrard Street,
Vancouver, V6Z 1Y6

Andrea Kleine-Punte
Research Audiologist
University Department
Otorhinolaryngology and Head and Neck
Surgery
Antwerp University, Belgium

Anthony Del Signore PHARM D MD
Resident
Otolaryngology and Head and Neck
Surgery
Mount Sinai School Of Medicine
New York, USA

Bert W O'Malley JR MD
Gabriel Tucker Professor and Chairman
Department of Otorhinolaryngology and
Head & Neck Surgery
Professor of Neurosurgery
Professor of Radiation Oncology
Professor of Dentistry
The University of Pennsylvania Health
System
3400 Spruce Street - 5 Ravdin
Philadelphia, PA 19104

Christian Pfeffer MD PHD
Research Fellow
Children's Hospital
Boston, MA, USA

Daniel H Coelho MD
Otology, Neurotology & Skull Base Surgery
Department of Otolaryngology - Head &
Neck Surgery
Virginia Commonwealth University
School of Medicine Richmond, VA USA

Dean M Toriumi MD
Professor
Division of Facial Plastic and
Reconstructive Surgery
Department of Otolaryngology and Head
& Neck Surgery
University of Illinois, Chicago

Dennis S Poe MD PHD
Associate Professor
Department of Otology and Laryngology
Harvard Medical School
Children's Hospital Boston, MA, USA

Fazil Apaydin MD
Professor
Department of Otorhinolaryngology
Ege University Medical Faculty, Bornova
35100, Izmir, Turkey

Frank Agada FRCS ED
Department of ENT, Head and Neck
Surgery
York Hospital
York, UK

Gerard P Reilly MB BCHIR
Department of ENT, Head and Neck
Surgery
York Hospital
York, UK

Gregory S Weinstein
Professor of Otorhinolaryngology
Head and Neck Surgery at the Hospital
University of Pennsylvania
Otorhinolaryngology
Head and Neck Surgery

Griet Mertens IAIN F HATHORN BSC, MBCHB,
DOHNS, PGCME, FRCSED (ORL-HNS)
Endoscopic Sinus and Skull Base Clinical
Fellow
St. Paul's Sinus Center, St. Paul's Hospital
Vancouver, British Columbia
Canada

Jason A Beyea MD PHD
PGY 4 - Otolaryngology Head and Neck
Surgery
University of Western Ontario
London Health Sciences Centre
800 Commissioners Road East
London, Ontario, Canada, N6A 5W9

Lorne S Parnes

Professor, Site Chief (University Hospital)
Professor, Department of Clinical Neuro-
logical Sciences
Schulich School of Medicine and Dentistry
University of Western Ontario
London
Ontario,Canada

Lucian Sulica MD

Director, Voice Disorders/Laryngology
Associate Professor
Department of Otorhinolaryngology
Weill Medical College of Cornell University
1305 York Avenue, 5th Floor
New York, NY 10021

Maurizio Barbara

Director Chair of Audiology
Sapienza University
Medicine and Psychology Faculty
Director From Sense Organs
UOC of Otolaryngology
St. Andrew's Hospital
Rome

Michael E. Hoffer CAPT MC USN

Director, Spatial Orientation Center
NMW EHR Clinical Champion
Department of Otolaryngology
Naval Medical Center San Diego
San Diego, CA 92134
(619) 532-8355

Niels Kokot MD

Assistant Professor
Department of Otolaryngology-Head and
Neck Surgery
Keck School of Medicine
University of Southern California
1520 San Pablo Street
Suite 4600
Los Angeles, CA 90033

Patrick C Angelos MD

Fellow, Facial Plastic and Reconstructive
Surgery
University of Illinois, Chicago

Paul Van de Heyning

Chairman
University Deptarment Otorhinolaryngol-
ogy and Head and Neck Surgery
Antwerp University Hospital (USA)
University of Antwerp, Belgium

Rodolfo Lugo Saldaña MD

Otolaryngologist
Associate Professor, Otolaryngology
Constitution ISSSTE Hospital, Monterrey
Snoring Clinic
Director, Nuevo León
México

Scott Rickert MD

Acting Director, Pediatric Otolaryngology
Director, Pediatric Voice Center
Assistant Professor
Department of Otolaryngology New York
University
Langone Medical Center

Simonetta Monini

Associate Professor of Audiology
Director of Audiology and Phoniatrics
(Center for the Facial Nerve Rehabilitation
Logopedic Phono)

Sumit K Agrawal MD

Assistant Professor
Department of Otolaryngology - Head
and Neck Surgery
Schulich School of Medicine and Dentistry
University of Western Ontario
London
Ontario, Canada

Thomas Kühnel

Prof. Dr. Med.
Consultant
ORL-Dept., Head and Neck Surgery,
University of Regensburg
Franz-Josef-Strauß-Allee 11
D-93042 Regensburg

Vivek Gurudutt

Assistant Professor
Otolaryngology
Mount Sinai Hospital
New York, USA

Yi-Ho Young MD, PHD

Professor
National Taiwan University Hospital
Taiwan, Japan

Preface

Otolaryngology—Head and Neck Surgery is a dynamic medical and surgical specialty characterized by rapid advances in its scientific foundation and of its therapeutic armamentarium. Simultaneously, there are novel technical and technological innovations that positively impact on patient care. Consequently, otolaryngology is constantly evolving as new knowledge comes forth, and new technologies become available. Recent examples of advances in otolaryngology include robotic surgery, implantable hearing aids, hybrid cochlear implant, vestibular evoked myogenic potential (VEMP) test and office-based laryngeal surgery, among others. The challenge for the busy clinician in the 21st century is to remain abreast of these ever expanding bodies of knowledge, surgical techniques, diagnostic test, imaging technology and prosthetics while being deeply immersed in their clinical practice. Ironically, this has become even more difficult with the explosion of technologies designed to put information at one's fingertips. It is with this in mind that we introduce this new annual periodical, Recent Advances in Otolaryngology—Head and Neck Surgery, to make it easy for the clinician to keep current with what is new. As its title suggests, it will cover all the subspecialties of otolaryngology. Due to its rapid publication cycle, the material will be current, topical and immediately relevant to the clinician. Reviews will emphasize clear artwork rendered in color to convey new concepts and surgical approaches. We have assembled an outstanding international editorial board to assist us in this exciting project. Similarly, invited authors are leaders in the field and have made seminal contributions in their topics. We hope that you will enjoy reading this new book as much as we have enjoyed assembling it.

Anil K Lalwani
Markus HF Pfister

Contents

Contents   **xv**

Chapter

1

TRANSTYMPANIC MEDICAL THERAPY

Michael E Hoffer and Daniel H Coelho

ABSTRACT

Transtympanic (TT) medical therapy is a technique in which medicine is delivered to the middle ear with the intention of treating inner ear disorders. This modality is attractive because it provides the ability to achieve a significant concentration of medicine in the inner ear while avoiding the systemic consequences of dosing the medicines by mouth or intravenous (IV). The therapy is also convenient in that it can be administered in an office setting. Despite these obvious advantages, a number of basic questions surround the use of this modality including the medicine of choice for each disorder, the ideal delivery device, the appropriate dose and dosing regimen, and the proper endpoint of therapy as well as the potential need for boosters. In this manuscript, we begin by examining the basic work that has been done on inner ear kinetics followed by a look at delivery devices. We then examine in detail the three most common disorders treated by TT therapy: Ménière's disease (MD), sudden sensorineural hearing loss (SSNHL) and tinnitus. With respect to MD, we examine the work on gentamicin and steroid therapy after a detailed discussion of the disorder. With sudden HL and tinnitus, we examine the controversies surrounding the use of steroids to treat these two disorders. TT medical therapy is becoming increasingly more common and is used to treat disorders where there are few other treatment options. As popularity increases, it is critically important to understand the science and the evidence that underscores this treatment modality.

INTRODUCTION

It is potentially beneficial to deliver medicines as close to the intended site of action as possible. Such a delivery achieves a higher concentration at the site of action while likely reducing systemic side effects. Eye drops and, for some disorders, local joint injections are two regularly utilized applications of this technology. Otolaryngologists treating ear disease have envied their ophthalmologic colleagues and spent a great deal of time and effort figuring out the best way to administer medicine as close to the inner ear as possible. Over the years, a variety of different terms have been adopted to describe such therapy including TT and intratympanic (IT). For the sake of this manuscript, these terms are synonyms and we will utilize the abbreviation TT to describe any application of medicine into the middle ear designed to work on the inner ear. There are a variety of other applications of TT technology including delivering gene products packaged in a virus with the intent of altering the gene activity of inner ear cells or delivering novel agents designed to promote cell growth or cell differentiation. While these are TT technologies, they are more speculative and go beyond the scope of this manuscript. In addition, the delivery of medicines directly to the inner ear (such as by a cochlear implant or during surgery) will also not be considered. Rather, we will confine ourselves to the more common and widely used medicines and disorders for which TT technology is usually employed. Despite a dedicated history of work in this area, several significant and essential questions have never been answered. Questions still exist about what disease entities should be treated with TT, the optimal mode of TT administration, the correct dose of medicine, the ideal dosing frequency, and the end point of therapy. In this manuscript, we will first examine the kinetics of drug delivery to the inner ear through the middle ear and then consider dosing technology since this topic applies equally to all the other sections of the manuscript. Then, we will examine a number of different disease entities and discuss TT medicines in these disorders. These disorders will include MD, SSNHL and tinnitus.

KINETICS

Inherent to the technique of TT medicine, application is the fact that the medicine must pass from the middle ear to the inner ear in order for the medicine to become active. In order for medicine to go from the middle ear to the inner ear, it must pass through the round window membrane (RWM). A number of factors govern the amount of medicine that passes through this membrane. Of course, the size of the particle is critical since no active transport across the round window has yet to be described. Also, of importance is the duration that the medicine is in contact with the round window. Depending on the delivery technique, this may or may not be equivalent to the duration that the medicine stays in the middle ear. Indeed, there are a number of techniques that attempt to control the presence of medicine at the round window over time. Another consideration is the concentration of the medicine at the round window. In this case, the delivery concentration and the amount of medicine already in the inner ear both have important contributions. Salt and colleagues described the steps involved in inner ear medicine transport.[1] In this work, Salt reported that the steps were: (1) Clearance of the medicine from the middle ear, (2) Permeability of the round window, and (3) Diffusion across the scala. As the medicine diffuses through the scala, there is clearance from the scala tympani, scale vestibulae, intrascala diffusion of medicine, and clearance from the vestiubule. The rate of clearance governs the concentration of medicine on the inner ear side. Because the speed of clearance cannot be changed, repeated or continuous dosing can result in higher levels but there seems to be a peak/ceiling in total inner ear concentration. Hoffer and colleagues used a small mammal model and demonstrated the patterns of uptake of gentamicin when medicine was administered to the middle ear via injection and via a sustained release vehicle.[2,3] Figure 1.1 is a model graph showing the data they obtained. As can be seen with either device, there is a large and rather quick uptake spike (at 2 hours or less) theoretically from the boost given by the pressure of the injection or the seating of the device right against the round window. This spike comes down and steady state peak levels occur between 18–24 hours with fall of by 48 hours (from a single injection) and persistence (at a slightly lower level) for as long as the sustained release is delivering medicines. Note should also be made that the error bars (discrepancy between absorption from one animal to the next) are quite large with TT injections. This is an important issue in TT medicine delivery. The inability to get a precise dosing level or rather the fact that imprecise dosing is the rule means that medicines with large therapeutic windows (work at a variety of dose levels) and low side effect profiles are the best choices for TT therapies. There are many reasons for this large difference in absorption into the inner ear. Amount of time the medicine comes in contact with the RWM, the shape of the round window niche and the presence of webs in that area

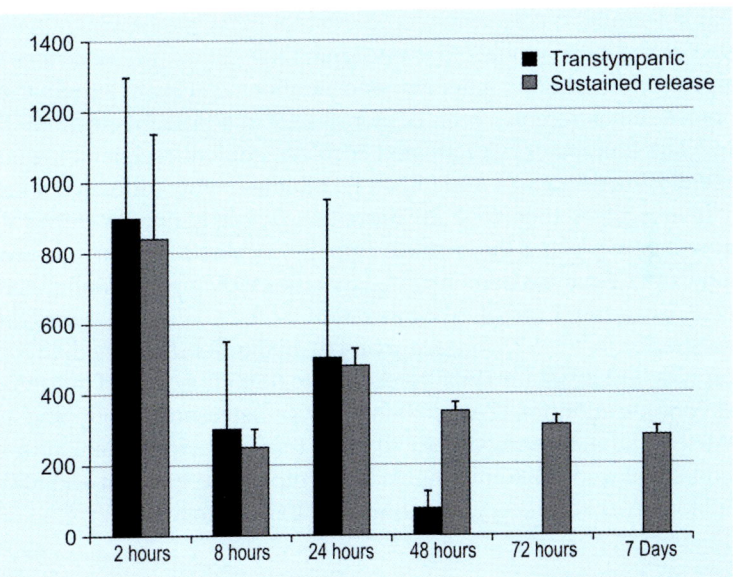

Fig. 1.1: Theoretical graph showing perilymph concentration of gentamicin after injection (dark bar) or via a sustained release device (light bar). Note the initial rapid rise for both modalities followed by a falling dose with stabilization at 24 hours. Virtually, all of the medicine given by injection is gone by 48 hours whereas the sustained release device can continue to deliver a consistent dose over time. Note should be made of the very large error bars particularly with the injection method

are all likely factors. In addition, Yoshioka demonstrated difference in the permeability of the RWM.[4] Their work suggested that almost 20% of RWM show poor or no absorption. Therefore, even with more precise control of the input of the medicine and maintenance in contact with the RWM, absorption may still vary. Also, important is the thin otic capsule in the mammalian models. Mikulec demonstrated that some of the middle ear medicine can actually absorb through the otic capsule in addition to the round window. This amount would vary from animal to animal and may or may not be important in humans due to our thicker otic capsules.[5] More recent work in this area suggested that sustained release devices differ from TT injections in other ways as well. Zou and colleagues studied the distribution of Gadolinium in the inner ear of rats after TT administration and found increase apex uptake after gelatin sponge administration as compared to simple TT injection.[6] The fate/distribution of medicine once entering the inner ear has been studied by a number of groups. Salt and colleagues demonstrated that the gradient for distribution of most drugs in the inner ear is determined by passive diffusion and as such the user has little control over medicine distribution.[7] Models in his lab confirmed Zou's observations that more apical distribution was likely to be facilitated by multiple injections or a sustained release vehicle. Clearance of the medicine from the inner ear has widely been accepted to occur via the blood and cerebrospinal fluid. However, Roehm demonstrated active detoxification of the cochlea via the spiral ganglion.[8] This detoxification was present with gentamicin as the active agent; it is unclear if a similar mechanism would exist for other medicines.

One of the philosophies that underpins the use of TT medicines is an attempt to achieve higher inner ear concentrations and lower systemic levels. This promise has recently been demonstrated in a brilliant study by Bird's group.[9] The investigators pretreated cochlear implant recipient with either IT of IV dexamethasone (4 mg/ml) 45–90 minutes before estimated sampling time. Investigators then took 20 micoliters of perilymph from the round window before placing the cochlear implant. A blood sample was taken at the same time. Analysis demonstrated that the median perilymph concentration was 0.016 mg/l for IV administration as compared to 1.4 mg/l for IT administration (a 260-fold increase over IV). In the blood, the median concentration was 0.12 mg/l for IV as compared to 0.003 mg/l for IT meaning the blood concentration for IT was 40-fold lower. This same group had previously used a similar methodology to show that methylprednisolone administered IT achieved a 126-fold higher perilymph concentration and a 33-fold lower blood concentration when compared to IV administration.[10]

DELIVERY DEVICES

A variety of methods have been utilized to deliver drug to the inner ear. We will confine ourselves for the purposes of this discussion to methods designed to deliver medicine to the middle ear. Generally, the techniques can be divided into those that do not control delivery and those that provide sustained release of medicine. We have already reviewed some of the experimental evidence examining the effects of delivery methods on the kinetics and distribution of the medicine in the inner ear. Much of this work has been done in small mammals or via mathematical simulation. In practice, on humans, many practitioners choose their delivery method based on empiric evidence, training, and past practice. With regards to "non-controlled" delivery, the medicine is simply injected into the middle ear either with a direct injection through the eardrum (with or without anesthesia and with or without a second hole) or a myringotomy tube is placed and medicine is injected into the tube (Fig. 1.2). There is likely little difference in the overall effectiveness of these routes. The myringotomy with tube option may be easier on the patient for subsequent injections but there are sporadic reports of an increased risk in persistent perforation.[11] As for the sustained release devices, there have been a number that have been used over time. Many groups fashioned catheters to insert through a myringotomy tube. This technique was standardized by the round window microcatheter which was inserted underneath the eardrum and had a head especially designed to fit into the round window niche. The catheter could be left in place for up to 2 weeks and was capable of delivering a continuous dose of medication.[12] At the same time, other groups were examining sponge like material from dissolvable pledgets that were placed entirely in the ear to wicks that were placed through the eardrums. Silverstein developed a microwick that was placed through the eardrum that allowed patients to self-dose medicines for inner ear disease.[13] More recently, groups have been looking at soft materials that can be preimpregnated or fully integrated with the medicine of choice.[14,15] An even newer approach is being pioneered by Otonomy (San Diego, CA) who has invented a thermally activate polymer for delivering medicines.[16]

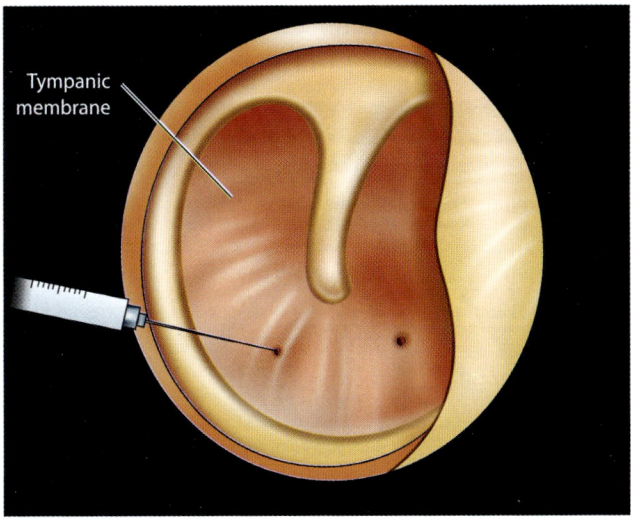

Fig. 1.2: Right ear

Despite extensive work in the area, none of the sustained release devices have yet proven absolutely reliable in terms of delivering a predicted dose to the middle ear. This is in part because, as mentioned earlier, the devices must deliver medicine to the RWM where local factors influence medicine delivery. The inability to deliver a precise dose places a theoretical limit on medicines that can be used for TT therapy. The medicines need to have a wide therapeutic window in case the amount delivered is on the low side and a low-side effect profile in case the amount delivered is on the high side. Interestingly, gentamicin, one of the most commonly used TT medicines has a wide therapeutic window but a narrow safety profile as higher dosages can lead to hearing loss (HL).

COMMON DISORDERS TREATED WITH TRANSTYMPANIC THERAPY

In the remainder of this manuscript, we will address the most common current clinical uses of TT medicines. While there are a number of potential uses of this type of therapy, by far, the three most common are in the treatment of MD, SSNHL and tinnitus. Many papers have been written on this subject—a "Pubmed" search of inner ear medicine yielded 1921 results from last 15 years alone. However, we must offer a few words of caution when reviewing the data. In actuality, there is a paucity of well-controlled studies and often conflicting outcomes. In this manuscript, we will try to summarize some of the most important and most recent work in each area. For the readers' reference, Table 1.1 shows the most common medicine preparations used in this therapy and Figure 1.2 is an image depicting one common method of instillation.

Meniere's Disease

Meniere's disease is a disease classically characterized by recurrent episodes of vertigo, fluctuating HL, low frequency tinnitus, and a sense of aural fullness. In reality, the presentation of MD is highly variable and

Table 1.1: The most common medicine preparations and indications		
Preparation	Indications	Comments
Gentamicin (40 mg/ml)—buffered to 26.7 mg/ml	Meniere's disease	Neutral Ph
Gentamicin (10 mg/ml)	Meniere's disease	Pediatric dosing vial
Methylprednisolone (125 mg/ml)	Meniere's disease/SSNHL/Tinnitus	Burns and is not stable
Dexamethasone (10 mg/ml)*	Meniere's disease/SSNHL/Tinnitus	Stable, stocked at most pharmacies
Dexamethasone (24 mg/ml)	Meniere's disease/SSNHL/Tinnitus	Stable, can be difficult to find
Note: All medicines injected in quantity of 0.3 – 1 ml *Doses of less than 10 mg/ml have been used by some authors			

its clinical course characterized by acute exacerbation and spontaneous remission. As no definitive objective tests are available to prove MD, the diagnosis is based on clinical presentation. To define the certainty of diagnosis of MD, the American Academy of Otolaryngology–Head and Neck Surgery (AAO-HNS) promulgated diagnostic and reporting guidelines, published in 1972, 1985, and 1995. Unfortunately, these criteria remain poorly or incorrectly used.[17]

The pathophysiology of MD is presumed to be aberrant fluid homeostasis leading to endolymphatic hydrops, but this may likely be too simplistic. Moreover, the variable nature of the disease has made it difficult to prospectively determine the efficacy of therapeutic intervention, and thus the treatment of MD is primarily empiric.[18] Absence of robust prospective, randomized, placebo-controlled studies has led to a variety of medical and surgical therapeutic interventions of uncertain value.[19,20] Given both a diagnostic and therapeutic void, the aims of management of MD are limited to (1) reducing the number and severity of acute attacks of vertigo; (2) aborting or ameliorating HL and tinnitus associated with such attacks; (3) alleviating any chronic symptoms (e.g., tinnitus and imbalance); and (4) preventing progression of the disease, in particular, the loss of hearing and balance that characterizes the disorder.[21] Some authors prefer the term "management" in lieu of "treatment" because currently, there is no known treatment option that adequately addresses all four of the above criteria.[18] MD should be considered a chronic condition for which interventions do not eliminate the underlying cause of disease. Moreover, no medical treatments appear to result in long-term preservation of hearing.[22] Despite the relative paucity of evidence-based research, current medical regimens can control disease (as defined by vertiginous attacks) in approximately 80% of patients.

As with other disorders of the inner ear, TT delivery has become an increasingly utilized tool in the management of MD. Those medicines delivered to the middle ear space generally can be categorized as either ablative (aminoglycosides) or immunomodulatory (steroids).

Aminoglycoside Ablation

The aim of ablative therapy is to stop the fluctuating malfunction of a diseased labyrinth. By creating a lasting, and perhaps more importantly, stable vestibular hypofunction, central compensation can finally occur. The aminoglycosides are toxic to the inner ear; streptomycin and gentamicin are selectively vestibulotoxic and destroy the endolymph-producing dark cells in the ampullary crista.[23] These properties can be used to treat vertigo associated with MD. First described in 1948, Fowler reported the used systemic streptomycin in the treatment of MD.[24] In 1956, Schuknecht described middle ear perfusion with streptomicin for the treatment of MD.[25] Streptomicin, with higher cochleotoxic properties than other aminoglycosides, was eventually replaced by gentamicin. Over the past 2 decades, TT gentamicin (TTG) has become an extremely common therapeutic options for the approximately 10% of patients with MD refractive to maximal medical treatment.

Gentamicin can be delivered to the middle ear via myringotomy, tympanostomy tube, microwick, or microcatheter. The exact method of introduction to the inner ear may come through the RWM itself, the annular ligament, or vascular channels.[26] Once in the inner ear, the mechanism of vestibulotoxicity remains incompletely understood. Only one histopathologic examination of the vestibular end organs has been reported, showing severe atrophy of the neuroepithelium of the semi-circular canal cristae ampullares with undifferentiated cells, fibrosis and edema of the stroma.[27]

The large number of published reports on the efficacy of intratympanic gentamicin (ITG) has led to near abandonment of surgical intervention.[28] As one of the first groups to follow the AAO-HNS guidelines, Kaasinen and colleagues followed 93 patients for 2 years reporting elimination of vertigo in 81%.[29] In 2001, Harner and colleagues reported a similar 82% rate of control at 2 years in 56 patients.[30] In 2004, Cohen-Kerem and colleagues synthesized the data in a meta-analysis reporting on 627 patients. They found Class A control in 74.7% of patients, and 92.7% Class B control.[31] However, a note of caution was raised—not a single acceptable double-blind or blinded prospective control trial was identified.[31] Variations in concentration, dose, frequency, and duration all limit standardization and comparison of results. Therefore, little consensus exists for the optimal protocols for delivery, even in the rare occurrence when outcomes measures are standardized. Cohen-Kerem's landmark article, despite prompting widespread use and numerous subsequent published reports on the use of ITG in MD, only two prospective, double-blind, placebo-controlled randomized clinical trials have been published.[32] Stokroos and colleagues compared 30 mg/ml buffered gentamicin to only buffer solution injected directly into the middle ear every 6 weeks until control of symptoms.[33] They found attacks had completely disappeared in the gentamicin group, and also that attacks significantly reduced in the placebo group as well. Neither group experienced significant changes in hearing. Postema et al. used 0.4 ml of 30 mg/ml gentamicin (versus placebo) through a previously placed tympanostomy tube weekly for 4 weeks.[34] Nine of 16 patients had complete control of vertigo after 1 year versus none in the placebo group. HL increased slightly (8.1 dB) in the gentamicin group, and one patient experienced a loss greater than 60 dB.

While easy to use, ITG should be used with caution. Wu and Minor followed 34 patients for greater than 2 years and reported a 15% rate of HL, including one patient with profound HL.[35] This study was not case-controlled but the authors conclude that the rates of HL were comparable to published rates seen in MD patients treated medically. Generally, patients with more advanced (higher stage) disease are more likely to have deterioration in hearing following ITG.[36] Given that 20% of patients develop bilateral disease, the risk of bilateral labyrinthine hypofunction during patient's lifetime is high. The resultant disequilibrium and oscillopsia can be incapacitating and irreversible.[37] Vestibular evoked myogenic potential testing may be useful in identifying patients with unilateral symptoms that actually have subclinical contralateral (bilateral) disease. In patients with bilateral MD, we favor the use of TT steroids, or nonablative surgery (e.g., endolymphatic sac decompression).

Great variability exists in described methods, dosage (single and cumulative), concentration, and duration of ITG administration. They can be grouped into five different techniques: (1) multiple daily dosing; (2) weekly dosing, usually for 4 weeks; (3) low-dose in which repeat injections are only given for persistent vertigo; (4) continuous microcatheter delivery; and (5) titration technique in which daily or weekly doses are given until change in vertigo symptoms or onset of HL.[32] In patients with unilateral MD, the authors prefer to use the low-dose method described by Driscoll et al.[38] Unbuffered gentamicin sulfate at a concentration of 40 mg/cc, is drawn into a 1-ml tuberculin syringe. A 3-1/2 inch, 25-gauge needle is attached, and approximately 0.5–0.75 ml is drawn up. At first, an air-release whole is made with the needle in the anterior/superior quadrant to allow for adequate injection of fluid into the middle ear space. Then, the gentamicin is injected through the posterior/superior quadrant into the middle ear space. Patients are then left supine for 30 minutes and instructed to keep water out of their ear for 2 weeks. Patients return in 1 month when an audiogram is obtained. Such intervention resulted in a 76% improvement in vertigo and no change in hearing at 4 years post-injection.[38] Approximately 15–20% of patients require a second ITG injection usually at 1 month interval; a third injection is rarely required. This low-dose method is rarely associated with HL.

Steroids

A strong body of research exists to support the role of immunologic dysfunction in the etiology of MD.[18] As early as the 1970s, McCabe recognized the role of steroids in the treatment of inner ear diseases.[39] Fifty percent of patients with MD have inhalant and/or food allergies and treating these allergies with immunotherapy and diet modification improved allergic and Ménière's symptoms when compared to controls.[40] Brooks showed circulating immune complexes in 54% of patients with MD.[41] Tomoda et al. reported up to 6% of all patients with MD may have an autoimmune etiology.[42] Other supportive evidence includes the presence of MD-like symptoms in other autoimmune disease (e.g., Cogan's Periarteritis nodosa), raised IgM complexes and C1q component of complement,[43] the presence of lymphatics and immunocompetent cells close the endolymphatic space, responsiveness to immunoglobulin E (IgE) therapy,[44] elevated antibodies directed against type II collagen in Ménière's patients compared to normal controls,[45] the presence of anti-endolymphatic sac autoantibodies in the serum of MD patients,[46] and IgG deposits found in the endolymphatic sacs of patients undergoing shunt surgery for MD.[47]

Steroid responsiveness in MD patients with increased rate of expression of certain human leukocyte antigens (HLA) further supports an immune mechanism. It is not therefore surprising that immunomodulatory medicines, mostly steroids, have been employed with varying success in the management of MD. In addition to immune and inflammatory regulation, corticosteroids are known to affect carbohydrate, electrolyte, protein, and lipid metabolism making exact physiologic effect impossible to gauge. Furthermore, the discovery of glucocorticoid receptors in the inner ear suggests that steroids may also affect fluid homeostasis.[48] Nonetheless, the use of steroids in MD is largely empiric, based on successes of this technique in patients with SSNHL, autoimmune HL, and tinnitus.[18] More recently, despite absence of strong evidence, TT application of steroids for MD has gained in popularity. Like ITG, the advantages are numerous including ease of administration, avoidance of surgery, contraindications to systemic therapy (e.g., patients with hypertension and diabetes), intolerance of systemic therapy (insomnia, gastrointestinal disturbances, etc.), salvage therapy when systemic treatment fails, and selection of the active ear for treatment.[49] Furthermore, concentrations of steroids in the inner ear following TT administration far exceed those seen in systemic administrations, theoretically further potentiating their efficacy.[50,51] Complications may include pain, short-lasting vertigo, otitis media, tympanic membrane perforation, vertigo (temporary or permanent), and HL.

As with ITG, optimal drug doses, schedule, duration, and means of delivery to the inner ear have yet to be standardized and reporting of complications has been inconsistent. In their review of TT steroids for MD, Phillips and Westerberg identified only one trial out of 235 articles with sufficient "low-risk of bias".[52] That trial, by Garduno-Anaya and colleagues found that 24 months after 5 consecutive days of once daily TT dexamethasone administration, patients had statistically significant improvement in vertigo compared with placebo controls.[53]

The relatively few prospective studies that have been conducted suggest that although vertigo symptoms may improve, hearing and tinnitus do not significantly change.[54-56] Silverstein and colleagues reported a 72% rate of substantial or complete vertigo control at 18 months, though not significantly different than TTG or endolymphatic sac decompression.[57,58] Lack of effect on hearing is in contrast to the anecdotal evidence that TT steroids are effective in reversing HL in SSNHL suggesting different pathophysiology for these two disorders.[18] In MD patients in whom hearing improvement/preservation is not of primary concern or those who have failed other medical therapies, TT steroid injection may provide substantial benefit prior to more aggressive surgical options. Clearly, more prospective and controlled studies are needed to fully understand and utilize this treatment option.

▌Sudden Sensorineural Hearing Loss

Steroids have long been postulated as an important treatment for sudden HL. This is despite the fact that true "level one" evidence of a significant beneficial effect has been difficult to produce.[59] Conlin and Parnes examined all of the work and concluded that there was no level one evidence supporting the use of oral steroids in sudden HL.[60] Nevertheless, there is work showing that oral steroids do have a beneficial effect.[61] In fact, recent studies report success rates over 60%.[62] Because of the common use of this medicine orally and the significant side effect profile of oral steroid use, many groups began investigating TT usage. Schuknecht is credited with one of the earliest uses of TT medicine in 1957.[25] His goal was to ablate function in MD. TT therapy enjoyed resurgence in popularity in the 1980s but for many years, the focus remained on MD. One of the earliest reports on steroids for HL was performed by Silverstein who concluded that, in a small group of patients, TT steroids were not better than placebo at treating HL.[58] Since that time, there has been a significant increase in interest and publications regarding TT steroids for HL. Yet, widely disparate management styles exist amongst practitioners in the use steroids for SSNHL.[63] There are several important factors to consider when analyzing the data for HL as follows: (1) The techniques utilized in different papers vary a great deal and so, direct methodological comparisons are very difficult; (2) The steroid chosen (usually dexamethasone vs. methylprednisolone) varies from study to study; (3) The actual dose, concentration, and dosing frequency vary from study to study, and (4) The definition of improvement in hearing is not standardized. In fact, a Cochran review was done in 2006, that conclude that TT steroids were of no proven benefit for sudden HL. In this review, the authors concluded that only two studies to date were of significant methodological value to be analyzed and one of these showed now benefit from TT steroids and a second showed a 32% improvement compared to over 60% for oral treatment.[64] As we examine some particular studies, it is important to remember that some publications will have occurred before this document was produced but many will have been performed after the Cochrane review.

One of the questions with respect to TT medicines, as work went forward, was the actual steroid of choice. Parnes studied this in detail in an animal model and found that hydrocortisone, methylprednisolone, and dexamethasone all showed greater cochlear fluid concentrations when administered transtympanically than orally. He further showed that methylprednisolone reached a higher concentration in one particular fluid compartment.[65] Despite these findings, the field remains divided on the steroid of choice. Many individuals use dexamethasone because it is easier to store (more stable), and does not burn as compared to methylprednisolone which is harder to store and burns a significant amount. Others use methylprednisolone believing that the higher concentration is necessary.

Initial work focused on using TT when oral steroids failed. Giancoli used a ventilation tube to administer steroids on four occasions over 10–14 days and demonstrated a 44% improvement in hearing in those who failed steroids.[66] Other studies using steroids for salvage have quoted success rates as high as 75% using steroids.[67] Other groups used devices as a salvage mechanism. Van Wijck and colleagues used a Silverstein Microwick to administer methylprednisolone twice a day for 3 weeks. This group showed that 66% of individuals improved and that 60% of these showed a return to baseline.[68] Most recently, a group from Taiwan conducted a double-blind placebo control trial on TT steroids {four injections of 0.5 ml dexamethasone (4 mg/ml) versus saline}. Forty-four percent of the individuals in the steroid group had an improvement in the pure tone average (PTA) of 10 dB or more with 30% of the group showing an improvement of 15 dB or better as compared to 11% and 7% for the saline group respectively.[69]

Overtime, the use of TT steroids as a primary modality (not simply after oral steroid failure) began to be adopted. The rationale for this was a higher concentration, the avoidance of systemic complications, and the perceived need to start TT therapy as soon as possible. A variety of approaches have been used for primary TT steroid therapy. Kopke and colleagues used a round window microcatheter to deliver steroids to the round window niche and showed improvement in 5/6 patients treated in under 6 weeks with 4/5 of those who improved returning to baseline hearing.[70] This study showed no improvement in those treated after 6 weeks and did result in one patient losing his hearing. Haynes and colleagues injected dexamethasone (24 mg/ml) and showed a 40% of patients improved (defined as PTA increase > 20 dB or > 20% speech discrimination improvement). This group showed no improvement in patients whose therapy started more than 5 weeks after the HL.[71] Battaglia and colleagues compared TT dexamethasone with oral steroids to IT dexamethasone alone and oral steroids alone and found that all three groups did better than observation alone, and that the combination therapy was overall the most successful option.[72] More recently, Zhou and colleagues examined the use of early TT therapy versus oral steroids in "poor prognosis" HL and demonstrated that approximately 45% of the TT group (given four injections of methylprednisolone over the first 7 days) showed a significant hearing improvement (defined as a 15 dB PTA improvement or 15% speech discrimination improvement). This percentage was significantly better than oral steroids.[73]

The need for more controlled data motivated a large number of investigators to conduct a large-scale, multi-institutional study of TT steroid treatment. In this novel study, the investigators performed a non-inferiority study of TT steroids (four doses of 40 mg/ml methylprednisolone over 14 days) versus oral prednisone (60 mg per day x 14 days with a 5-day taper). The study showed an average PTA improvement of 30 dB for both groups and concluded that TT therapy was not inferior to oral steroids.[74] Overtime, there has been little level one evidence which shows that oral steroids or TT steroids are better than no treatment for sudden HL. The weight of published evidence does, however, suggest that steroid treatment may have a benefit with an acceptable risk profile. As a result, most individuals who manage this disorder give oral and/or TT therapy. The protocols utilized vary and depend on location, training, and personal philosophy and there is almost no evidence to support the use of one technique over any other. The authors of this article use slightly different practices. At Navy Medical Center San Diego, we treat sudden HL with 10–14 days of oral steroids (60 mg prednisone q 9 AM) along with three TT injections of 0.3 ml dexamethasone (10 mg/ml) with a 27-gauge needle. At Virginia Commonwealth University, the practice is to use 1 mg/kg of prednisone one daily x 10 days along with a TT injection of 0.6 ml of dexamethasone (24 mg/ml) injected one time and repeated two more times weekly if the audiogram done 1 week after the first injections shows an improvement in PTA or speech discrimination. We do not routinely use anesthesia for these injections. We space the injections 2 weeks apart and give a fourth injection for those who partially respond. Individuals with contraindications to oral steroids receive the injections alone.

Tinnitus

As the popularity of TT therapy for MD and HL increased, it was natural to begin to think about the therapy for tinnitus alone. This thought grew from the observations of many investigators that in some patients, steroids did not resolve all of the MD symptoms or the HL but did reduce or eliminate the tinnitus. Since there was no other universally effective medical option, tinnitus became an independent rationale for TT therapy in many clinics. While it may seem convenient to think of TT treatment of tinnitus in much the same way as HL, that would not be entirely accurate. There are definite similarities including the lack of good high-level research reports and the difficulty in comparing studies due to differences in delivery methods, particular steroid used, dosing, and concentration. But, there are fundamental differences including a much more difficult set of outcome measures to assess. First of all, many of the outcomes in tinnitus treatment are much more subjective in nature and the range of responses is variable from elimination to reduction in either severity, frequency, or both. There are a variety of different scales that can be used to judge response to therapy and the best scale has yet to be determined. In addition, tinnitus differs from HL by the fact that, unlike steroid for HL, there is no (evidence based or not) accepted oral medicine for tinnitus. Most importantly, tinnitus is multifactorial in nature. It is possible that some tinnitus etiologies may respond to TT therapy, while others may not.[75] Unfortunately, accurately characterizing tinnitus etiologies is difficult and often not included in studies, so this makes assessing the success of TT therapy even more difficult.

Many of the tinnitus outcomes are referred to in papers discussing the treatment of HL or MD. As such, there is a relative paucity of articles that deal with mainly tinnitus. One of the first, and still one of the largest, series in which the primary aim was examining control of tinnitus was the landmark article by Sakata and Itoh who used a sustained release device to deliver 2–4 mg of dexamethasone to 3,978 ears in 3,041 patients.[76] Tinnitus was improved in 75% of patients and the response was dependent on the etiology with hydrops patients responding better than for noise or drug induced tinnitus. Since that publication, there have been mixed results on the effectiveness of steroids for controlling tinnitus in the literature. Cesarini's group used a set of diagnostic tests to try to limit their patient population to subjective idiopathic tinnitus of cochlear origin.[77] Their study showed a 34% elimination and a 40% reduction of tinnitus in a group of 50 patients treated with 4 mg dexamethasone given to the middle ear three times daily for 3 months. Several years later, She's group demonstrated significant improvement in those treated with either TT dexamethasone or TT methylprednisolone.[78] While these studies advocated TT injections, other studies found the injections no better than control. Araujo's group gave patients either 0.5 ml of 4 mg/ml dexamethasone via TT injection once per week for 4 weeks or saline in the same manner and found no difference in the outcome of the two groups.[79] There was some "placebo like" improvement in approximately 30% of the patients in both groups. More recently, Topak's group studied TT injections in 59 patients with subjective tinnitus.[80] The patients were divided into an active group (three injections of methylprednisolone one per week for three weeks) or a control group (three injections of saline one per week for 3 weeks). There was no significant difference between the outcome in the two groups and both groups improved from baseline only in subjective loudness. Again, the effectiveness of TT injections for tinnitus is difficult to compare because all of these studies use different dosing regimens. At the current time, we do not utilize TT steroids for tinnitus alone in our clinic unless we are treating the tinnitus in combination with a sudden HL or MD.

CONCLUSION

Transtympanic medical therapy is an appealing option for ear disease. The therapy allows us to largely target the ear avoiding systemic effects of medicine and obtaining high concentrations of medicine in the inner ear. The therapy is commonly used for disorders where other treatments are not entirely effective including MD, SSNHL, and tinnitus. The use of TTG for MD and the use of TT steroids for SSNHL seem to have the most favorable support in the literature. Nevertheless, despite years of study, there are few high-quality level one studies supporting the use of this treatment modality for any disorder. Moreover, despite some success, the best method of dosing the medicine, the best dosing regimen, and the end point of therapy have not been well-worked out for any disorder with any medicine. There continues to be significant work on developing delivery devices that more precisely control drug delivery. At the same time, it remains imperative that basic science continues to study this modality. Science should not limit itself to the current medicines being used in the clinic, but should study other opportunities to utilize this therapy in patients.

Disclaimer: The views expressed in this article are those of the authors and do not necessarily reflect the official policy or position of the Department of the Navy, Department of Defense, or the U.S. Government.

REFERENCES

1. Salt AN, Gill RM, Plontke SK. Dependence of hearing changes on the dose of intratympanically applied gentamicin: a meta-analysis using mathematical simulations of clinical drug delivery protocols. Laryngoscope. 2008;118(10):1793-800. Available from: PM:18806480
2. Hoffer ME, Allen K, Kopke RD, et al. transtympanic versus sustained-release administration of gentamicin: kinetics, morphology, and function. Laryngoscope. 2001a;111(8):1343-57. Available from: PM:11568567
3. Hoffer ME, Allen K, Gottshall K, et al. The early kinetics of gentamicin uptake into the inner ear. Int Tinnitus J. 2002;8(1):27-9. Available from: PM:14763232
4. Yoshioka M, Naganawa S, Sone M, et al. Individual differences in the permeability of the round window: evaluating the movement of intratympanic gadolinium into the inner ear. Otol Neurotol. 2009;30(5):645-8. Available from: PM:19415042
5. Mikulec AA, Plontke SK, Hartsock JJ, et al. Entry of substances into perilymph through the bone of the otic capsule after intratympanic applications in guinea pigs: implications for local drug delivery in humans. Otol Neurotol. 2009;30(2):131-8. Available from: PM:19180674
6. Zou J, Ramadan UA, Pyykko I. Gadolinium uptake in the rat inner ear perilymph evaluated with 4.7 T MRI: a comparison between transtympanic injection and gelatin sponge-based diffusion through the round window membrane. Otol Neurotol. 2010;31(4):637-41. Available from: PM:20142794
7. Salt AN, Plontke SK. Principles of local drug delivery to the inner ear. Audiol Neurotol. 2009;14(6):350-360. Available from: PM:19923805
8. Roehm P, Hoffer M, Balaban CD. Gentamicin uptake in the chinchilla inner ear. Hear Res. 2007;230(1-2):43-52. Available from: PM:17616288
9. Bird PA, Murray DP, Zhang M, et al. Intratympanic versus intravenous delivery of dexamethasone and dexamethasone sodium phosphate to cochlear perilymph. Otol Neurotol. 2011;32(6):933-6. Available from: PM:21725263
10. Bird PA, Begg EJ, Zhang M, et al. Intratympanic versus intravenous delivery of methylprednisolone to cochlear perilymph. Otol Neurotol. 2007;28(8):1124-30. Available from: PM:18043438
11. Rutt AL, Hawkshaw MJ, Sataloff RT. Incidence of tympanic membrane perforation after intratympanic steroid treatment through myringotomy tubes. Ear Nose Throat J. 2011;90(4):E21. Available from: PM:21500156
12. Hoffer ME, Kopke RD, Weisskopf P, et al. Use of the round window microcatheter in the treatment of Ménière's disease. Laryngoscope. 2001b;111(11 Pt 1):2046-9. Available from: PM:11801994
13. Silverstein H, Thompson J, Rosenberg SI, et al. Silverstein MicroWick. Otolaryngol Clin North Am. 2004;37(5):1019-34. Available from: PM:15474108
14. Borden RC, Saunders JE, Berryhill WE, et al. Hyaluronic acid hydrogel sustains the delivery of dexamethasone across the round window membrane. Audiol Neurootol. 2011;16(1):1-11. Available from: PM:20431286

15. Xu L, Heldrich J, Wang H, et al. A controlled and sustained local gentamicin delivery system for inner ear applications. Otol Neurotol. 2010;31(7):1115-21. Available from: PM:20616758

16. Wang X, Dellamary L, Fernandez R, et al. Dose-dependent sustained release of dexamethasone in inner ear cochlear fluids using a novel local delivery approach. Audiol Neurootol. 2009;14(6):393-401. Available from: PM:19923809

17. Thorp MA, Shehab ZP, Bance ML, et al. The AAO-HNS Committee on Hearing and Equilibrium guidelines for the diagnosis and evaluation of therapy in Ménière's disease: have they been applied in the published literature of the last decade? Clin Otolaryngol Allied Sci. 2003;28(3):173-6. Available from: PM:12755750

18. Coelho DH, Lalwani AK. Medical management of Ménière's disease. Laryngoscope. 2008;118(6):1099-108. Available from: PM:18418279

19. Antonio SM, Friedman R. Ménière's Disease. In: Jackler RK, Brackmann DE (Eds). Neurotology. Philadelphia:Elsevier; 2005. pp. 621-38.

20. Thorp MA, Shehab ZP, Bance ML, et al. Does evidence-based medicine exist in the treatment of Ménière's disease? A critical review of the last decade of publications. Clin Otolaryngol Allied Sci. 2000;25(6):456-60. Available from: PM:11122279

21. Thirlwall AS, Kundu S. Diuretics for Ménière's disease or syndrome. Cochrane Database Syst Rev. 2006;3:CD003599. Available from: PM:16856015

22. Kinney SE, Sandridge SA, Newman CW. Long-term effects of Ménière's disease on hearing and quality of life. Am J Otol. 1997;18(1):67-73. Available from: PM:8989954

23. Black FO, Pesznecker SC. Vestibular ototoxicity. Clinical considerations. Otolaryngol Clin North Am. 1993;26(5):713-36. Available from: PM:8233485

24. Fowler EP, Jr. Streptomycin treatment of vertigo. Trans Am Acad Ophthalmol Otolaryngol. 1948;52:293-301. Available from: PM:18915191

25. Schuknecht HF. Ablation therapy for the relief of Ménière's disease. Laryngoscope. 1956;66(7):859-70. Available from: PM:13358249

26. Hirsch BE, Kamerer DB. Intratympanic gentamicin therapy for Ménière's disease. Am J Otol. 1997;18(1):44-51. Available from: PM:8989951

27. Ishiyama G, Lopez I, Baloh RW, et al. Histopathology of the vestibular end organs after intratympanic gentamicin failure for Ménière's disease. Acta Otolaryngol. 2007;127(1):34-40. Available from: PM:17364327

28. De BL, Stokroos R, Kingma H. Intratympanic gentamicin therapy for intractable Ménière's disease. Acta Otolaryngol. 2007;127(6):605-12. Available from: PM:17503229

29. Kaasinen S, Pyykko I, Ishizaki H, et al. Intratympanic gentamicin in Ménière's disease. Acta Otolaryngol. 1998;118(3):294-8. Available from: PM:9655201

30. Harner SG, Driscoll CL, Facer GW, et al. Long-term follow-up of transtympanic gentamicin for Ménière's syndrome. Otol Neurotol. 2001;22(2):210-4. Available from: PM:11300271

31. Cohen-Kerem R, Kisilevsky V, Einarson TR, et al. Intratympanic gentamicin for Ménière's disease: a meta-analysis. Laryngoscope. 2004;114(12):2085-91. Available from: PM:15564826

32. Pullens B, van Benthem PP. Intratympanic gentamicin for Ménière's disease or syndrome. Cochrane Database Syst Rev. 2011;(3):CD008234. Available from: PM:21412917

33. Stokroos R, Kingma H. Selective vestibular ablation by intratympanic gentamicin in patients with unilateral active Ménière's disease: a prospective, double-blind, placebo-controlled, randomized clinical trial. Acta Otolaryngol. 2004;124(2):172-5. Available from: PM:15072419

34. Postema RJ, Kingma CM, Wit HP, et al. Intratympanic gentamicin therapy for control of vertigo in unilateral Ménière's disease: a prospective, double-blind, randomized, placebo-controlled trial. Acta Otolaryngol. 2008;128(8):876-80. Available from: PM:18607963

35. Wu IC, Minor LB. Long-term hearing outcome in patients receiving intratympanic gentamicin for Ménière's disease. Laryngoscope. 2003;113(5):815-20. Available from: PM:12792316

36. Silverstein H, Wazen J, Van Ess MJ, et al. Intratympanic gentamicin treatment of patients with Ménière's disease with normal hearing. Otolaryngol Head Neck Surg. 2010;142(4):570-5. Available from: PM:20304280

37. Peterson WM, Isaacson JE. Current management of Ménière's disease in an only hearing ear. Otol Neurotol. 2007;28(5):696-9. Available from: PM:17468673

38. Driscoll CL, Kasperbauer JL, Facer GW, et al. Low-dose intratympanic gentamicin and the treatment of Ménière's disease: preliminary results. Laryngoscope. 1997;107(1):83-9. Available from: PM:9001270

39. McCabe BF. Autoimmune sensorineural hearing loss. Ann Otol Rhinol Laryngol. 1979;88(5 Pt 1):585-9. Available from: PM:496191

40. Derebery MJ. The role of allergy in Ménière's disease. Otolaryngol Clin North Am. 1997;30(6):1007-16. Available from: PM:9386237

41. Brookes GB. Circulating immune complexes in Ménière's disease. Arch Otolaryngol Head Neck Surg. 1986;112(5):536-40. Available from: PM:3485438

42. Tomoda K, Suzuka Y, Iwai H, et al. Ménière's disease and autoimmunity: clinical study and survey. Acta Otolaryngol Suppl. 1993;500:31-4. Available from: PM:8452018

43. Evans KL, Baldwin DL, Bainbridge D, et al. Immune status in patients with Ménière's disease. Arch.Otorhinolaryngol. 1988;245(5):287-92. Available from: PM:3245800

44. Siebenhaar F, Kuhn W, Zuberbier T, et al. Successful treatment of cutaneous mastocytosis and Ménière's disease with anti-IgE therapy. J Allergy Clin Immunol. 2007;120(1):213-5. Available from: PM:17544095

45. Yoshino K, Ohashi T, Urushibata T, et al. Antibodies of type II collagen and immune complexes in Ménière's disease. Acta Otolaryngol Suppl. 1996;522;79-85. Available from: PM:8740816

46. Alleman AM, Dornhoffer JL, Arenberg IK, et al. Demonstration of auto-antibodies to the endolymphatic sac in Ménière's disease. Laryngoscope. 1997;107(2):211-5. Available from: PM:9023245

47. Dornhoffer JL, Waner M, Arenberg IK, et al. Immunoperoxidase study of the endolymphatic sac in Ménière's disease. Laryngoscop. 1993:103(9):1027-34. Available from: PM:8361306

48. Rarey KE, Curtis LM, ten Cate WJ. Tissue specific levels of glucocorticoid receptor within the rat inner ear. Hear Res. 1993;64(2):205-10. Available from: PM:8432691

49. Doyle KJ, Bauch C, Battista R, et al. Intratympanic steroid treatment: a review. Otol.Neurotol. 2004;25(6):1034-9. Available from: PM:15547441

50. Chandrasekhar SS, Rubinstein RY, Kwartler JA, et al. Dexamethasone pharmacokinetics in the inner ear: comparison of route of administration and use of facilitating agents. Otolaryngol Head Neck Surg. 2000;122(4):521-8. Available from: PM:10740171

51. Parnes LS, Sun AH, Freeman DJ. Corticosteroid pharmacokinetics in the inner ear fluids: an animal study followed by clinical application. Laryngoscope. 1999a;109(7 Pt 2):1-17. Available from: PM:10399889

52. Phillips JS, Westerberg B. Intratympanic steroids for Ménière's disease or syndrome. Cochrane Database Syst Rev. 2011;(7):CD008514. Available from: PM:21735432

53. Garduno-Anaya MA, Couthino De TH, Hinojosa-Gonzalez R, et al. Dexamethasone inner ear perfusion by intratympanic injection in unilateral Ménière's disease: a two-year prospective, placebo-controlled, double-blind, randomized trial. Otolaryngol Head Neck Surg. 2005;133(2):285-94. Available from: PM:16087029

54. Arriaga MA, Goldman S. Hearing results of intratympanic steroid treatment of endolymphatic hydrops. Laryngoscope. 1998;108(11 Pt 1):1682-5. Available from: PM:9818826

55. Barrs DM. Intratympanic injections of dexamethasone for long-term control of vertigo. Laryngoscope; 2004;114(11):1910-4. Available from: PM:15510013

56. Hirvonen TP, Peltomaa M, Ylikoski J. Intratympanic and systemic dexamethasone for Ménière's disease. ORL J Otorhinolaryngol Relat Spec. 2000;62(3):117-20. Available from: PM:10810254

57. Sennaroglu L, Sennaroglu G, Gursel B, et al. Intratympanic dexamethasone, intratympanic gentamicin, and endolymphatic sac surgery for intractable vertigo in Ménière's disease. Otolaryngol Head Neck Surg. 2001;125(5):537-43. Available from: PM:11700457

58. Silverstein H, Isaacson JE, Olds MJ, et al. Dexamethasone inner ear perfusion for the treatment of Ménière's disease: a prospective, randomized, double-blind, crossover trial. Am J Otol. 1998;19(2):196-201. Available from: PM:9520056

59. Labus J, Breil J, Stutzer H, et al. Meta-analysis for the effect of medical therapy vs. placebo on recovery of idiopathic sudden hearing loss. Laryngoscop. 2010;120(9):1863-71. Available from: PM:20803741

60. Conlin AE, Parnes LS. Treatment of sudden sensorineural hearing loss: II. A Meta-analysis. Arch Otolaryngol Head Neck Surg. 2007;133(6):582-6. Available from: PM:17576909

61. Zadeh MH, Storper IS, Spitzer JB. Diagnosis and treatment of sudden-onset sensorineural hearing loss: a study of 51 patients. Otolaryngol Head Neck Surg. 2003;128(1):92-8. Available from: PM:12574765

62. Alimoglu Y, Inci E, Edizer DT, et al. Efficacy comparison of oral steroid, intratympanic steroid, hyperbaric oxygen and oral steroid + hyperbaric

oxygen treatments in idiopathic sudden sensorineural hearing loss cases. Eur Arch Otorhinolaryngol. 2011. Available from: PM:21431435

63. Coelho DH, Thacker LR, Hsu DW. Variability in the management of idiopathic sudden sensorineural hearing loss. Otolaryngol Head Neck Surg. 2011. Available from: PM:21690271

64. Wei BP, Mubiru S, O'Leary S. Steroids for idiopathic sudden sensorineural hearing loss. Cochrane Database Syst Rev. 2006;(1):CD003998. Available from: PM:16437471

65. Parnes LS, Sun AH, Freeman DJ. Corticosteroid pharmacokinetics in the inner ear fluids: an animal study followed by clinical application. Laryngoscope. 1999b;109(7 Pt 2):1-17. Available from: PM:10399889

66. Gianoli GJ, Li JC. transtympanic steroids for treatment of sudden hearing loss. Otolaryngol Head Neck Surg. 2001;125(3):142-6. Available from: PM:11555744

67. Dallan I, Bruschini L, Nacci A, et al. transtympanic steroids as a salvage therapy in sudden hearing loss: preliminary results. ORL J Otorhinolaryngol Relat Spec. 2006;68(5):247-52. Available from: PM:16679810

68. Van WF, Staecker H, Keithley E, et al. Local perfusion of the tumor necrosis factor alpha blocker infliximab to the inner ear improves autoimmune neurosensory hearing loss. Audiol Neurootol. 2006;11(6):357-65. Available from: PM:16988499

69. Wu HP, Chou YF, Yu SH, et al. Intratympanic steroid injections as a salvage treatment for sudden sensorineural hearing loss: a randomized, double-blind, placebo-controlled study. Otol Neurotol. 2011;32(5):774-9. Available from: PM:21646929

70. Kopke RD, Hoffer ME, Wester D, et al. Targeted topical steroid therapy in sudden sensorineural hearing loss. Otol Neurotol. 2001;22(4):475-9. Available from: PM:11449103

71. Haynes DS, O'Malley M, Cohen S, et al. Intratympanic dexamethasone for sudden sensorineural hearing loss after failure of systemic therapy. Laryngoscope. 2007;117(1):3-15. Available from: PM:17202923

72. Battaglia A, Burchette R, Cueva R. Combination therapy (intratympanic dexamethasone + high-dose prednisone taper) for the treatment of idiopathic sudden sensorineural hearing loss. Otol Neurotol. 2008;29(4):453-60. Available from: PM:18401285

73. Zhou Y, Zheng H, Zhang Q, et al. Early transtympanic steroid injection in patients with 'poor prognosis' idiopathic sensorineural sudden hearing loss. ORL J Otorhinolaryngol Relat Spec. 2011;73(1):31-7. Available from: PM:21124045

74. Rauch SD, Halpin CF, Antonelli PJ, et al. Oral vs intratympanic corticosteroid therapy for idiopathic sudden sensorineural hearing loss: a randomized trial. JAMA. 2011;305(20):2071-9. Available from: PM:21610239

75. Shulman A, Goldstein B. Principles of tinnitology: tinnitus diagnosis and treatment a tinnitus-targeted therapy. Int Tinnitus J. 2010;16(1):73-85. Available from: PM:21609918

76. Sakata E, Ito Y, Itoh A. Clinical experiences of steroid targeting therapy to inner ear for control of tinnitus. Int Tinnitus J. 1997:3(2):117-21. Available from: PM:10753373

77. Cesarani A, Capobianco S, Soi D, et al. Intratympanic dexamethasone treatment for control of subjective idiopathic tinnitus: our clinical experience. Int Tinnitus J. 2002;8(2):111-4. Available from: PM:14763222

78. She W, Dai Y, Du X, et al. Treatment of subjective tinnitus: a comparative clinical study of intratympanic steroid injection vs. oral carbamazepine. Med Sci Monit. 2009;15(6):I35-9. Available from: PM:19478715

79. Araujo MF, Oliveira CA, Bahmad FM, Jr. Intratympanic dexamethasone injections as a treatment for severe, disabling tinnitus: does it work? Arch Otolaryngol Head Neck Surg. 2005;131(2):113-7. Available from: PM:15723941

80. Topak M, Sahin-Yilmaz A, Ozdoganoglu T, et al. Intratympanic methylprednisolone injections for subjective tinnitus. J Laryngol Otol. 2009;123(11):1221-5. Available from: PM:19640315

Chapter

2

BONE CONDUCTING HEARING AID SOLUTIONS

F Agada and PG Reilly

ABSTRACT

Hearing loss is a common disability and traditionally, a conventional air conduction hearing aid has been the mainstay of rehabilitation. However, for various reasons, a significant number of patients are unable to derive benefit from these. Bone conduction aids provide an alternative means of rehabilitation. These are available for use on a head band or via implantable devices. This chapter discussed the use of such aids. The BAHA and a newer transcutaneous bone conduction aid using magnets to hold the device in place have significantly increased the range of options available to patients.

INTRODUCTION

Hearing impairment is a common disease with a wide variety of causes. Most patients who have a hearing disability have an abnormality of cochlear function and can be treated by use of a conventional air conduction hearing aid. However, a significant number of patients have a conductive cause for their hearing loss. Many of these patients can also be treated with conventional aids but a proportion do not tolerate the presence of a mould or insert in the ear canal and so alternative means of hearing rehabilitation must be considered. A further group of patients do not have an ear canal either because of congenital or acquired external auditory canal stenosis and so cannot wear a conventional air conduction aid at all.

Sound can be transmitted directly to the cochlea by bone conduction, thus bypassing the ear canal and middle ear. Hearing aids designed to transmit sound directly to the cochlea have existed for many years. These are available as sound transducers that are held against the head by a steel spring, or concealed in a pair of spectacles, so that the earpieces are pressed against the skin and bone behind the ears. These types of aids, while often providing good hearing rehabilitation, are uncomfortable to wear and can be associated with a risk of developing skin complications.

More recently, the concept of implanting a titanium fixture into the bone of the skull by osseointegration was developed. This allowed for a bone conduction hearing aid to be attached directly to the bone via a transcutaneous abutment. In the last few years, a device has been developed which relies on insertion of a titanium plate containing two rare earth magnets into the bone of the skull and then using magnetic attraction to hold the hearing aid in place on the overlying skin.

MECHANISM OF BONE CONDUCTION HEARING

Sound can be transmitted to the cochlea in three ways:

1. Firstly, vibration of the bone of the skull is coupled to the soft tissues of the ear canal and so, vibrations will be induced in the air within the canal and then transmitted externally and also to the cochlea via the tympanic membrane and ossicular chain. Bone conduction by this route increases when the ear canal is occluded.
2. In a similar manner, when the bone of the skull vibrates, some of the sound energy will be transferred directly to the ossicular chain and then on to the cochlea. This element will be reduced if there is middle ear pathology that reduces the mobility of the ossicles, or if there is discontinuity of the ossicular chain.
3. The third route depends on alternate compression and expansion of the cochlear shell by vibratory forces on the bone, thus producing inner ear fluid displacement (this depends on the differing size and shape of the cochlear scalae).

Tonndorf[1] has provided a good description of the mechanism of bone conduction.

BONE CONDUCTION HEARING AIDS

Until the 1980s, patients who needed amplification to provide hearing rehabilitation had to use a mechanical transducer held against the soft tissues adjacent to the ear by a steel spring headband. These aids provide good hearing results in those with conductive hearing loss, but the discomfort caused by the pressure of the band means that many patients are unable to tolerate the aid for more than a short while. Many patients are also unhappy with cosmetic aspects. An alternative is to have the transducer fitted to a pair of sturdy spectacles but these can cause similar levels of discomfort and are unpopular in those patients who do not otherwise need to wear spectacles.

BONE ANCHORED HEARING AIDS

In 1950, Per-Ingvar Brånemark discovered that titanium chambers implanted into the bone of rats became firmly fixed to the bone so that removal became impossible.

Brånemark's work on dental implants in animals during the 1960s showed that if titanium screws were placed in bone and left unloaded for 3–6 months, then the bone would grow in close apposition with the screws and holds them firmly in place. He coined the term "osseointegration" for this process.

In 1977, Anders Tjelstrom began to implant titanium fixtures in humans and his work led to development of the fixtures that are in current use for bone-anchored hearing aids.

Bone anchored hearing aid technology was developed by the Swedish firm Nobelpharma later came to be known as Nobel Biocare and then Entific. Cochlear™ now markets and continues to develop the devices. BAHA® is the registered trademark of the Cochlear™ company. The first commercially available implantable hearing aid system became commercially available in 1987.

The U.S. Food and Drug Administration (FDA) licensed BAHA® in 1997. Lustig et al.[2] evaluated the U.S. experience of the first 40 patients implanted with the BAHA® in 12 tertiary referral medical centers. They found that the BAHA® provided a reliable and predictable adjunct for auditory rehabilitation in appropriately selected patients, offering a means of dramatically improving hearing thresholds in patients with conductive or mixed hearing loss who are otherwise unable to benefit from traditional hearing aids. Patient responses to the implant were uniformly satisfactory.

Oticon™ have recently entered the market and supply similar implants but a different sound processor.

BAHA®

BAHA® is the trade name for the bone anchored hearing aid system currently available from Cochlear™. It consists of a titanium flange fixture (screw) which is inserted into the bone of the skull adjacent to the ear and which osseointegrates. An abutment is attached transcutaneously. The hearing aids fit on to the abutment by "snap coupling".

There are currently three BAHA® aids available that are of differing power. These are the BP100, BAHA Intenso and BAHA Cordell. Selection of the type of aid depends on cochlear reserve. The BP100 is suitable for patients whose cochlear reserve is better than 45 dB, whereas the Intenso is suitable for up to 55 dB and the Cordelle II up to 65 dB.

Indications for BAHA®

Most patients with hearing loss are able to wear conventional hearing aids that provide appropriate amplification and good cosmesis. However, a small group are either unable to wear such aids or find that if they do, they develop problems such as discharge from the ear which limits hearing aid use (Table 2.1).

Table 2.1: Indications for BAHA
Auricular atresia
Chronic ear discharge
Conductive hearing loss when surgical restoration of hearing is not advised
Otosclerosis
Trauma
Single-sided deafness

FDA approval has been granted for patients with conductive and mixed hearing bilateral losses, and single-sided deafness. It is not currently approved for children under 5 years old, but these children can use the "soft band" elastic band with an attached BAHA® processor.

Patient Selection

Audiometry should reveal that a potential patient has adequate cochlear reserve to benefit from the appropriate aid once the fittings are implanted. A trial of the aid on a headband is useful because it can demonstrate to the patient what level of amplification and sound quality can be expected with the implanted aid.

It is also important to check for conditions that may affect bone quality. These include local infection, previous irradiation, diabetes mellitus and smoking history. Apart from local infection, none of these are absolute contraindications but patients should be warned that healing of the skin flaps and osseointegration may take longer than usual.

It is also important that the patient understands the need for daily care of the skin around the abutment. It is advisable to clean the area around the abutment daily. Those patients with poor personal hygiene may not be good candidates. Potential patients who are not able to care for the area themselves must have a carer willing and able to fulfill the role.

Surgical Procedure

The surgical procedure is relatively straightforward but does require specialized instruments to drill and countersink an appropriate site for the implant (Figs 2.1A to I).

Surgery can be carried out either under general or local anesthesia. In the former, it is useful to infiltrate the skin and subcutaneous tissue with epinephrine (1%) with lidocaine (1:100,000) to aid hemostasis.

The site of the intended implant is marked allowing sufficient room behind the pinna so that the hearing aid will not touch it when worn.

Crucial to success of the procedure is creation of an area of thin non-hair bearing skin around the transcutaneous abutment. A variety of techniques have been described including use of an electric dermatome to raise a split skin graft with removal of the soft tissues down to the periosteum or use of a

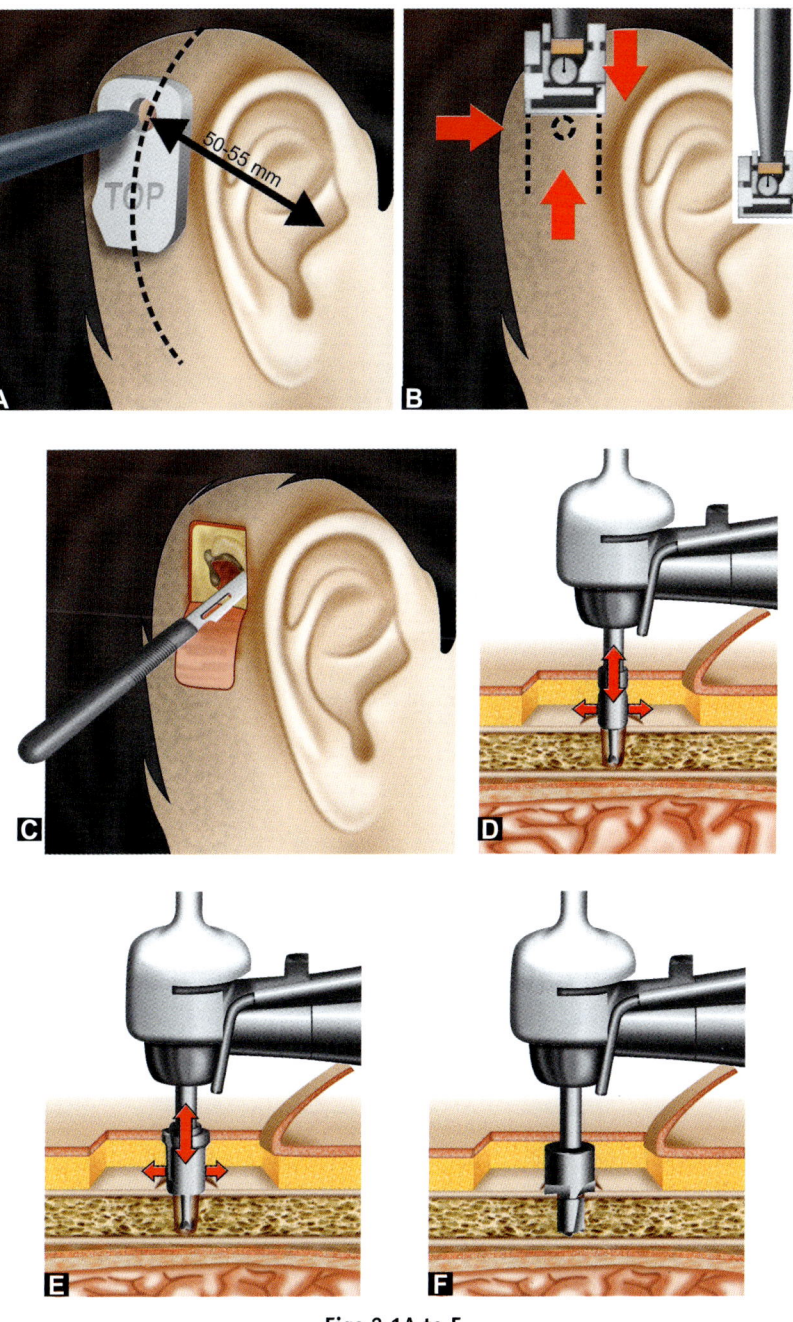

Figs 2.1A to F

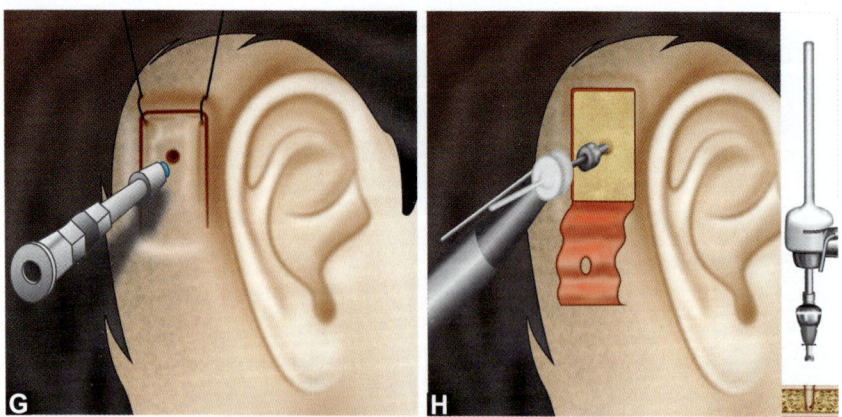

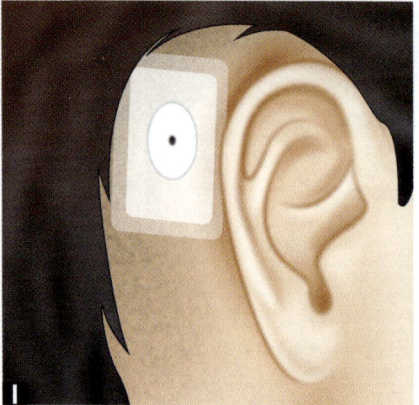

Figs 2.1G to I

Figs 2.1A to I: The stages of BAHA surgery. (A) The intended site for the abutment is measured about 50–55 mm from the ear canal; (B) Split-thickness skin flap is raised using a dermatome; (C) Soft tissue is excised down to periosteum; (D) A 3-mm hole is first drilled into the bone; (E) The drill-hole is deepened to 4 mm; (F) A countersink is used to widen the hole; (G) The skin flap replaced, and perforated; (H) The abutment is self-tapped into the hole in the bone via the perforation in the skin; (I) Skin dressing in place

linear incision (single vertical incision) which allows the soft tissues including hair follicle to be excised for an area of about 3 cm from the implant.

A 3-mm hole is drilled in the bone of the skull taking care to avoid heating of the bone by using constant irrigation with normal saline. If bone is encountered in the depths of the hole then the hole is deepened to 4 mm. The hole is then widened and countersunk. The self-tapping, factory assembled, flange fixture and abutment are then inserted at low speed; again, using appropriate irrigation until a preset tightness is achieved (usually 30–40 Ncm).

The skin or graft is perforated to accommodate the abutment and then sutured in place.

When implanting children, most surgeons perform surgery as a two-stage procedure, implanting the flange fixture as the first stage and then attaching the abutment and thinning the skin as the second stage. Some surgeons advocate placing a second fixture close to the first that can be used if the first fitting fails to osseointegrate or is subsequently damaged by trauma.

About 3 months after surgery, osseointegration should be secure enough to allow the hearing aid to be fitted. The choice of aid depends on the cochlear reserve (Figs 2.2A to C).

Complications of Surgery

These are rare but include damage to the dura or lateral sinus.

Late Complications

Skin reactions around the abutment are common. Badran et al.[3] found that 21% of implanted patients suffered from skin reactions. These complications can be minimized by careful surgical techniques to ensure that the adjacent skin is thin and hairless but it is also important that the patients understand the importance of adequate hygiene. They should be instructed in how to clean the area around the abutment using a soft toothbrush and if necessary, dental floss to ensure that there is no build-up of debris between the abutment and the skin. If skin reactions do occur, they can often be treated with topical antibiotics.

Loosening of the flange fixture can occur as a late complication and may result in the fixture becoming detached.

Previously, the abutment and flange fixture were supplied as separate components. Once the flange fixture had been inserted, the abutment was attached and tightened. Loosening of the abutment from the flange fixture occasionally occurred, but this is now less common as the two components are attached to each other during the manufacturing process.

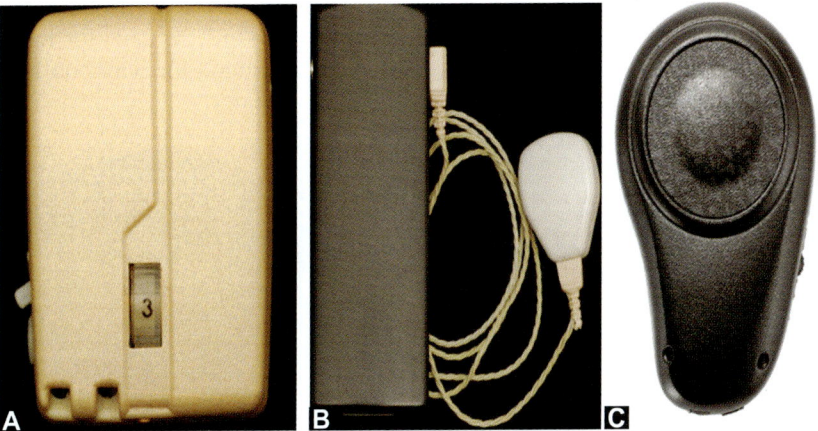

Figs 2.2A to C: Showing BAHA Divino, Cordelle II and Oticon Ponto hearing aids
Source: Courtesy of Cochlear™ and Oticon

Results

The functional outcomes of surgery depend on the indications for which the BAHA was implanted.

A recent study by Mace et al.[4] showed that bone-anchored hearing aid usage and satisfaction levels as assessed by the Glasgow Benefit Inventory were high with a median total score of + 33.3.

NEW DEVELOPMENTS IN IMPLANTABLE BONE CONDUCTION HEARING AIDS

Sophono Alpha 1 System

While BAHA provides good hearing rehabilitation for selected patients, it is associated with a high incidence of skin complications, varying from mild irritation around the implant to formation of granulation tissue and overgrowth of soft tissue sometimes requiring revision surgery.[5,6]

The Alpha 1 system was developed in Germany and was made available in 2006 (Figs 2.3A to C). The device is now distributed by Sophono Inc (Boulder, Colorado). FDA approval was given in June 2011. The FDA approval includes indication for single-sided deafness. The device works via magnetic coupling and acoustic transmission between implanted and external magnets.

Implantation is a single-stage procedure, involving surgical implantation of a magnetic plate to the skull with titanium screws (Fig. 2.4).

The plate is completely buried beneath the skin without any external protrusion, thus skin reaction is minimal and there are no aesthetic concerns. The hearing aid is held in place by magnetic attraction.

The Sophono Alpha 1 system has functional and aesthetic advantages and the postoperative results from the first UK Sophono implanted patients are very encouraging.

Key advantages of Sophono Alpha 1 can be summarized as absence of a percutaneous abutment, minimal skin complications and no need for long-term wound care.[7] Figure 2.5 shows audiological criteria for Sophono in a chart.

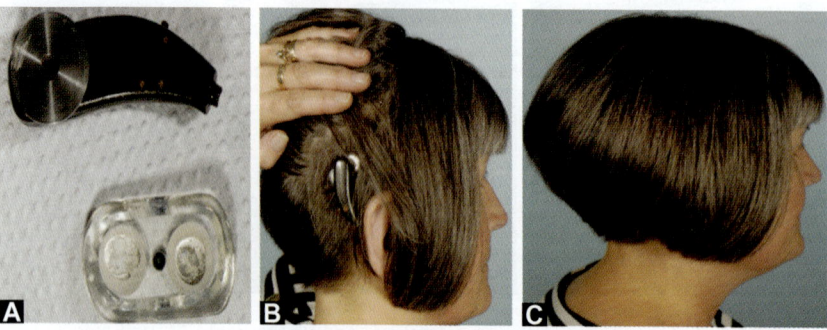

Figs 2.3A to C: Sophono Alpha 1 hearing aid on a patient

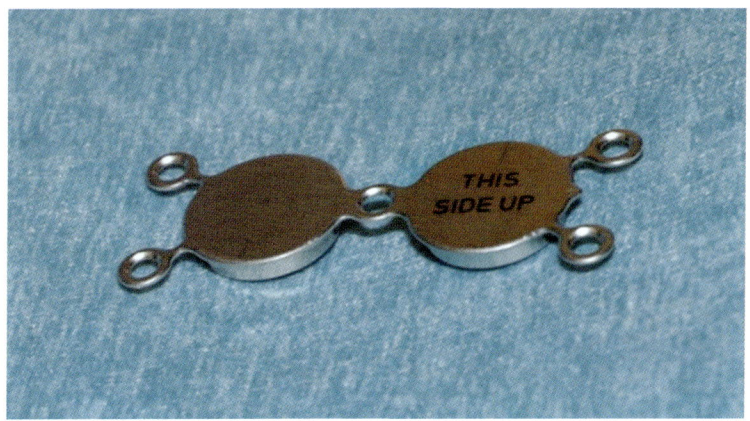

Fig. 2.4: Magnetic implant for Sophono Alpha 1

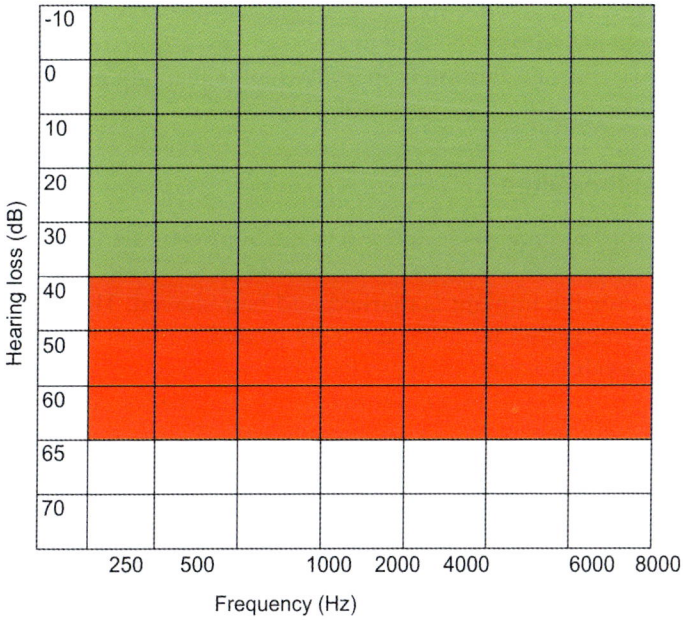

Fig. 2.5: Audiological criteria for Sophono in a chart. Sophono implant is indicated for patients with bone conduction up to 40 dB (Green shade); while BAHA can be implanted in patients with BC up to 65 dB (Green + Red shade)

Indications for Sophono

Patients who are suitable and are keen to use a BAHA, but are worried about the cosmetic appearance of an external abutment or are unable to care for the skin flap, will find the Sophono Alpha 1 implant an appropriate alternative. The selection criteria are outlined in Table 2.2.

Table 2.2: The Sophono implant is best for a patient who meets the following criteria
1. Pure conductive hearing loss
2. Mixed loss up to 45 dB sensory neural hearing loss
3. Single-sided deafness
4. Medical indications (i.e., chronic otitis media, congenital aural atresia, otitis external)

Patient Selection

Patient consideration for a Sophono implant is similar to that of BAHA; however, Sophono implants are recommended for individuals with better cochlear reserve. The bone conduction should not be worse than 45 dB measured at 0.5 kHz, 1 kHz, 2 kHz, and 3 kHz whereas with BAHA, patients with sensorineural thresholds of up to 65 dB can be fitted.

It can be fitted in children over 5 years of age. The FDA approval includes patients with single-side deafness (Table 2.2).

A relative contraindication is an individual who might need serial MRI scan.

Surgical Procedure

The procedure is single stage and can be performed under local or general anesthesia.

The site for the implant is marked and hair shaved. The thickness of the scalp is measured by using a needle passed through the skin to the bone. The depth of penetration can then be measured.

A 5-cm bow-shaped incision is made 7.5 cm superior and posterior to the external auditory canal at an angle of 45°. The incision is deepened through skin and periosteum, and the flap is raised anteriorly.

The wells to accommodate the magnets are drilled using a 4-mm cutting burr. The implant is secured to the skull with 2-mm diameter, 4-mm long maxillofacial bone screws (Figs 2.6A to F).

The flap can be thinned to approximately 4-mm, if necessary.

The flap is replaced and wound sutured. After about 4 weeks, the external bone vibrating audio processor that attaches magnetically over the implant can be fitted.

Our results in York suggest that for patients with conductive hearing loss or single-sided deafness, hearing rehabilitation is good with minimal complications.

Complications of Surgery

Intraoperative complications are rare; we have outlined our complications in Table 2.3.

Recent Advances in Otolaryngology – Head and Neck Surgery

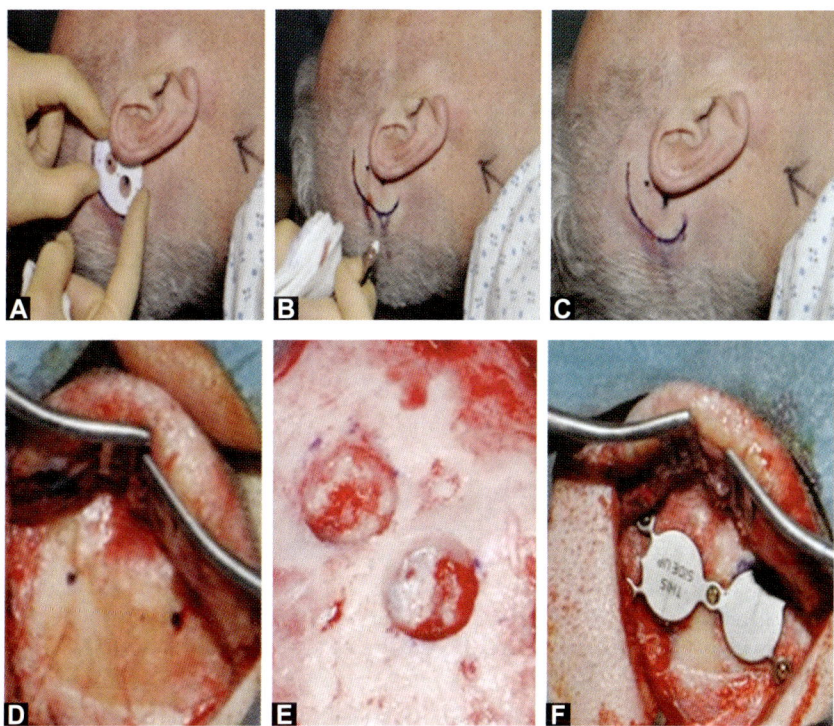

Figs 2.6A to F: Stages of surgery for Sophono Alpha 1 implant; (A) A template is used to mark the site. To use the template it must be above the frankfurt line. Methylene blue injected after marking. The aim is to stain the periosteum for the drilling of the well that comes later; (B) Local anesthetic used (the whole of the bed—we use 2% lignocane and 1 in 80,000 adrenaline); (C) A skin incision is made through skin and periosteum. This flap is raised anteriorly; (D) Methylene blue used to mark the center of the implant well site; (E) The implant well is drilled using a 4-mm cutting Burr; (F) The implant is put in place and held by six 4-mm screws. The flap is put back in place and wound closed with Novafil 4/0

Table 2.3: Complications of Sophono		
	York (13)	*Recklinghausen (57)*
Surgical complications	0	0
Wound problems	0	0
Skin redness (pressure)	1	4
Any other complications	0	0

SUMMARY

There are currently several options for hearing rehabilitation for patients with hearing loss who are unable to wear conventional air conduction hearings aids including BAHA®, Oticon® Ponto and Sophono Alpha 1.

ACKNOWLEDGMENTS

1. We are grateful to Mr. Mike Pringle, the medical photographer at York Teaching Hospital who kindly helped with the intraoperative and postoperative pictures.
2. We acknowledge Cochlear™ and Oticon who have provided us with some illustrations, and have kindly agreed their use in this publication.
3. We express gratitude to all our patients who have supported this publication by kindly giving permission for the use of their intraoperative and postoperative clinical pictures.

REFERENCES

1. Tonndorf J. Bone conduction. Studies in experimental animals. Acta Otolaryngol. 1966;Suppl 213:1+.
2. Lustig LR, Arts HA, Brackmann DE, et al. Hearing rehabilitation using the BAHA bone-anchored hearing aid: results in 40 patients. Otol Neurotol. 2001;22(3):328-34.
3. Badran K, Arya AK, Bunstone D, et al. Long-term complications of bone-anchored hearings aids: a 14-year experience. J Laryngol Otol. 2009;123(2):170-6.
4. Mace AT, Isa A, Cooke LD. Patient quality of life with bone-anchored hearing aid: 10-year experience in Glasgow, Scotland. J Laryngol Otol. 2009;123(9):964-8.
5. de Wolf MJ, Hol MK, Mylanus EA, et al. Bone-anchored hearing aid surgery in older adults: implant loss and skin reactions. Ann Otol Rhinol Laryngol. 2009;118(7):525-31.
6. Doshi J, Karagama Y, Buckley D, et al. Observational study of bone-anchored hearing aid infection rates using different post-operative dressings. J Laryngol Otol. 2006;120(10):842-4.
7. Siegert R. Partially implantable bone conduction hearing aids without a percutaneous abutment (Otomag): technique and preliminary clinical results. Adv Otorhinolaryngol. 2011;71:41-6.

SUPERIOR SEMICIRCULAR CANAL DEHISCENCE SYNDROME: EVALUATION AND MANAGEMENT

Jason A Beyea, Lorne S Parnes, Sumit K Agrawal

ABSTRACT

The superior semicircular canal dehiscence (SSCD) syndrome was first described by Minor et al. in 1998. The underlying pathophysiology is caused by a dehiscence of the bone overlying the superior semicircular canal. This permits the labyrinth to respond to sound and pressure changes. Symptoms can include Tullio phenomenon, pressure-induced vertigo, chronic disequilibrium, hearing loss, autophony, pulsatile tinnitus, and hyperacusis of bone conducted sounds. Physical examination includes presentation of auditory tones and tragal compression to evaluate for the presence of evoked eye movements in the plane of the superior semicircular canal. Audiometry may show a low-frequency conductive hearing loss with bone conduction thresholds less than 0 dB. Vestibular evoked myogenic potentials may demonstrate a reduced response threshold on the affected side. Computed tomography with 0.5 mm collimation and oblique reformats in the plane of the superior semicircular canal is used to evaluate for the presence of a bony dehiscence. Management is first directed at trigger avoidance. For those whom conservative management is not successful, surgical management is offered. Canal plugging is superior to resurfacing. This can be performed through either a transmastoid or middle cranial fossa approach. This chapter details the transmastoid approach.

INTRODUCTION

The superior semicircular canal dehiscence syndrome was first described by Minor et al.[1] Studies on cadaveric temporal bones have found a dehiscence of the overlying bone of the SSC in 0.5% of specimens.[2] In an additional 1.4% of specimens, the bone coverage was less than 0.1 mm, such that it might appear dehiscent even on ultra-high resolution computed tomography of the temporal bone. Despite the high radiographic and histological prevalence, the clinical prevalence is much lower.

PATHOPHYSIOLOGY

The underlying pathophysiology is related to an opening in the bone that overlies the SSC. This creates a third mobile window (the first and second being the oval and round windows) into the inner ear. As a result, the membranous labyrinth responds to sound and pressure changes.

Excitation

Excitation of the superior canal occurs with application of positive pressure in the external auditory canal (EAC), Valsalva's maneuver against pinched nostrils and presentation of loud sound to the ear.[2] Positive pressure to the EAC and Valsalva against pinched nostrils create a positive pressure gradient from the middle to the inner ear, the pressure is released through the dehiscence over the superior canal and resultant utriculofugal flow in the superior canal is excitatory. The mechanism of loud sound-induced excitation has been postulated to occur through a different mechanism, which may be due to rectified stapes motion, excitation/inhibition asymmetry and/or vestibular nerve afferent phase-locking.[2]

Inhibition

Inhibition of the superior canal occurs with creation of negative pressure in the EAC, Valsalva's maneuver against a closed glottis and jugular venous compression. These stimuli create a positive pressure gradient from the middle cranial fossa to the inner ear at the dehiscence, the pressure is released at the round or oval windows, and the resultant utriculopetal flow in the superior canal is inhibitory.

Nystagmus

The resultant eye movements (Figs 3.1A and B) typically align themselves with the plane of the affected SSC. With eyes in center gaze, excitation of the right SSC (tone presentation to right ear) results in slow phase nystagmus directed upwards with a torsional rotation of the superior pole of the eyes toward the patient's left side.[3] Fast phase nystagmus is directed downwards with a torsional rotation of the superior pole of the eyes toward the patient's right side. Conversely, excitation of the left SSC (tone presentation to the left ear) results in slow phase nystagmus directed upwards with a torsional rotation of the superior pole of the eyes toward the patient's right side. Fast phase nystagmus is directed downwards with a torsional rotation of the superior pole of the eyes toward the patient's left side. The

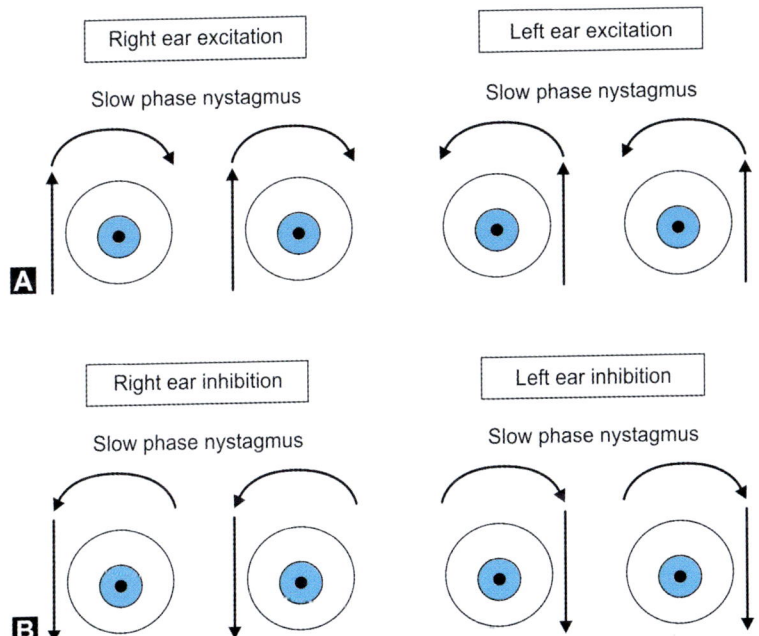

Figs 3.1A and B: Slow phase nystagmus upon excitation (A) and inhibition (B) of the superior semicircular canal in neutral gaze position. Excitation of the superior canal is caused by application of positive pressure in the EAC, Valsalva's maneuver against pinched nostrils, and presentation of loud sound to the ear. Conversely, inhibition of the superior canal is caused by creation of negative pressure in the EAC, Valsalva's maneuver against a closed glottis, and jugular venous compression. This figure demonstrates slow phase nystagmus only in neutral gaze. For excitation of a given ear with gaze towards that ipsilateral ear, nystagmus is purely upward. For excitation of a given ear with gaze towards the contralateral ear, nystagmus is purely torsional with the superior pole of the eyes beating towards the contralateral ear. For inhibition of a given ear with gaze towards that ipsilateral ear, nystagmus is purely downward. For inhibition of a given ear with gaze towards the contralateral ear, nystagmus is purely torsional with the superior pole of the eyes beating towards the ipsilateral ear

presence of the torsional and vertical components of the nystagmus is dependent on direction of gaze [(neutral, right and left gaze) Fig. 3.1].

Origin of Bony Dehiscence

Dehiscence of the bone overlying the SSC is presumed to arise from reduction of the normal thickening of bone over the superior canal which occurs during the first 3 postnatal years,[2] although this postnatal developmental cause of SSCD remains controversial. Tsunoda and Terasaki [2002] used a computer simulation model to propose that SSCD arises during the fetal developmental period.[4] Wang and Parnes [2010] described a case of bilateral SSCD in a patient with external, middle, and inner ear abnormalities, providing support to a congenital etiology.[5] In contrast, a recent retrospective radiological series of temporal bone

CT scans demonstrated a statistically significant increase in superior canal dehiscence with increasing age,[6] lending support to an acquired cause. Precipitating events of the SSCD syndrome remain speculative. These include direct trauma, activities that produced changes in middle ear or intracranial pressure[7] and systemic bony demineralization which occurred with increasing age.[6]

SYMPTOMS

This syndrome can include vestibular and audiologic symptoms (Table 3.1). Vestibular symptoms manifest as vertigo, oscillopsia, chronic disequilibrium and motion intolerance.[1] Minor [2005] reported that 60 (92%) of 65 patients with superior canal dehiscence had vestibular symptoms that were attributed to the dehiscence of the superior canal. In this same series, 54 (83%) had loud sound-induced vertigo and 44 (68%) had pressure-induced (induced by coughing, sneezing, straining) vertigo.[8] The Tullio phenomenon (brief transient vertigo

Table 3.1: Signs, symptoms and investigation findings in superior semicircular canal dehiscence syndrome

Symptoms	Percentage of Patients Affected
Tullio phenomenon	83% (54/65)[8]
Hearing loss	82% (9/11)[9]
Aural fullness	80% (4/5)[10]
Pressure-induced vertigo	68% (44/65)[8]
Autophony	60% (39/65)[8]
Hyperacusis of bone conducted sounds	52% (34/65)[8]
Pulsatile tinnitus	27% (3/11)[9]
Signs	
Sound-evoked eye movements	77% (46/60)[8]
256 Hz tuning fork heard at lateral malleolus	75% (3/4)[11]
Valsalva-evoked eye movements	70% (42/60)[8]
External auditory canal applied pressure-evoked eye movements	43% (26/60)[8]
Sound-evoked head tilt in plane of SSC	18% (11/60)[8]
Investigations	
VEMP—Lowered threshold	91% (32/35)[12]
Audiogram—Air-bone gap ≥ 10 dB at 250 Hz	72% (38/53)[8]
Audiogram—Depressed bone conduction < 0 dB	67% (2/3)[13]
Audiogram—Acoustic reflexes absent	11% (2/18)[12]

Abbreviations: SSC = Superior Semicircular Canal, VEMP = Vestibular-Evoked Myogenic Potential

induced by loud sounds) often is characteristic of this syndrome. A complete focused history includes a search for other causes of vestibular symptoms.

Associated auditory symptoms include hearing loss, autophony and hyperacusis of bone conducted sounds such as the sound of the patient's own footsteps and their eyes moving in their orbits.[8,14] In the series of Minor [2005],[8] 39 patients (60%) had autophony and 34 patients (52%) had hyperacusis of bone conducted sounds.

Interestingly, SSCD can present purely as a conductive hearing loss (CHL), without associated vestibular symptoms.[15] In this manner, SSCD can mimic otosclerosis. Patients may undergo failed middle ear surgery for a presumed otosclerosis.[16] A key distinguishing factor is the presence of the acoustic reflex in patients with SSCD,[16] whereas this will typically be absent in patients with otosclerosis.[17] Furthermore, Röösli et al. [2008] highlighted the role of obtaining a CT scan prior to revision of stapes surgery to identify abnormalities, such as SSCD, and to avoid performance of unnecessary surgeries.[18] These findings emphasize the importance of screening patients with suspected otosclerosis for vestibular symptoms. SSCD should be on the clinician's differential diagnosis of CHL.

An explanation for the variability in symptomatology experienced by different patients has been proposed by Pfammatter et al. [2010].[19] These investigators found that patients with both vestibular and cochlear symptoms had significantly larger dehiscences of the superior canal (mean of 4.1 mm) than those with only vestibular or cochlear symptoms (mean of 1.9 mm) ($p < 0.001$).

PHYSICAL EXAMINATION

Sound or pressure evoked eye movements should be observed in the absence of visual fixation,[3] as visual fixation can suppress the nystagmus of labyrinthine origin. However, the torsional nystagmus component is poorly inhibited by visual fixation,[20] as point fixation can only suppress the vertical and horizontal components of the nystagmus. Avoidance of visual fixation suppression can be achieved with the use of infrared video equipment or Frenzel's glasses.[3] Cremer et al. [2000] recommended assessment of evoked eye movements during presentation of tones (125 Hz to 6 kHz, intensity of 110 dB HL), Valsalva's maneuvers and tragal compression. Direction of the evoked nystagmus will be as previously described (Fig. 3.1).[3] Minor [2005] found that of patients with vestibular signs associated with SSCD, 82% had sound-evoked eye movements, 75% had Valsalva-evoked eye movements and 45% had EAC pressure-evoked eye movements.[8] Furthermore, a tilt of the head in the plane of the superior canal evoked by sound was detected in 20% of these patients. In dehiscences greater than or equal to 5 mm, nystagmus evoked by tone presentation aligns between the plane of the superior and horizontal canals.[14] Weber 512 Hz tuning fork will lateralize to the affected ear and a low-frequency tuning fork (128 and 256 Hz) placed on the lateral malleolus of the ankle may be heard by the patient.[11,21] The evaluation should include a complete head and neck examination, Dix-Hallpike and a focused neurological examination.

INVESTIGATIONS

Audiometry typically reveals a low frequency CHL on the affected side, with normal word recognition and intact acoustic reflexes.[1,22,23a,b] Bone conduction thresholds may be less than 0 dB HL. Tympanometry demonstrates normal pressure.[7] As noted, the intact acoustic reflexes may be the significant clue that differentiates SSCD from otosclerotic CHL.[24]

Routine electronystagmography fails to identify objective abnormal findings, but the patient may report vertigo with the application of pressure to the EAC.[25] Caloric testing will typically be normal.[26]

Vestibular evoked myogenic potentials (VEMPs) are enhanced in SSCD, displaying a reduced response threshold on the affected side.[8,23] Pfammatter et al. [2010] demonstrated that with a bone dehiscence of greater than or equal to 2.5 mm, the VEMP threshold was more often lowered ($\leq$ 80 dB SPL) than if the dehiscence was less than 2.5 mm (p = 0.009).[19] The VEMP responses typically reported for SSCD syndrome are cervical VEMPs, as electromyography is recorded from the sternocleidomastoid muscle. Ocular VEMPs, measured from electrodes placed on the cheek below the eye, have been shown to be equally useful in diagnosis and follow-up of SSCD syndrome,[27] but demonstrate better test-retest reliability than cervical VEMPs.[28] Our center currently uses cervical VEMPs.

High-resolution CT scanning is necessary to accurately diagnose the bony dehiscence. The use of 0.5 mm collimation and oblique reformats in the plane of the SSC has been demonstrated to improve specificity and positive predictive value (PPV) of a finding of dehiscence.[29] Belden et al. [2003] found that the PPV of an apparent dehiscence in SSCD was 50% with 1.0 mm collimation using coronal and transverse images, which improved to 93% with 0.5 mm collimation and CT reformatting in the plane of the SSC. An example of pre- and postoperative CT findings in a patient with left SSCD syndrome is shown in Figures 3.2A and B. New technology using Cone-Beam Volumetric Tomography holds promise for improved diagnostic accuracy related to its ability to provide greater information content and spatial resolution compared to Multi-Slice Computed Tomography.[30]

DIAGNOSIS

Figure 3.3 describes our diagnostic algorithm. SSCD syndrome is diagnosed by the presence of vestibular and/or audiologic symptoms characteristic of the syndrome, evoked eye movements in the plane of the affected SSC, and radiological confirmation of bony dehiscence over the SSC.[8] A low frequency CHL and normal word recognition on audiometry, the presence of intact acoustic reflexes and lowered thresholds on VEMP testing aid in the diagnosis.

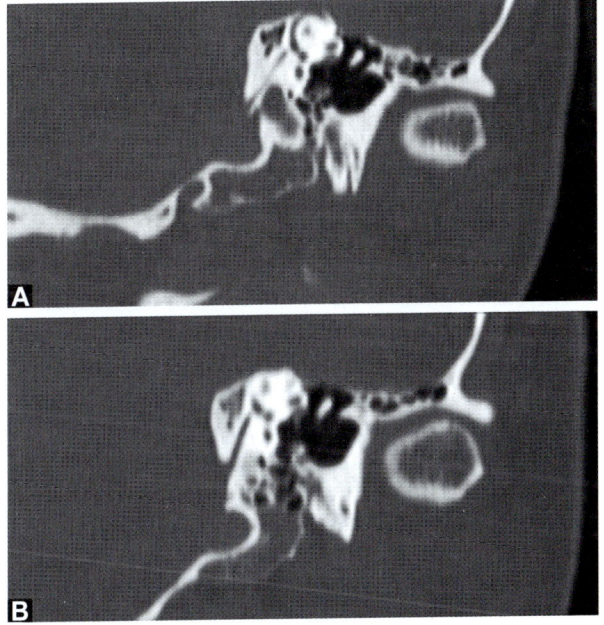

Figs 3.2A and B: A Patient's CT scan with 0.625 mm collimation, following oblique refor-matting. (A) Left superior semicircular canal dehiscence; (B) Postoperative CT scan from the patient in A. The patient has undergone a transmastoid approach superior semicircular canal occlusion

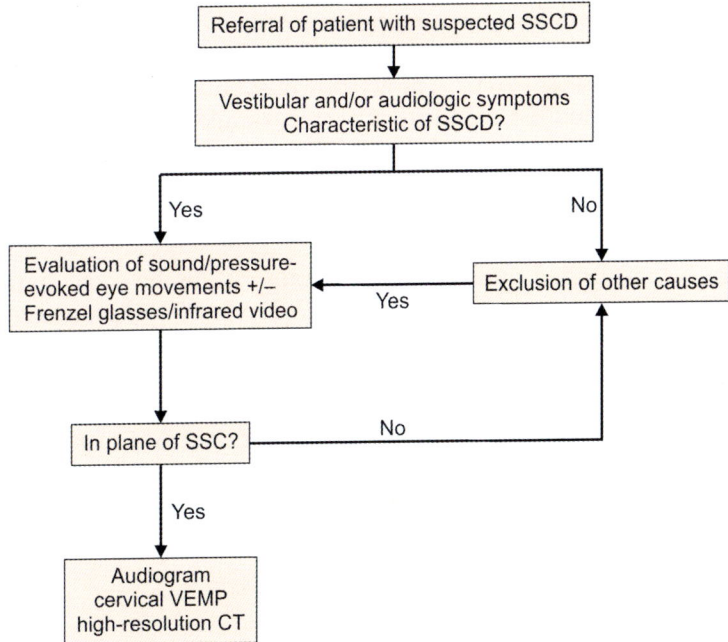

Fig. 3.3: Our diagnostic algorithm for superior semicircular canal dehiscence syndrome

Differential Diagnosis

Careful consideration of the presenting symptoms of SSCD syndrome permits formulation of a broad differential diagnosis. A history of transient vertigo raises the possibility of benign paroxysmal positional vertigo (BPPV). This can be distinguished from SSCD syndrome by the absence of audiologic symptoms, the absence of sound/pressure-evoked nystagmus, a positive Dix-Hallpike and the presence of bony coverage of the superior canal on CT scan. Otosclerosis also presents with a CHL, but can be distinguished based on the absence of vestibular symptoms on history, the absence of acoustic reflexes and the presence of bony coverage of the superior canal on CT scan. Patulous Eustachian tube shares with SSCD the symptom of autophony. Poe [2007] noted in his series that the patients with patulous Eustachian tube had autophony of their breathing, whereas those with SSCD syndrome did not.[31] Clinical evaluation for respiratory excursion of the tympanic membrane and a high-resolution CT scan will further clarify the diagnosis. In addition to SSCD, a labyrinthine fistula can be caused by post-traumatic leakage of perilymph from the inner to the middle ear and from disruption of the labyrinthine bone caused by cholesteatoma or chronic otitis media.[23a] Clinical history, the direction of evoked eye movements, and CT scan findings will distinguish these pathologies from SSCD.[23a] Finally, migraine-associated vertigo should be considered. Migraine-related vertigo (MV) is the most common cause of spontaneous non-positional episodic vertigo.[32] Brief MV attacks lasting seconds with possible migraine-associated symptoms of hearing loss, tinnitus and aural fullness can be difficult to distinguish from SSCD on clinical history. Typically, noise or Valsalva-precipitated vertigo is not present in MV.[32] The absence of sound and pressure-evoked eye movements and the presence of bony coverage of the superior canal on CT scan will distinguish MV from SSCD.

MANAGEMENT

Figure 3.4 describes our management algorithm. In most patients, control of symptoms is achieved by avoidance of symptom-evoking sound and pressure stimuli.[33] A conscientious patient can often avoid their distinct triggers. Only after attempted trigger avoidance and in the presence of debilitating vestibular or auditory symptoms should surgical management be pursued. The dizziness handicap inventory (DHI) can be used to quantify the disability that SSCD syndrome is causing for the patient and to evaluate postoperative response to surgery.[34]

Surgical Management

Surgical management of SSCD syndrome is through resurfacing or plugging of the SSC. Resurfacing is typically performed through a middle

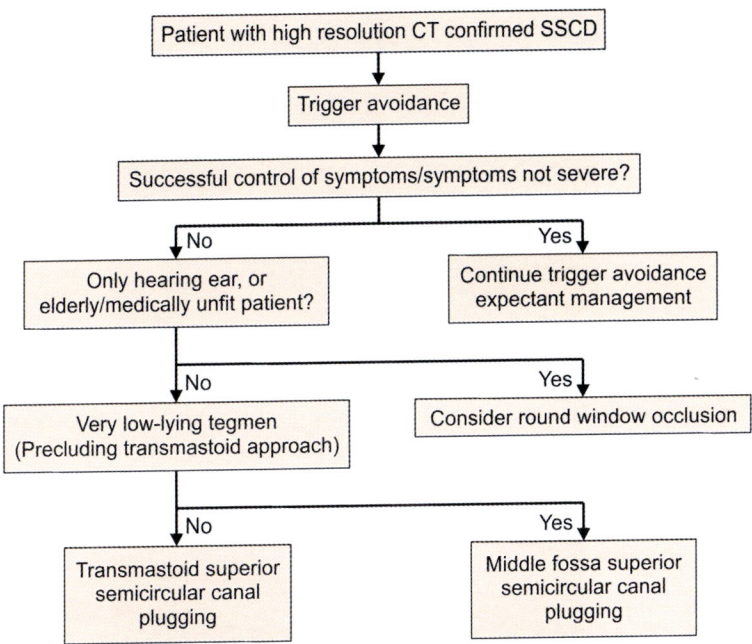

Fig. 3.4: Our management algorithm for superior semicircular canal dehiscence syndrome

fossa approach,[8] although recently transmastoid resurfacing has been described.[10,35] Plugging is performed through a middle fossa[1] or transmastoid[22,24,36] approach. A recent meta-analysis[37] has demonstrated the superiority of canal plugging or capping (with hydroxyapatite cement) over resurfacing for resolution of symptoms.

The transmastoid approach to SSC plugging has become our surgical approach of choice. This approach has the advantages of obviating a craniotomy, avoidance of temporal lobe retraction, familiarity of the approach for experienced otologists and the ability to occlude the canal without manipulating the defect.[24] In the minority of patients with a very low-lying tegmen, the middle fossa approach would be considered (Fig. 3.4). We use bone dust for canal plugging, as opposed to bone wax, as bone dust has been shown to promote less inflammation and to demonstrate improved osteogenesis.[38] Briefly, a 5–6 cm postauricular incision is made, a standard mastoidectomy is performed and the horizontal canal is visualized (Fig. 3.5). Bone between the horizontal canal and tegmen is carefully drilled layer by layer with a small diamond burr to blue-line the superior canal on both sides of the dehiscence (Fig. 3.6). The dura over the canal is gently mobilized, but not elevated, to verify the dehiscence (Fig. 3.7). Care must be taken as dural elevation may cause injury to the inner ear. A 1 x 3 mm endosteal island is made on both the ampulated and nonampulated sides of the canal, and gently elevated with a fine 90° hook to visualize the membranous labyrinth. Bone pâté (dry bone dust and fibrinogen sealant) is gently

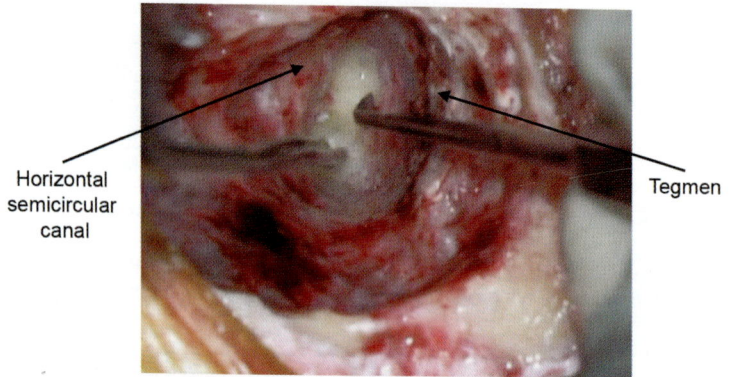

Horizontal
semicircular
canal

Tegmen

Fig. 3.5: Standard mastoidectomy has been completed and the horizontal canal is visualized

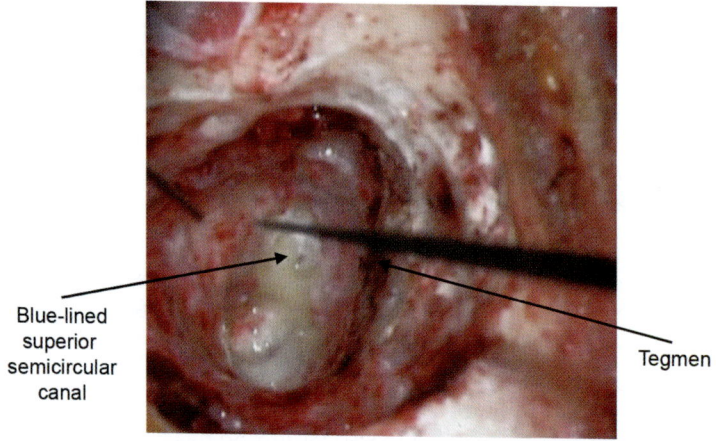

Blue-lined
superior
semicircular
canal

Tegmen

Fig. 3.6: The superior semicircular canal has been blue-lined on both sides of the dehiscence

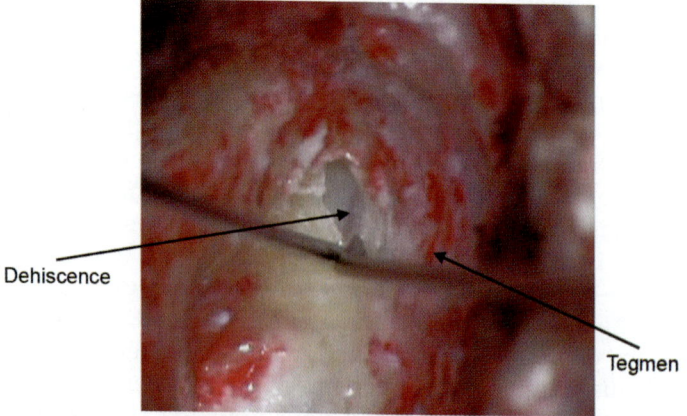

Dehiscence

Tegmen

Fig. 3.7: The dura is gently mobilized to verify the dehiscence

packed into both fenestrations (Fig. 3.8). This occludes the canal and isolates the dehiscent region. The occlusions are covered with temporalis fascia and fibrinogen sealant to protect against perilymph leakage.

In patients whose SSCD ear is their only hearing ear and/or their only ear with vestibular function, or who are elderly/medically unfit for transmastoid semicircular canal occlusion, consideration is given to a round window occlusion. Patching of the round window theoretically dampens the hypercompliance of the round and oval windows, and makes the inner ear less sensitive to sound and pressure.[39] This approach is minimally invasive and does not preclude future transmastoid/middle fossa procedures for the patient if round window occlusion is unsuccessful. To date we have treated three patients with round window occlusion. These patients have demonstrated short-term relief or significant improvement of pulsatile tinnitus, autophony and hyperacusis of bone conducted sounds. At present, the long-term success of this procedure is not known. This procedure has been previously described by Silverstein and Van Ess [2009].[39] Our technical approach to round window occlusion is as follows. A standard tympanomeatal flap is elevated through an endaural approach. The round window membrane is visualized and the superficial layer is removed with a 90° pick. Overhanging bone from the round window niche is removed with a diamond burr. A small piece of temporalis fascia is harvested and used to plug the round window (Figs 3.9A and B). Fibrin sealant is dispensed over the fascia and round window. The tympanomeatal flap is returned to its native position and thrombin sponge is placed in the EAC.

OUTCOME

Most outcome literature on SSCD surgical repair is from series that used a middle cranial fossa approach. Complete vestibular symptom

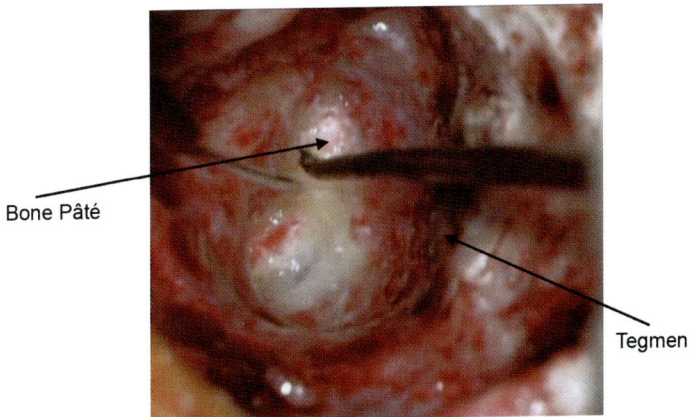

Fig. 3.8: Bone pâté is packed gently into both fenestrations to occlude the canal and isolate the dehiscent region

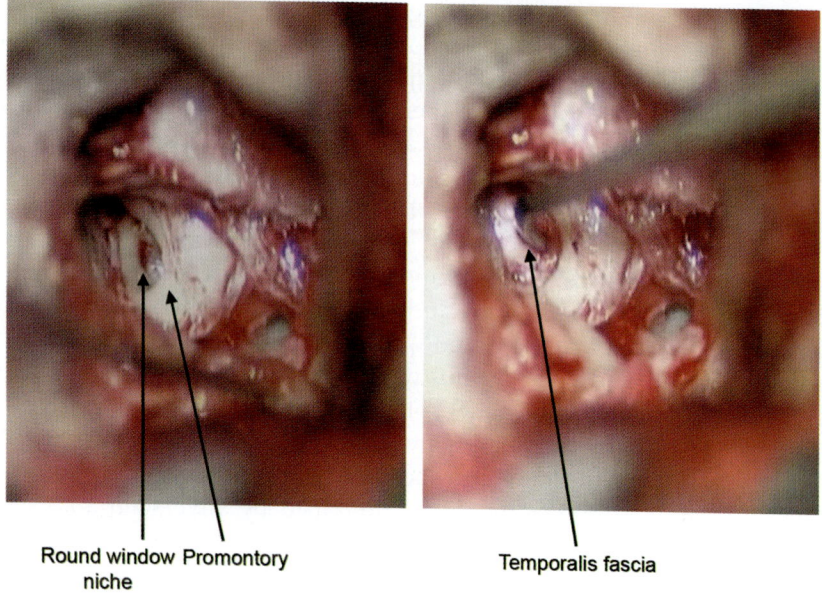

Round window Promontory
niche   Temporalis fascia

Figs 3.9A and B: (A) Through an endaural approach, a standard tympanomeatal flap is elevated and the round window membrane is visualized; (B) A small piece of temporalis fascia is used to plug the round window

and sign resolution occurs more often in patients who underwent SSCD plugging (8 out of 9) versus resurfacing (7 out of 11).[8] This is supported by the meta-analysis of Vlastarakos et al. [2009][37] who demonstrated success rates of 32/33, 8/16, and 14/15 for plugging, resurfacing, and capping with hydroxyapatite-cement, respectively. Delayed failures of resurfacing procedures can be caused by bone graft resorption.[40] Of note, SSCD plugging produces a significant postoperative reduction in DHI scores,[34] highlighting the usefulness of pre- and postoperative DHI testing.

Our previous report [Agrawal and Parnes, 2008] of three cases of transmastoid SSC occlusion has now been substantiated by a further 12 cases in which symptoms have improved or abated [unpublished data].[24] One of our patient's vestibular symptoms did not improve postoperatively. All patients had either unchanged or improved pure-tone thresholds compared to preoperative thresholds. As previously discussed, high-resolution preoperative imaging cannot be overemphasized. We have had one case in which a dehiscence was recognized on the CT scan, but was not identified intraoperatively. Table 3.2 describes the publications in the literature to date which used a transmastoid SSC plugging approach. Of published cases, 19 of 20 ears demonstrated significant or complete resolution of sound- and pressure-induced symptoms.

Table 3.2: Transmastoid approach superior semicircular canal dehiscence plugging

Authors	Number of ears	Occlusion material	Resolution of sound/ pressure- induced symptoms?	Postoperative hearing status
Fiorino et al. 2010[36]	6	Bone dust and Fibrin glue	6/6 complete	5 unchanged 1 moderate CHL*
Deschenes et al. 2009[41]	3	Bone dust and bone wax	3/3 complete	2 improved 1 unchanged
Kirtane et al. 2009[42]	1	Bone pâté	1/1 complete	1 mild low- frequency SNHL
Teixido et al. 2008[43]	5	2 perichondrium 3 bone wax	4/5 significant or complete	1 improved 4 unchanged
Agrawal and Parnes 2008,[24] plus 13 unpublished cases	16	Bone dust and fibrinogen sealant	15/16 significant or complete	2 improved 14 unchanged
Brantberg et al. 2001[22]	2	Temporalis fascia	2/2 complete	1 unchanged 1 hearing loss

Abbreviations: CHL = Conductive Hearing Loss, SNHL = Sensorineural Hearing Loss
*Attributed to a middle ear effusion. Ventilation tube insertion resulted in recovery to preoperative levels.

Limb et al. [2006] found that middle fossa repair of SSCD was not associated with sensorineural hearing loss (SNHL), and a small group of patients demonstrated postoperative improvement in CHL.[44] The risk of SNHL is higher in patients who have previously undergone inner ear surgery.[44] SSCD plugging results in reduced function in the surgically repaired canal, but typically does not impair the function of the other two ipsilateral semicircular canals.[45] Interestingly, VEMP thresholds have been found to normalize after corrective surgical plugging of the SSCD.[27]

SUMMARY

Diagnosis of SSCD is based on the presence of vestibular and/or audiologic symptoms characteristic of the syndrome, evoked eye movements in the plane of the affected SSC and high-resolution CT confirmation of bony dehiscence over the SSC. Most patients with SSCD syndrome can be adequately managed without surgical intervention through trigger avoidance. For those who undergo surgical management, canal plugging is superior to resurfacing. This can be performed through either a transmastoid or middle cranial fossa approach.

REFERENCES

1. Minor LB, Solomon D, Zinreich JS, et al. Sound- and/or pressure-induced vertigo due to bone dehiscence of the superior semicircular canal. Arch Otolaryngol Head Neck Surg. 1998;124(3):249-58.
2. Carey JP, Minor LB, Nager GT. Dehiscence or thinning of bone overlying the superior semicircular canal in a temporal bone survey. Arch Otolaryngol Head Neck Surg. 2000;126(2):137-47.
3. Cremer PD, Minor LB, Carey JP, et al. Eye movements in patients with superior canal dehiscence syndrome align with the abnormal canal. Neurology. 2000;55(12):1833-41.
4. Tsunoda A, Terasaki O. Dehiscence of the bony roof of the superior semicircular canal in the middle cranial fossa. J Laryngol Otol. 2002;116:514-8.
5. Wang JR, Parnes LS. Superior semicircular canal dehiscence associated with external, middle, and inner ear abnormalities. Laryngoscope. 2010;120:390-3.
6. Nadgir RN, Ozonoff A, Devaiah AK, et al. Superior semicircular canal dehiscence: congenital or acquired condition? Am J Neuroradiol. 2011;32:947-9.
7. Banerjee A, Whyte A, Atlas MD. Superior canal dehiscence: review of a new condition. Clin Otolaryngol. 2005;30(1):9-15.
8. Minor LB. Clinical manifestations of superior semicircular canal dehiscence. Laryngoscope. 2005;115:1717-27.
9. Chi FL, Ren DD, Dai CF. Variety of audiologic manifestations in patients with superior semicircular canal dehiscence. Otol Neurotol. 2010;31:2-10.
10. Teixido M, Seymour PE, Kung B, et al. Transmastoid Middle Fossa Craniotomy Repair of Superior Semicircular Canal Dehiscence Using a Soft Tissue Graft. Otol Neurotol. 2011 Jun 8. [Epub ahead of print].
11. Watson SRD, Halmagyi GM, Coltebach JG. Vestibular hypersensitivity to sound (Tullio phenomenon): structural and functional assessment. Neurology. 2000;54:722-8.
12. Zhou G, Gopen Q, Poe DS. Clinical and diagnostic characterization of canal dehiscence syndrome: a great otologic mimicker. Otol Neurotol. 2007;28:920-6.
13. Streubel SO, Cremer PD, Carey JP, et al. Vestibular-evoked myogenic potentials in the diagnosis of superior canal dehiscence syndrome. Acta Otolaryngol Suppl. 2001;545:41-9.
14. Minor LB, Cremer PD, Carey JP, et al. Symptoms and signs in superior canal dehiscence syndrome. Ann N Y Acad Sci. 2001;942:259-73.
15. Mikulec AA, McKenna MJ, Ramsey MJ, et al. Superior semicircular canal dehiscence presenting as conductive hearing loss without vertigo. Otol Neurotol. 2004;25:121-9.
16. Li PM, Bergeron C, Monfared A, et al. Superior semicircular canal dehiscence diagnosed after failed stapedotomy for conductive hearing loss. Am J Otolaryngol. 2010 Sep 29. [Epub ahead of print].
17. Shahnaz N, Bork K, Polka L, et al. Energy reflectance and tympanometry in normal and otosclerotic ears. Ear Hear. 2009;30:219-33.
18. Röösli C, Hoffmann A, Treumann T, et al. Significance of computed tomography evaluation before revision stapes surgery. HNO. 2008;56:895-900.

19. Pfammatter A, Darrouzet V, Gartner M, et al. A superior semicircular canal dehiscence syndrome multicenter study: is there an association between size and symptoms? Otol Neurotol. 2010;31:447-54.
20. Maire R, Duvoisin B. Localization of static positional nystagmus with the ocular fixation test. Laryngoscope. 1999;109:606-12.
21. Halmagyi GM, Aw ST, McGarvie LA, et al. Superior semicircular canal dehiscence simulating otosclerosis. J Laryngol Otol. 2003;117:553-7.
22. Brantberg K, Bergenius J, Mendel L, et al. Symptoms, findings and treatment in patients with dehiscence of the superior semicircular canal. Acta Otolaryngol. 2001;121:68-75.
23a. Minor LB. Labyrinthine fistulae: pathobiology and management. Curr Opin Otolaryngol Head Neck Surg. 2003;11:340-6.
23b. Minor LB, Carey JP, Cremer PD, et al. Dehiscence of bone overlying the superior canal as a cause of apparent conductive hearing loss. Otol Neurotol. 2003;24:270-8.
24. Agrawal SK, Parnes LS. Transmastoid superior semicircular canal occlusion. Otol Neurotol. 2008;29(3):363-7.
25. Mong A, Loevner LA, Solomon D, et al. Sound- and pressure-induced vertigo associated with dehiscence of the roof of the superior semicircular canal. AJNR Am J Neuroradiol. 1999;20:1973-5.
26. Brantberg K, Bergenius J, Tribukait A. Vestibular-evoked myogenic potentials in patients with dehiscence of the superior semicircular canal. Acta Otolaryngol. 1999;119(6):633-40.
27. Welgampola MS, Myrie OA, Minor LB, et al. Vestibular-evoked myogenic potential thresholds normalize on plugging superior canal dehiscence. Neurology. 2008;70:464-72.
28. Nguyen KD, Welgampola MS, Carey JP. Test-retest reliability and age-related characteristics of the ocular and cervical vestibular evoked myogenic potential tests. Otol Neurotol. 2010;31:793-802.
29. Belden CJ, Weg N, Minor LB, et al. CT evaluation of bone dehiscence of the superior semicircular canal as a cause of sound- and/or pressure-induced vertigo. Radiology. 2003;226:337-43.
30. Penninger RT, Tavassolie TS, Carey JP. Cone-Beam Volumetric Tomography for Applications in the Temporal Bone. Otol Neurotol. 2011 Feb 8. [Epub ahead of print].
31. Poe DS. Diagnosis and management of the patulous eustachian tube. Otol Neurotol. 2007;28:668-77.
32. Eggers SD. Migraine-related vertigo: diagnosis and treatment. Curr Pain Headache Rep. 2007;11(3):217-26.
33. Minor LB. Superior canal dehiscence syndrome. Am J Otol. 2000;21:9-19.
34. Crane BT, Minor LB, Carey JP. Superior canal dehiscence plugging reduces dizziness handicap. Laryngoscope. 2008;118:1809-13.
35. Amoodi HA, Makki FM, McNeil M, et al. Transmastoid resurfacing of superior semicircular canal dehiscence. Laryngoscope. 2011;121:1117-23.
36. Fiorino F, Barbieri F, Pizzini FB, et al. A dehiscent superior semicircular canal may be plugged and resurfaced via the transmastoid route. Otol Neurotol. 2010;31:136-9.

37. Vlastarakos PV, Proikas K, Tavoulari E, et al. Efficacy assessment and complications of surgical management for superior semicircular canal dehiscence: a meta-analysis of published interventional studies. Eur Arch Otorhinolaryngol. 2009;266(2):177-86.

38. Kim TH, Nam BH, Park CI. Histologic Changes of Lateral Semicircular Canal after Transection and Occlusion with Various Materials in Chinchillas. Korean J Otolaryngol-Head Neck Surg. 2002;45:318-21.

39. Silverstein H, Van Ess MJ. Complete round window niche occlusion for superior semicircular canal dehiscence syndrome: a minimally invasive approach. Ear Nose Throat J. 2009;88:1042-56.

40. Friedland DR, Michel MA. Cranial thickness in superior canal dehiscence syndrome: implications for canal resurfacing surgery. Otol Neurotol. 2006;27:346-54.

41. Deschenes GR, Hsu DP, Megerian CA. Outpatient repair of superior semicircular canal dehiscence via the transmastoid approach. Laryngoscope. 2009;119(9):1765-9.

42. Kirtane MV, Sharma A, Satwalekar D. Transmastoid repair of superior semicircular canal dehiscence. J Laryngol Otol. 2009;123:356-8.

43. Teixido MT, Artz GJ, Kung BC. Clinical experience with symptomatic superior canal dehiscence in a single neurotologic practice. Otolaryngol Head Neck Surg. 2008;139:405-13.

44. Limb CJ, Carey JP, Srireddy S, et al. Auditory function in patients with surgically treated superior semicircular canal dehiscence. Otol Neurotol. 2006;27:969-80.

45. Carey JP, Migliaccio AA, Minor LB. Semicircular canal function before and after surgery for superior canal dehiscence. Otol Neurotol. 2007;28:356-64.

Chapter

4

IMPLANTABLE HEARING AIDS

Maurizio Barbara, Simonetta Monini

ABSTRACT

The major active middle ear implants (AMEI) for rehabilitation of different types of hearing loss are presented. Selection criteria are also particularly stressed, including a thorough audiological assessment, especially based on free-field speech audiometric tests under aided and unaided conditions. Both partially- and fully-implantable devices are taken into considerations with remarks on surgical steps needed for their application. A final, preliminary algorithm is also presented with the aim to direct the audiologist/otologist for the best available option.

Active middle ear implants (AMEI) have recently implemented the armamentarium for the rehabilitation of different types of hearing loss (HL). Until now, in many postoperative instances where the functional recovery is not fully or at all achieved by standard otological procedures, leaving a residual conductive or mixed HL, bone- or magnetically-anchored devices — treated elsewhere in this Volume — have been widely accepted and used since several years. Their application would encompass:

* Non-otological procedures, hence with no risks of surgery-related hearing worsening;
* Fairly good outcome;
* But, in the most used device, an external abutment visible also when it is not in function.

Additional systems have recently been introduced for treatment of conductive or mixed type of HL, by performing surgical procedures much resembling standard otological techniques. Although an appropriate validation for being considered in all cases a valid alternative — either to standard otological approaches or to conventional hearing aids (HAs) — is still needed, AMEI surgery is surely foreseen as one of the most promising otologic applications for the forthcoming years.

Before describing each single device and application in the different clinical settings, it is worth to linger over the factors that contribute to the selection of an AMEI from both surgeon's and patient's viewpoint.

INDICATIONS FOR ACTIVE MIDDLE EAR IMPLANT

Conventional middle ear surgery may provide an adequate solution for purely conductive HL such as the case of initial stages of otosclerosis or chronic otitis media with eardrum perforation and/or ossicular chain interruption. Nevertheless, apart from potential life-threatening situations (e.g. cholesteatoma), it is common attitude to inform the patient that the HL associated with chronic ear disease can also find a solution by either bone- or air-conductive conventional HA. However, these latters are usually contraindicated or inappropriate in case of discharging eardrum perforation or in presence of particular postoperative sequels such as a wide meatoplasty after radical mastoidectomy or blind-sac closure of the external auditory canal after subtotal or total petrosectomy.

Conversely, conventional HA surely represent a logical solution in case of sensorineural HL. However, difficulties are not uncommonly reported by HA wearers, partly attributable to technical limitations of the devices such as:

- Limited high-frequency amplification affecting speech understanding in noisy environment;
- Distortion and feedback, related to the diseased organ causing the impairment, i.e. the cochlea, when receiving external and amplified sounds;
- Occlusion effect and discomfort, when suffering from chronic inflammation or irritation or collapse of the external auditory canal, or wax overproduction and cumulation;
- Daily social attitudes, such as working in a humid, dusty environment, need for wearing mobile phone accessories (bluetooth), wearing sun- or eyeglasses, or stethoscopes (doctors);
- Inesthetism or stigma usually displayed even with last-generation miniaturized HA.

These are part of the reasons why only a small percentage of potential candidates actually owns a HA, and an even smaller percentage wears it regularly.

On the ground of these premises, the advent of alternative solutions for rehabilitation of a hearing deficit, even though necessitating a surgical procedure, but consisting in less visible and oftentimes better performing devices, has warmly been welcomed by the hearing-impaired population.[1]

For the time being, the available AMEI may cover most of the needs and can be distinguished according to:

- Type of HL [conductive, mixed or sensorineural hearing loss (SNHL)]
- Visibility (partially- or fully-implantable)
- Mode of stimulation (electromagnetic, piezoelectric).

Needless to say, the audiological evaluation and indication is of utmost importance if one wants to predict a fairly good chance of positive outcome. This is particularly true when the hearing-impaired subject has never experienced a HA. In fact, if it is true that HA cannot guarantee the best hearing solution in all cases, a minimum 1–2 months HA trial should be mandatory before excluding to choose it for his/her hearing problem. This is particularly true for most of the high-frequency, bilateral SNHL, when the hearing impairment displays only under certain listening circumstances, such as with background noise.

When considering the HL range suggested from the different AMEI companies, the moderate-to-severe losses are generally the most indicated (Figs 4.1A to C). As it will be shown later, also worse degrees of HL can obtain substantial benefit from an AMEI. So, in conclusion, the basic audiological principles should include:

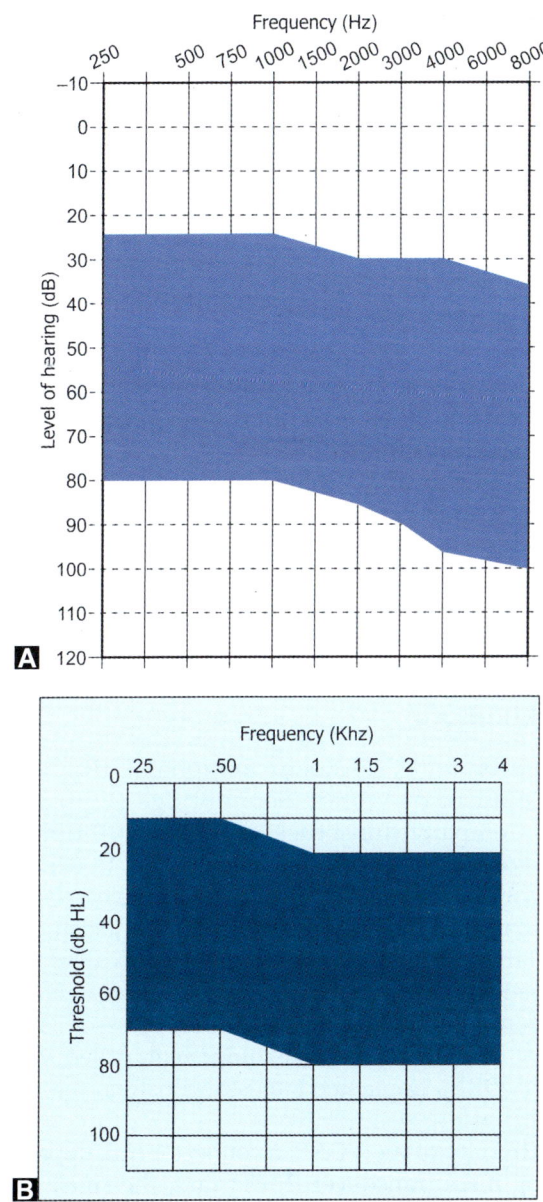

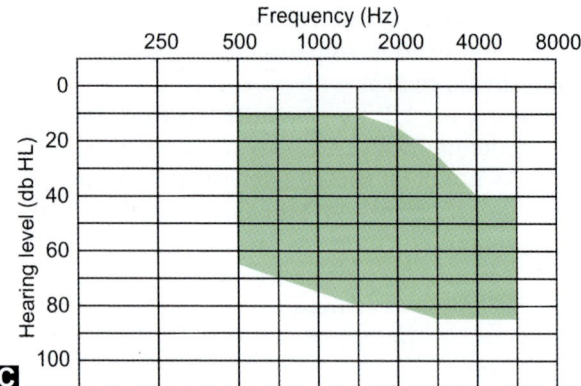

Figs 4.1A to C: The shaded areas represent frequency and intensity ranges of each device's indication, as advised by the Company. From left to right: Esteem®, Carina, Vibrant SoundBridge

1. Suitable audiometric thresholds.
2. Prior HA use or trial.

In case of pure SNHL, a perfect middle ear condition and function is also needed, as desumed by impedance audiometric testing.

The major advantage of an AMEI in respect to conventional HA is to drive a mechanoelectric stimulus directly to the ossicular chain or part of it, instead of having an amplified sound delivered by the HA speaker. Theoretically, but also in patient's opinion, this would provide a clearer and more natural sound listening.

Basically, two devices may presently cover the whole typology of hearing deficit, from the conductive to mixed and SNHL, and they will be the first to be treated in this survey.

VIBRANT SOUNDBRIDGE

Formerly owned by an US company Symphonix (R), today, production and development of Vibrant SoundBridge (VSB) are supported by the Med El Company (Innsbruck, Austria). VSB function is based on the general concept of middle ear devices, i.e. to drive directly the ossicular chain or its elements, in this case via an electromagnetic principle, in order to induce the minimal ossicular displacement needed for cochlear stimulation [1 micron displacement equivalent to 120 dB SPL (sound pressure level) output].

The VSB is composed of an external AudioProcessor (AP) that is kept in magnetic contact with an internal component, called vibrating ossicular prosthesis (VORP), implanted subcutaneously in the retro-auricular region (Fig. 4.2).

From one extremity of the VORP, a connector link departs, ending up with the floating mass transducer (FMT) unit, the small active component which, placed in contact with the ossicular chain, drives it directly,

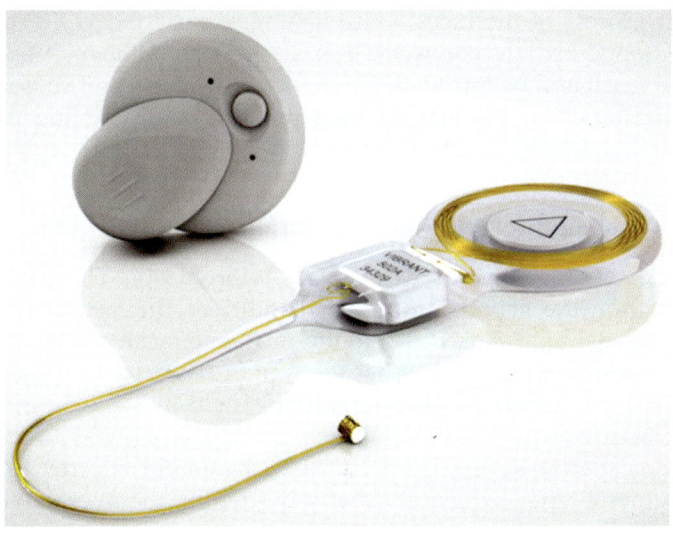

Fig. 4.2: The two VSB components: the external AudioProcessor (top left) and the VORP-FMT complex

creating a vibratory movement and generating a sound wave through the cochlea. The AP presently contains the following components: two microphones, signal processing electronics, telemetry coil, battery and a magnet that allows keeping it in position over the VORP, which receives the amplitude modulated signal. The receiver unit of the VORP contains a demodulator circuit filter that tailors an appropriate signal for the FMT, especially limiting an overstimulating output. The FMT (2.3 mm long, 1.6 mm large, 25 mg of weight) is a solenoid including two coils wound around a hermetically-sealed titanium alloy bobbin-shaped housing and a set of silicone elastomer springs, all further protected by a thin coating of medical-grade epoxy.

On the grounds of clinical indication (type and degree of HL), the surgical procedure will be considering various FMT positions:

1. Incus-Vibroplasty
2. Stapes- or footplate-Vibroplasty
3. Round Window (RW)-Vibroplasty

The surgical time is approximately 2 hours for any procedure.

Vibrant SoundBridge for Sensorineural Hearing Loss (Incus-Vibroplasty)

Via a superiorly-extended retroauricular incision, the lateral supratemporal and mastoid bone surfaces are exposed. After preparing a musculoperiosteal flap, a shallow well is drilled superiorly for the VORP antenna. A cortical mastoidectomy with posterior tympanotomy, slightly more extended in the superior part, is then carried out in order to totally expose the long process of the incus. Once having secured the VORP upon its supratemporal bed, the connector link is advanced in the mastoidectomy cavity to reach and be introduced into the facial recess and subsequently hooked/crimped to the incudal long process, finally having the FMT parallel to the stapes.[2]

Vibrant SoundBridge for Conductive/Mixed Hearing Loss

The first steps are similar to the incus-vibroplasty. The other steps depend upon the actual middle ear conditions. In case of tympano-plasty sequels, for a closed technique the same facial recess approach is used in order to visualize either the oval or RW area. In the first case, the FMT is placed on the stapes footplate, held in place by the stapes superstructure or cartilage/fascia assemblage. If a RW-vibroplasty is planned, a specific surgical procedure is carried out in order to expose the RW membrane—which is usually hidden by the overhanging RW superior lip—as well as to create the room to properly accommodate the FMT (Figs 4.3A to C).

This procedure is performed with 1–2 mm diamond burrs and modest, but continuous irrigation.

When the postoperative picture is derived from an open technique, then the skin flap lying over the mastoidectomy bowl is raised, possibly in continuity, ending up with the exposure of the promontory with the RW niche, which is prepared according to the above mentioned proce-dure.

The FMT is placed with one of the two flat extremities toward the RW membrane, interposing fascial tissue for coupling optimization. Inferiorly, the FMT is then sustained by fascia and/or cartilage.

At the end of vibroplasty surgery, bioengineers in the operating room

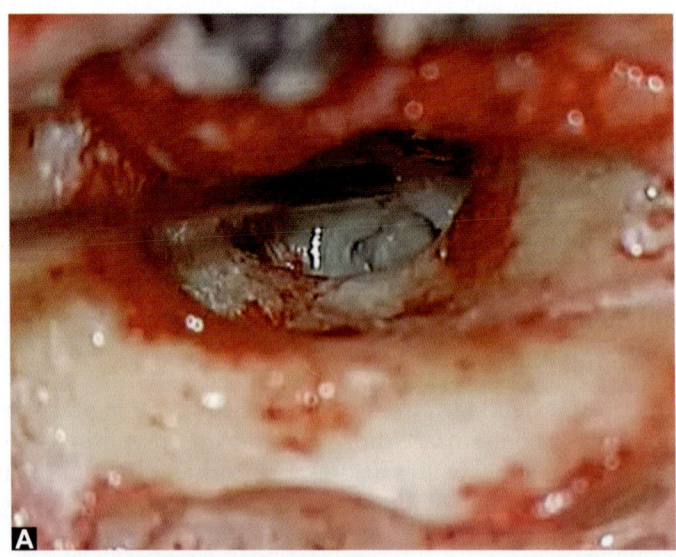

Recent Advances in Otolaryngology – Head and Neck Surgery

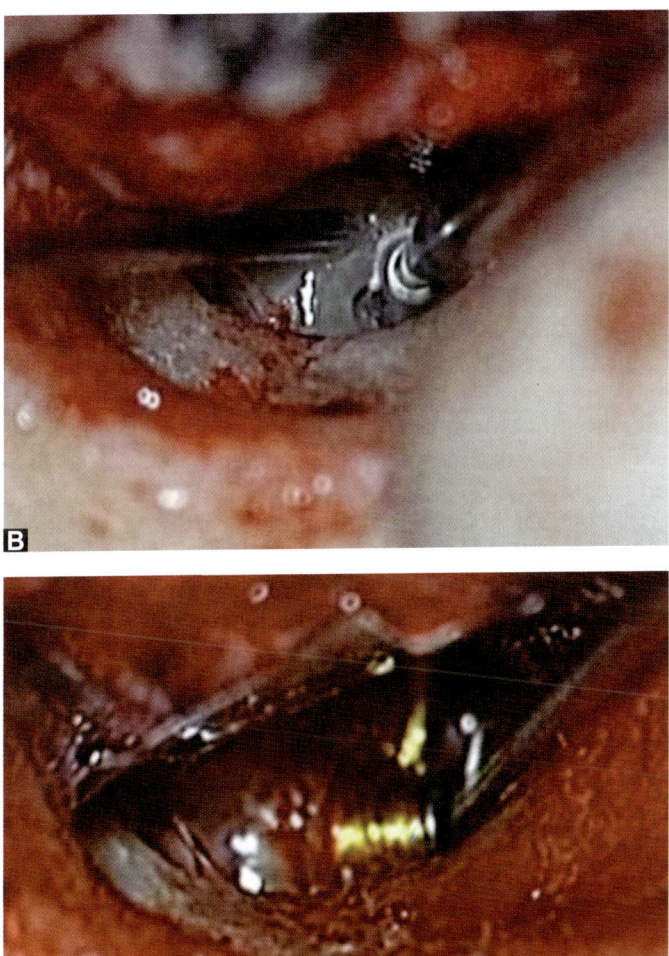

Figs 4.3A to C: Round window preparation for Vibroplasty. (A) Through the posterior tympanotomy, the promontory with the round window niche is visualized; (B) A 0.5 diamond burr is used to remove part of the superior round window lip and expose the round window membrane; (C) The FMT, with interposed fascia, is placed over the round window membrane

help the surgeon to ascertain that the FMT has been appropriately placed, via device-stimulated Cochlear Action Potential recording.

Several reports have highlighted the long-term efficacy of incus-vibroplasty for SNHL, especially for those cases with normal or near-normal low frequencies.[3,4] More recently, a few studies have reported better speech recognition score in VSB implanted as compared to conventional HA performances.[5,6]

MIDDLE EAR TRANSDUCER AND CARINA

They represent the partially- and fully-implantable devices of the same Company (Otologics, Boulder, Ca, USA), with very close similarities between them.

The middle ear transducer (MET®) has first been proposed for pure SNHL.[7] It is composed of an external magnetic component containing the battery, the sound processor and the microphone, placed retroauricularly in connection with the internal component, consisting of a receiver from which the connector cable departs, ending with a fine tip to be placed on the incus body. According to an electromagnetic mechanism, the entire ossicular chain is driven, thus determining cochlear stimulation.

Carina® represents the fully-implantable version of Otologics' device. The main difference from MET is the invisibility, obtained by hiding underneath the skin also the microphone, other than the electronic components and the transducer.[8]

Surgery consists in a partial, superior cortical mastoidectomy to expose the posterior epitympanum with full visualization of the incus body. A metallic bracket is then screwed to the surrounding cortical bone to support the advancement of the coupling rod toward the incus body (Fig. 4.4).

The fully-implantable version (Carina) also carries a further component, i.e. the microphone, implanted and placed in a subcutaneous pouch at the level of the mastoid tip. Carina needs to be daily recharged for about 60 minutes.

The Carina device has recently been proposed and applied for conductive or mixed HL, by using modified tip endings to be coupled either to

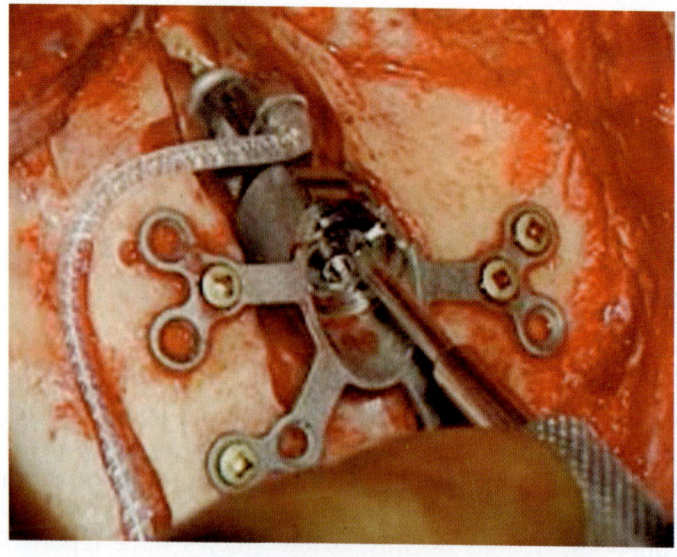

Fig. 4.4: The metallic bracket holding the cable ending up with the tip to be placed on the incus body of a MET (or Carina), in a right ear

the stapes or to the footplate or to the RW membrane. In particular, its application has been advocated in case of bilateral aural atresia, with an earlier implantation in comparison with a bone-anchored HA that is generally not advised before 6–7 years of age.

ESTEEM®

It represents a fully-implantable system developed in US (EnvoyMedical, St. Paul, MN). Presently, it is the only FDA-approved fully-implantable device (since March 2010). The main feature is that it does not need a microphone, this latter being played by the normal eardrum which, hit by the external sound, transmits the signal to the ossicular chain and, hence, to the cochlea. The Esteem® is composed of a titanium case containing the sound processor and the battery, and of two transducers to be assembled in contact with two ossicles, i.e. the sensor to the incus body, the driver to the stapes capitulum. For the best performance and for avoiding mechanical feedback, these two ossicles need to be separated. According to FDA guidelines, the Esteem® device is indicated in case of bilateral (better symmetric), nonprogressive SNHL of moderate-to-severe degree, with at least 40% speech discrimination, age older than 18 years and a normal middle ear function, as evaluated through impedance audiometry. The EnvoyMedical Company contraindicates this implant in case of allergy, abnormal tubal function or chronic naso-paranasal pathology, as well as of tendency to keloids or staphylococcal infections. One major drawback for the Esteem® is the additional conductive HL due to ossicular discontinuation, that makes inidoneous or useless to wear a conventional HA in the operated ear. Moreover, the battery, which does not need to be recharged, has a duration between 5 years and 9 years and necessitates another, though simpler surgery, to be replaced. As for the other AMEI, magnetic resonance imaging (MRI) is discouraged. So, this implant cannot be indicated in subjects needing periodical MRI for any reason. Owing to the actual dimensions of the two transducers, the mastoidectomy cavity needs to be large enough. In this regard, before selecting a subject for an Esteem® implantation, a high resolution CT scan should show a distance of at least 22 mm between the stapes capitulum and the anterior wall of the sigmoid sinus; and at least 4 mm from the tegmen tympani to the scutum.

Differently from both VSB and Otologics devices, Esteem® works according to piezoelectric principle, i.e. the peculiarity of some crystals to generate a current when they are deformed and, likewise, to be deformed by a current. Basically, a sound entering the ear canal, impacts the eardrum-malleus-amputated incus complex, i.e. the sheer microphone of the Esteem® that induces vibration of the sensor piezotransducer (PZT), thus promoting an electrical signal that reaches the SP (sound processor). The signal is then processed and fitted for each patient's need and sent back to the driver PZT, attached to the stapes head, where it induces a vibratory movement to the stapes and an amplified sound to the cochlea (Fig. 4.5).

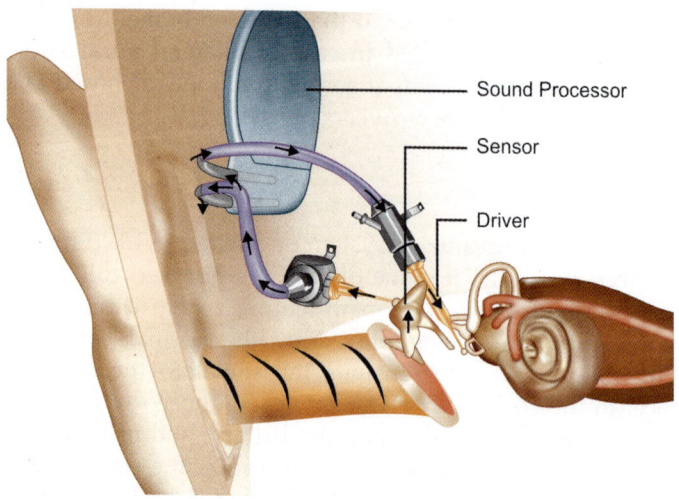

Fig. 4.5: Schematic drawing of an implanted Esteem® AMEI

Sound Processor

Sensor

Driver

Esteem® Surgery

After shaving the supero-postauricular region and infiltrating local anesthetic with vasoconstrictors, a lazy-S shaped incision is performed, followed by an ample musculo-periosteal flap (Palva's flap) which is anteriorly raised and kept in place by self-retaining retractors, in order to expose the squamous and mastoid portions of the temporal bone (TB) (Figs 4.6A and B).

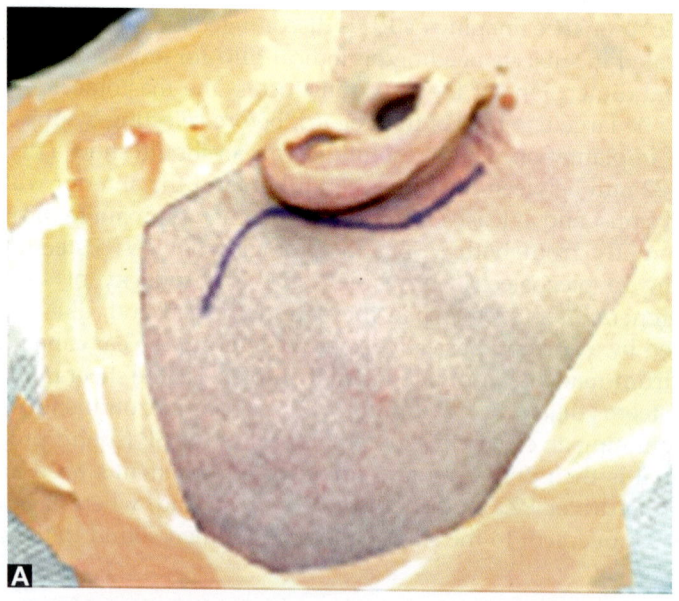

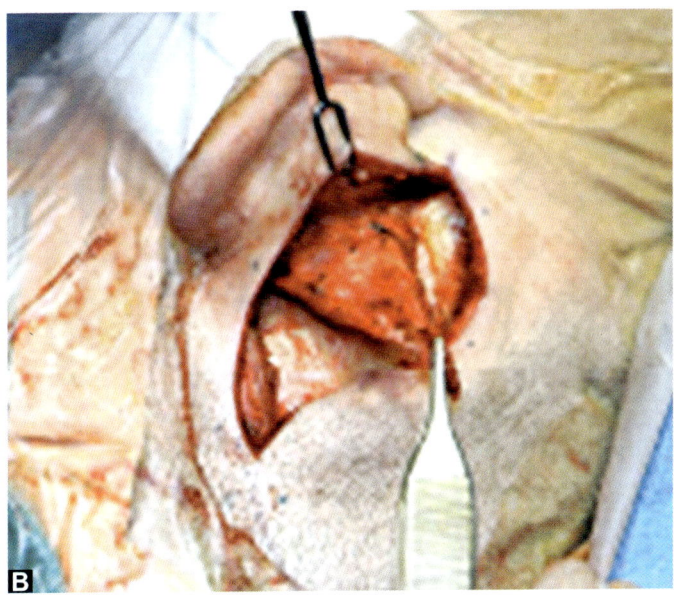

Figs 4.6A and B: Esteem® surgery in a right ear. (A) Lazy-S retroauricular incision; (B) Palva's flap

At the level of the squamous TB, with a 6 mm cutting burr and high-speed drill, a bony well is drilled for housing the SP that, due to its thickness (6.4 mm), can never be completely hidden in this depth. An enlarged mastoidectomy is then performed, by exposing the mastoid tegmen, the sino-dural angle and the mastoid tip area, followed by a wide posterior tympanotomy that must leave the posterior buttress intact, and should be extended inferiorly, giving rise to a trapezoidal area. In fact, enough space is needed in order to carry out the final phases of cementing; for achieving this goal, the chorda tympani is regularly sacrificed. The possibility of taste disturbance, therefore, should always be mentioned in the informed consent to the patient. The following surgical steps are addressed to the ossicular chain. Through the facial recess, at first mucosa is scraped away from the incudostapedial (IS) joint that is then separated before performing the section of 1–2 mm of the incudal long process, via a surgical laser (Fig. 4.7).

Afterward, with specially-forged tab microknives, the stapes capitulum is freed from the mucosa in order to allow the pre-coat with EnvoyCem (bioglass cement) (Figs 4.8A and B).

The two transducers are then anchored to Glasscock's stabilizers for facilitating their manipulation finalized to an appropriate placement on the incus body (sensor) and on the pre-coated stapes capitulum (driver). Once in place, the transducers are stabilized within the mastoidectomy bowl by hydroxyapatite cement (Fig. 4.9). The final surgical steps consist in firmly attaching the driver tip to the pre-coated stapes capitulum, while a neo-joint is created between the sensor tip and the incus body.

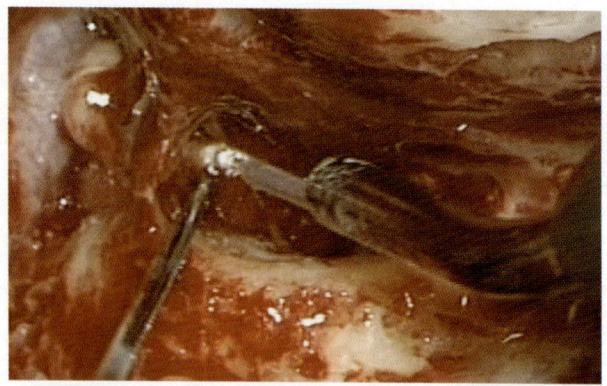

Fig. 4.7: Esteem® surgery in a right ear. After exposing the whole incudal long process, and disarticulation of the IS joint, the long process is amputated via laser beam

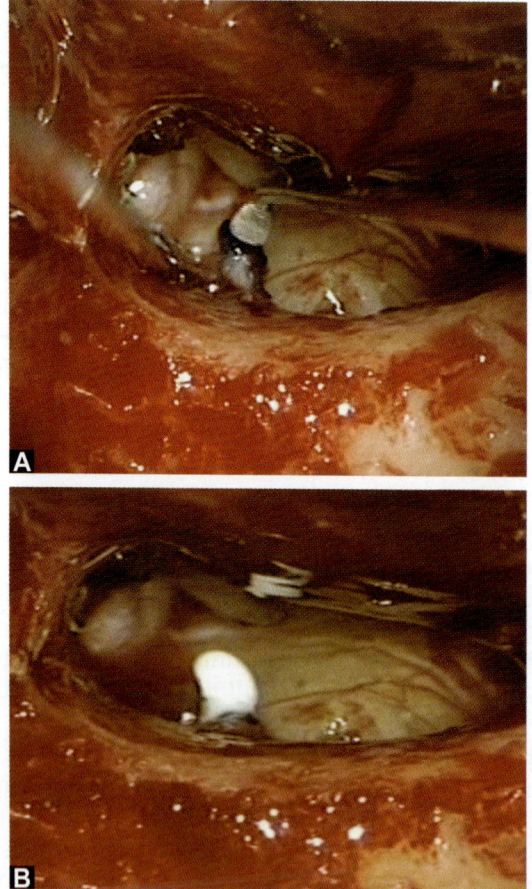

Figs 4.8A and B: Esteem® surgery. (A) With a tab knife, mucoperiosteum is scraped away from the stapes capitulum; (B) A drop of bioglass cement (EnvoyCem) is placed on the naked stapes capitulum to form the pre-coat

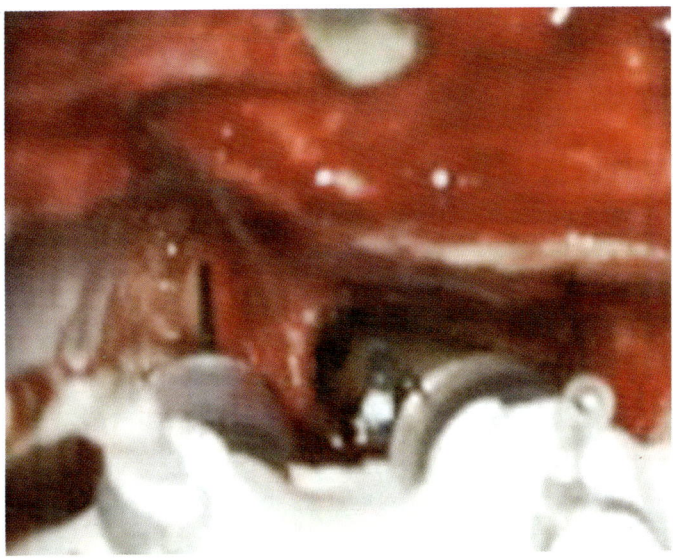

Fig. 4.9: Esteem® surgery. The body of the two transducers is immobilized within the mastoidectomy bowl with hydroxyapatite cement (MedCem) and the tips are precisely placed on the incus body (sensor) and the pre-coated stapes head (driver)

During and after surgery, field clinical engineers in the operating theater help the surgeon to check the integrity of each implanted component as well as the appropriateness of placement for optimizing the functional outcome, by using Laser Doppler Vibrometry with a dedicated software.

Surgery for replacing the battery can be performed either via the previous incision or, better, approaching the case from behind with an L-shaped incision, thus avoiding to inadvertently damage the leads that depart anteriorly from the SP itself.

Preliminary reports on Esteem® have been particularly encouraging, highlighting its possible efficacy also in severe-to-profound SNHL.[9,10]

MAXUM

This is a semi-implantable device that has been recently reproposed as behind-the-ear or completely-in-the-canal AMEI from the Ototronix Company (Houston, TX, USA). Similarly to VSB and the Otologics devices, MAXUM works according to the direct drive of the ossicular chain via an electromagnetic system. In both models, there is an external component that occupies the external auditory canal for almost its entirety, putting its tip in close proximity to the eardrum. The internal component is instead implanted following a simple procedure (Figs 4.10A to C) which includes the following:

1. Tympano-meatal flap with exposure of the IS joint.
2. IS disarticulation and placement of the magnet ring on the stapes capitulum.
3. Fixation with cement and replacement of the tympano-meatal flap.

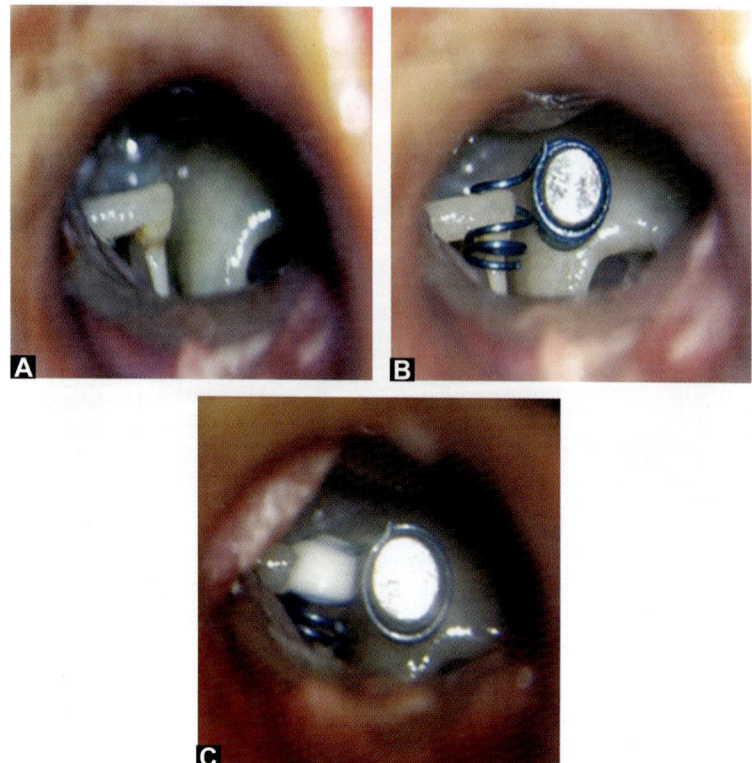

Figs 4.10A to C: Maxum surgery. (A) After performing a tympano-meatal flap, the middle ear is visualized with the IS joint; (B) After IS disarticulation, the magnet ring is placed on the stapes capitulum; (C) Further stabilization is achieved by placing a droplet of cement

RETROX

This device has been introduced since almost a decade but it seems not to have had the hoped success, although addressed to a very common type of HL, such as the so-called 'ski-slope' SNHL. In fact, contrary to the other AMEI that can be proposed for moderate-to-severe SNHL, its audiological indication is for those losses that include frequencies above 1000 Hz, i.e. in subjects who, more than hearing-impaired, refer the difficulty to listen under particular situations, such as in noisy environment. As a matter of fact, Retrox is a conventional HA with the following peculiarities:

- Minor surgical procedure
- Unoccluded external ear canal
- Discreet visibility

Similarly to bone conductive implantable devices, the candidate can be preliminarily assessed via a tester that reproduces the efficacy of the device so that the patient may experience directly the eventual functional result.

The few scientific reports present in the literature have highlighted practical advantages due to Retrox implantation for resolution of high-pitch-HL related difficulties, such as speech discrimination in noise.[11,12]

Retrox Surgery

The procedure is carried out under local anesthesia, as outpatient or day-hospital setting. By means of specific instrumentation, a sort of retroauricular piercing is performed from the retroauricular crease into the external auditory canal (Figs 4.11A to C).

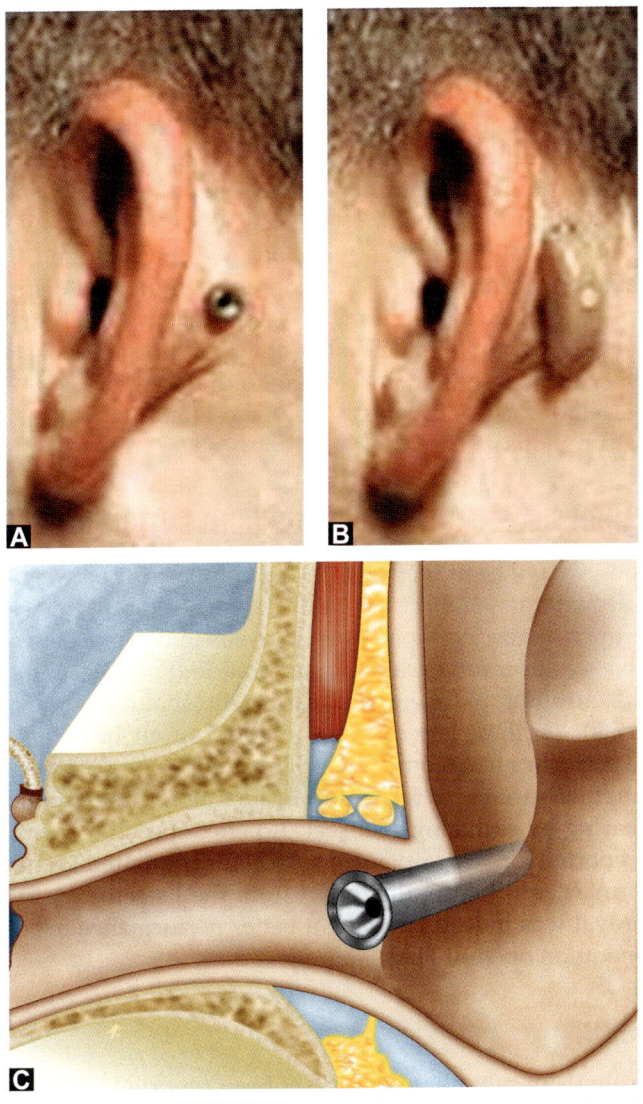

Figs 4.11A to C: Retrox hearing aid. (A) The titanium tube is placed in the retroauricular crease; (B) The Retrox hearing aid is placed on the titanium tube; (C) Schematic drawing showing the "piercing" surgery

IMAGING AND ACTIVE MIDDLE EAR IMPLANTS

A computed-tomographic (CT) imaging study is usually carried out before every AMEI surgery for additional diagnostic purposes, especially for sequels from previous middle ear surgery. For some device, moreover, a thorough study of eventual anatomic limitations is mandatory and plays a crucial role as inclusion criterion for AMEI application. This is particularly true for the devices that are still bulky, like the Esteem®, that is today contraindicated in case of a limited mastoid pneumatization, with a distance between stapes capitulum and anterior wall of the sigmoid sinus inferior to 22 mm. Also for the Otologic device a recent report has been advising not to perform surgery when the dura-meatal distance is inferior to 5 mm.[13]

Another issue to be taken into consideration is the safety when performing MRI in an AMEI implanted patient in terms of linear and torsional forces, heating, implant magnetization and image artefacts.[14] For Maxum device no major disturbances were experienced when using an open 0.3-T MRI on implanted volunteers.[15] Wagner et al. have recently tested in the laboratory various types of FMT coupling and the effects of undergoing exposure to 1.5-T MRI, observing potential displacements especially for nonfixed applications (RW Vibroplasty) and some effect on the transfer function of the device. For other AMEI, such as Esteem®, the Company's rule is absolutely forbidding to undergo any MRI exam and therefore excludes as candidate anyone who would need it periodically for his/her previous disease.

ACTIVE MIDDLE EAR IMPLANT VERSUS CONVENTIONAL HEARING AID

A few studies have been focusing on the comparison between different AMEI and conventional HA.[16] When considering this issue, which is surely of utmost importance, a clear distinction needs to be done between AMEI that involve postoperative hearing deterioration (Esteem®) and those that are not affecting the preoperative hearing threshold level (Vibrant and MET/Carina). For these latter, in fact, it would surely be easier and more reliable to perform such a comparison, switching on and off the implanted device. Another variable to take into consideration is the duration, if any, of HA wearing by each single subject. A better speech recognition score has been reported for VSB implanted subjects as compared to conventional HA performances.[5,6,17] Also, the report from the Esteem® trial that led to FDA approval was indeed stressing a better performance in comparison to last-generation open-fit HAs.[9]

CONCLUSION

On the grounds of what has previously been reported, there are several AMEI options to choose according to several factors including:
• Type of HL, whether conductive, mixed or purely sensorineural;

- Degree of HL, especially in case of mixed and SNHL;
- Frequential range mainly affected;
- Patient's compliance to undergo a surgical procedure, under local or general anesthesia, or of short or long duration and
- Availability (or reimbursement) by the hospital or National Health System.

Another additional factor is the single surgeon's decision to follow his/her AMEI protocol since, as evidenced by this review, for some types of HL more than one solution would be possible. In the Center for Implantable Hearing Devices at Sapienza University, Sant'Andrea Hospital, in Rome, a flowchart has been developed for driving a patient to one or another solution alternative to conventional HA (Fig. 4.12). This flowchart is obviously taking into account also the bone-anchored devices that are presented elsewhere in this issue.

From this flowchart, it is evident the major role played by:

- A thorough audiological work-out, mainly by speech and free-field pure tone audiometry under aided and unaided conditions, and
- Pre-testing of the device, when available (BAHA, Sophono). This latter is generally used also when planning an AMEI device for conductive or mixed HL.

The personal experience of the last 5 years, with more than 100 implanted devices, is nowadays privileging:

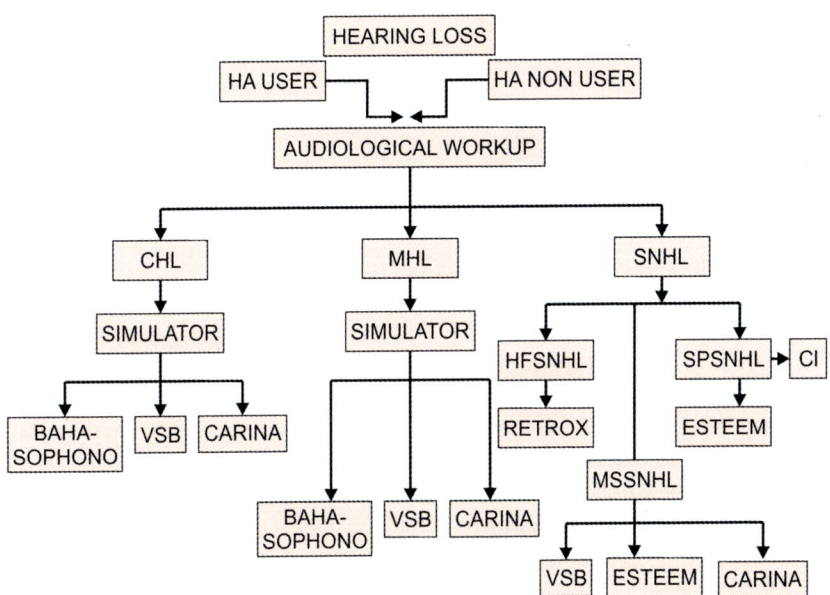

Fig. 4.12: Flowchart for selection of an implantable device
(CHL: conductive hearing loss; MHL: mixed hearing loss; SNHL: sensorineural hearing loss; HFSNHL: high-frequency sensorineural hearing loss; MSSNHL: moderate-to-severe sensorineural hearing loss; SPSNHL: severe-to-profound sensorineural hearing loss)

- VSB for conductive or mixed HL, after a positive pre-test with BAHA or Sophono simulator,[18] applied on the RW in case of open tympanoplasty sequels;
- Esteem® for SNHL, replaced by the VSB in case of a limited mastoid size.

More cases and longer follow-up are, however, needed in order to confirm such a strategy or rather modify it with different options.

REFERENCES

1. Wolf-Magele A, Schnabl J, Woellner T, et al. Active middle ear implantation in elderly people: a retrospective study. Otol Neurotol. 2011;32:805-11.
2. Pok SM, Schlogel M, Boheim K. Clinical experience with the active middle ear implant Vibrant SoundBridge in sensorineural hearing loss. Adv Otorhinolaryngol. 2010;69:51-8.
3. Bernardeschi D, Hoffman C, Benchaa T, et al. Functional results of Vibrant Soundbridge middle ear implants in conductive and mixed hearing loss. Audiol Neurootol. 2011;13:381-7.
4. Mosnier I, Sterkers O, Bouccara D, et al. Benefit of the Vibrant Soundbridge device in patients implanted for 5 to 8 years. Ear Hear. 2008;29(2):281-4.
5. Truy E, Philibert P, Vesson JF, et al. Vibrant SoundBridge versus conventional hearing aid in sensorineural high frequency hearing loss: a prospective study. Otol Neurootol. 2008;29:684-7.
6. Boeheim K, Pok SM, Schloegel M, et al. Active middle ear implant compared with open-fit hearing aid in sloping high frequency sensorineural hearing loss. Otol Neurootol. 2010;31:424-9.
7. Jenkins HA, Niparko JK, Slattery WH, et al. Otologics middle ear transducer ossicular stimulator: performance results with varying degrees of sensorineural hearing loss. Acta Otolaryngol. 2004;124:391-4.
8. Bruschini L, Forlì F, Passetti S, et al. Fully implantable Otologics MET Carina device for the treatment of sensorineural and mixed hearing loss: audio-otological results. Acta Otolaryngol. 2010;130:1147-53.
9. Kraus EM, Shohet JA, Catalano PJ. Envoy Esteem totally implantable hearing system: phase 2 trial, 1 year hearing result. Otolaryngol Head Neck Surgery. 2011;145:100-9.
10. Barbara M, Biagini M, Monini S. The totally implantable middle ear device Esteem for rehabilitation of severe sensorineural hearing loss. Acta Otolaryngol. 2011;131:399-404.
11. Barbara M, Bandiera G, Serra B, et al. Digital hearing aids for high-frequency sensorineural hearing loss: preliminary experience with Retrox device. Acta Otolaryngol Stock. 2005;125:693-6.
12. Van Damme JP, Jamart J, Garin P. Comparison between new and old generation Retrox auditory implants. B-ENT. 2010;6:1-8.
13. Kontorinis G, Lenarz T, Schwab B. Anatomic limitations of middle ear transducer and carina middle ear implant. Laryngoscope. 2010;120:2289-93.
14. Wagner JH, Ernst A, Todt I. Magnet resonance imaging safety of Vibrant SoundBridge system: a review. Otol Neurotol. 2011;32:1040-8.

15. Dyer RK jr, Nakmali D, Dormer KJ. Magnetic resonance imaging compatibility and safety of the Soundtec direct system. Laryngoscope. 2006;116:1321-33.
16. Tringali S, Perrot X, Berger P, et al. Otologics middle ear transducers with contralateral conventional hearing aid in severe sensorineural hearing loss. Otol Neurootol. 2010;31:630-6.
17. Sziklai I, Szilvassy J. Functional gain and speech understanding obtained by Vibrant SoundBridge or open-fit hearing aid. Acta Otolaryngol. 2011;131:426-33.
18. Cote' M, Deguine O, Calmels MN, et al. BAHA or MEDEL Vibrant Sound-Bridge: results and criteria of decision. Cochlear Implants Int. 2011;12(Suppl 1):S130-2.

Chapter

5

ELECTRIC ACOUSTIC STIMULATION AND HEARING PRESERVATION: ATRAUMATIC SURGICAL TECHNIQUES AND OUTCOME

Paul Van de Heyning, Griet Mertens, Andrea Kleine Punte

FROM COCHLEAR IMPLANTATION TO ELECTRIC ACOUSTIC STIMULATION

Hearing rehabilitation by cochlear implantation (CI) for bilateral severe to profound sensorineural hearing loss (SNHL) has been universally accepted as the method of choice, providing increased speech perception and improving quality of life. CI procedure was deemed to lead to a complete loss of preoperative acoustic hearing. Nevertheless, the minimal required preoperatively hearing loss in order to warrant CI decreased progressively over the last decade from 120 dB (500–1,000–2,000 Hz average); 0% speech recognition at 65 dB to 85 dB (500–1,000–2,000 Hz average), and 40% at 85 dB. The broadening of inclusion criteria for CIs due to the improved results of speech perception particularly in noise, and improved sound quality with CIs for adults[1] and children.[2]

The feasibility to preserve preoperative low frequency hearing when performing CI in the scala tympani (ST) gave rise to the concept of electric acoustic stimulation (EAS).[3]

Patients suffering from severe-, mid- and high-frequency SNHL with functional residual low frequency hearing (RLFH), are considered candidates for EAS treatment (Fig. 5.1). Mid- and high-frequency hearing is realized by electrical stimulation through the CI. Low frequency hearing is achieved by natural air conduction in case of normal to mild loss hearing levels, or with acoustic amplification through an hearing aid (HA) in case of mild to moderate hearing loss.[3] Electric and acoustic stimulation in the same ear has reduced the gap between prosthetic HA rehabilitation and CI. With EAS, the clinical demand for less traumatic surgical techniques and electrodes that induce minimal damage to cochlear structures has increased.

This paper describes the history and the developments of hearing preservation (HP) surgery for CI, and the current indications for EAS. Outcomes of HP, speech perception, and subjective outcomes with EAS will be discussed.

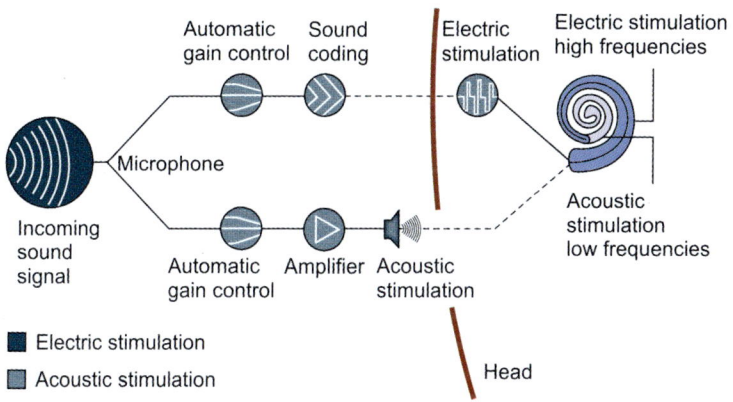

Fig. 5.1: Signal processing in electric acoustic stimulation

Source: Reprint from Van de Heyning P, Punte AK. Electric acoustic stimulation: a new era in prosthetic hearing rehabilitation. Adv Otorhinolaryngol. 2010;67:1-5.

THE HISTORY OF HEARING PRESERVATION COCHLEAR IMPLANTATION

The simultaneous use of electric and acoustic stimulation for patients with RLFH was first introduced by von Ilberg et al.[4] The first patient was successfully implanted for EAS with a partial insertion of the electrode array in the ST. This patient could preserve meaningful hearing at the low frequencies. This experience stimulated comprehensive clinical, surgical, technological and fundamental research efforts with the aim to find the most suitable surgical implantation technique and electrode design to maximize the chances of preserving RLFH for EAS. Meanwhile, many centers reported one year follow-up results of EAS showing stable preserved residual hearing in many patients combined with encouraging speech perception results and hearing capabilities.[5-8]

The importance attributed by the patients to their RLFH subjectively has been supported by evidence at different levels. The acoustical basics are provided by the perceived fine structure of the low frequency acoustic signal. On the other hand, the majority of speech algorithms only consider the envelope of the signal. Low frequency hearing supports music perception; recognition of male versus female voices, and adds to the tonality and prosody of speech.

Technically, the microphone of the behind the ear processor picks up the incoming sound. The sound is filtered in low frequency bands for acoustic stimulation and mid-and high-frequency bands for electric stimulation (ES). The edge frequency dividing the two is defined by the audiologist, and corresponds with the steep slope of the audiogram. Better results are achieved if the acoustic and electric frequency ranges are only slightly overlapping.[9] The low frequencies are processed and amplified, if necessary, by the EAS audio-processor and acoustically fed into the ear canal through the earmold. The mid-and-high frequencies are further processed by the audio processor, and sent by the coil to the internal part of the CI which electrically activates the corresponding intracochlear electrodes (Fig. 5.1). The first series of EAS patients received two separate devices—the acoustic HA and the CI. Both parts are now integrated in one processing unit, improving the comfort and acceptance of the patient.[10] The current EAS systems available are DUET 2 from Med-El GmbH and Hybrid Freedom from Cochlear LTD (Figs 5.2A to C).

Regarding terminology, different situations have to be considered which are described with different terms in literature concerning EAS; (1) EAS: electric and acoustic stimulation in the same ear, and (2) Bimodal stimulation: ES by CI in one ear and acoustic hearing via HA in the contralateral ear. However, in speech pathology and audiology, the term bimodal is more commonly referred to the meaning of combined sign language and auditory communication. Often, EAS users also use a contralateral HA, or have contralateral residual hearing, and this has to be described as such.

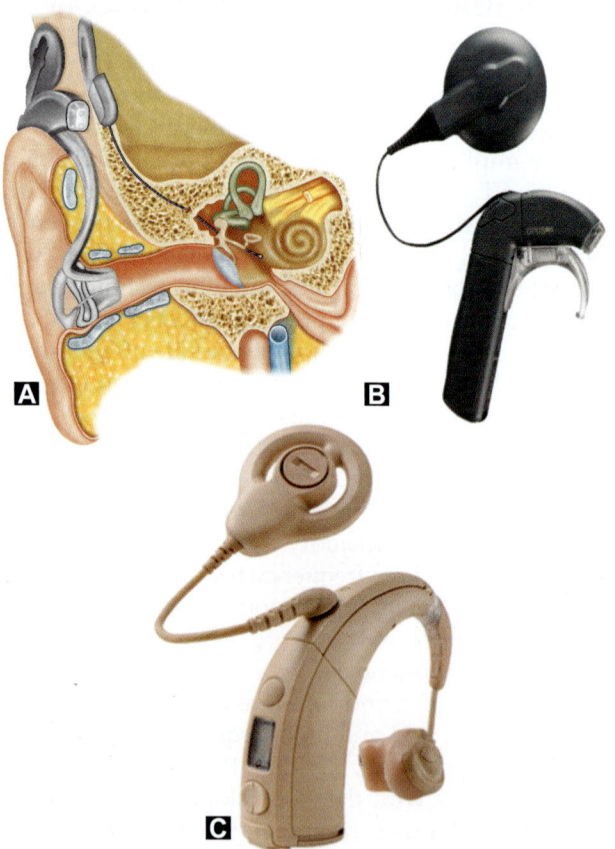

Figs 5.2A to C: (A) A cross-section of the EAS system; (B) Duet 2 audioprocessor of the Med-ElTM EAS system; (C) Hybrid audioprocessor of the Cochlear™ EAS system
Source: Courtesy of Med-EL GmbH, and Courtesy of Cochlear Ltd

INDICATIONS AND CRITERIA FOR EAS

The current audiological criteria for pure tone thresholds for EAS are illustrated in Figure 5.3. If there is any doubt whether dead regions influence the measured thresholds, a TEN test (threshold equalizing noise) should be performed.[11] Besides the criteria for pure tone thresholds, preoperative speech should be maximally 60% at 65 dB SPL in the best-aided condition. With these criteria, an improvement of speech recognition will be obtained in the vast majority of the patients even in the case where residual hearing is lost postoperatively.

Along with the audiogram and speech recognition results, there are some additional criteria for EAS candidacy. There should not be a significant progressive hearing loss. This progression has been defined as not more than 10 dB on two frequencies, and not more than 15 dB on one frequency over 1-year time period.[12] Other contraindications are autoimmune inner-ear disease or hearing loss as a result of meningitis or otosclerosis, or of any other ossification of the cochlea. There should not be malformation of the cochlea either. The maximum air-bone gap is 15 dB. There should also be no other contraindications in using acoustic amplification devices in the EAS ear if the preoperative low frequency threshold demands acoustic amplification.

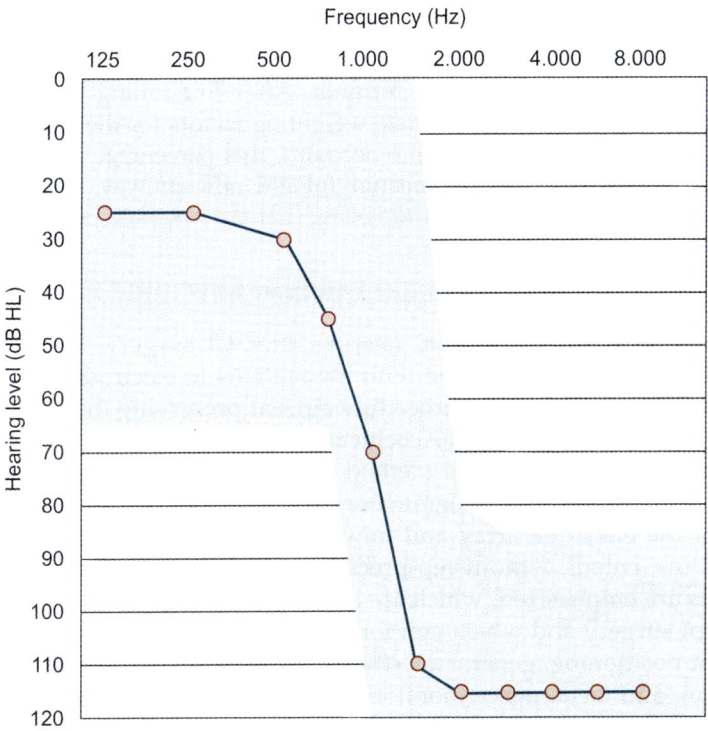

Fig. 5.3: Gray area depicts the hearing thresholds indicated for EAS. Black line indicates an example of hearing thresholds considered for EAS treatment

DEFINING RESIDUAL HEARING FOR EAS

A new classification system is required to describe and grade the residual hearing in partial deafness (PD). This will allow grading the degree of HP, and allow for better comparison between patient groups and between studies. The current audiometric indices, e.g. Fletcher index are based on mid-and-high frequencies from 500 Hz up to 4,000 Hz, and are inapt be used for the purpose of EAS and HP.

Skarzynski et al.[12,13] proposed a grading system per measured frequency in which the degree of residual hearing (RH) is divided in classes from A to E (≤ 30, ≤ 50, ≤ 70, ≤ 90 and > 90 dB). Accordingly, the RH in Figure 5.3. is described as AAABDE. Moreover, methods are being looked for to integrate the amount of preoperative hearing in the appreciation on hearing loss and its impact on hearing capabilities.[14]

Alternatives published in different studies compare postoperative to preoperative average and individual thresholds of 125 Hz, 250 Hz, 500 Hz and 1000 Hz. This average is used in Table 5.1.

Current authors are looking for a method that defines RH by using a percentage.

$$RH\,(\%) = \frac{1}{N} * \sum_{i=125}^{8000} RH\,(\%)_i$$

An example of an audiogram in a person with 41,07% RH is shown in Figures 5.4A and B. As also shown in this Figure, there is a positive linear correlation between RH(%) preoperative and RH(%) 12 months postoperative, using this preliminary formula. After fine-tuning this formula (taking transitions and appropriate weighting factors for the low and the inter-octave frequency bands into account), this percentage can quantify 'preserved hearing' in a more meaningful and efficient way.

It is recommended for the time being that the raw data be reported

HEARING PRESERVATION COCHLEAR IMPLANT SURGERY

In order to preserve residual hearing after CI surgery, several EAS surgical techniques combined with innovations in electrode design are realized. The EAS surgical procedure aims at preserving the anatomical structures and preserving the cochlear function. To achieve these goals, a minimal invasive surgical method is combined with drug treatment to prevent intracochlear inflammatory reaction resulting from the insertion of the electrode array and unwanted blood and debris. The total procedure entails a multistep-procedure. Those medical and surgical aspects are emphasized, which are different from the standard cochlear implant surgery and which aim for conserving the preoperative RFLH. Patient positioning, general anesthesia, localization of the implant, skin incision, and facial nerve monitoring are similar in EAS as in classical CI surgical procedure. In order to be less traumatic to the intracochlear structures and hence to avoid postimplantation hearing loss, particular care is taken in the design of electrodes with less traumatic physical

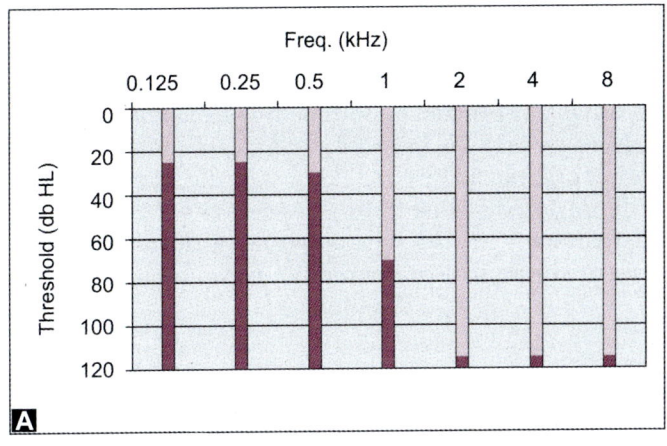

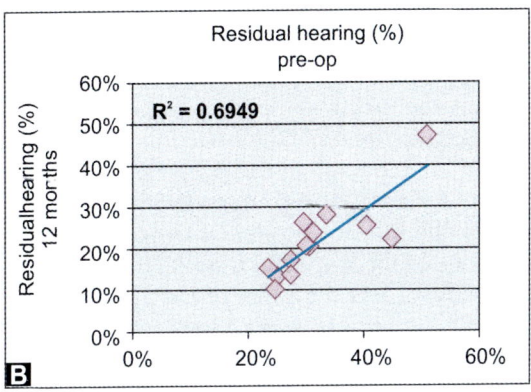

Figs 5.4A and B: (A) Shows an audiogram in a person with 41,07% RH, calculated with the preliminary formula of the current authors; (B) Shows a positive linear correlation between RH(%) preoperative and RH(%) 12 months postoperative, using the formula

characteristics, and with different insertion depths for HP surgery. The described technique is the current authors' preference based on world-wide research efforts of many teams among which are one anatomical work[15] on temporal bone experiments[16,17] on cochleostomy surgical technique;[18,19,8] one round window (RW) approach,[20] and one of the numerous panel discussions on this topic last several years as well as based on our own experience.[5,21,6] However, the authors emphasize that all aspects are subject to critical appraisal and that EAS is a fast evolving field with different views.

Step 1: Pre-incision Measures

At the time of the induction of the anesthesia, antibiotic prophylaxis and systemic corticosteroid medication are given. Typically, the antibiotic prophylaxis consists of second generation cephalosporins during 24 hours, but regional antimicrobial resistance patterns and otological conditions may lead to other schemes, e.g. amoxyclav or to a prolongation perorally, in a therapeutic schedule of 8 days. The corticosteroid treatment aims at reducing or preventing intracochlear inflammatory reactions, as well as prevent apoptotic triggering when the ST is opened and the electrode array is inserted. Many variations are used but most often, methylprednisolone 1 mg/kg bw or dexamethasone 0.1 mg/kg bw are administered systemically. Discussion exists whether the corticosteroid treatment should start a couple of days before the surgery, and has to be continued for another 2 weeks to outweigh the adverse effects.

▌Step 2: Posterior Tympanotomy

A standard mastoidectomy, with identification of the short process of the incus, is performed. Optionally, bone dust can be collected at this stage with a bone filter in case the bone dust is used at the end of the surgery mixed with fibrin glue to bone pâté. Undercutting the cortical margins may help to retain the electrode lead in place later on in the surgery. Extreme care is taken to preserve the insertion of the short process of the incus by leaving a bone bridge to the posterior tympanotomy. A posterior tympanotomy is created with appropriately sized diamond burrs visualizing clearly the inferior border of the promontory inferiorly; the pyramidal eminence of the stapedial muscle; the RW niche and the bony facial canal posteriorly, and the canal of the chorda tympani anteriorly. This implicates a wider exposure than in most standard CI approaches. Particular care is taken to remove all bone dust particles in the middle ear and attic, and between the crura of the stapes as well as in the oval window niche and the incus, in order to avoid conductive hearing loss postoperatively.

▌Step 3: Endosteum Exposure at the Cochleostomy Site or Round ▌Window Membrane Exposure

A choice is made to perform a cochleostomy site (CS) or a RW electrode insertion. In this phase, the endosteum of the ST or the round window membrane (RWM) is exposed without opening the ST and avoiding a perilymphatic leak at this stage. The choice between RW or CS is based on individual anatomical variations allowing for a better exposure of the RW or of the inferior side of the promontory; also, the preference and experience of the surgeon, the choice of electrodes and insertion depth can determine this choice. Currently, the RW approach is mostly used if feasible.

Cochleostomy approach (Fig. 5.5): The location of the cochleostomy is anatomically inferior; 2–4 mm anterior to the inferior margin of the RW, and not extending more lateral than the upper margin of the RW niche. The drilling is done with a low speed rotating 1.0 mm diamond burr from inferior to superior direction after removing the overlying mucosa. By refraining from drilling in a lateral direction, fracturing of the osseous

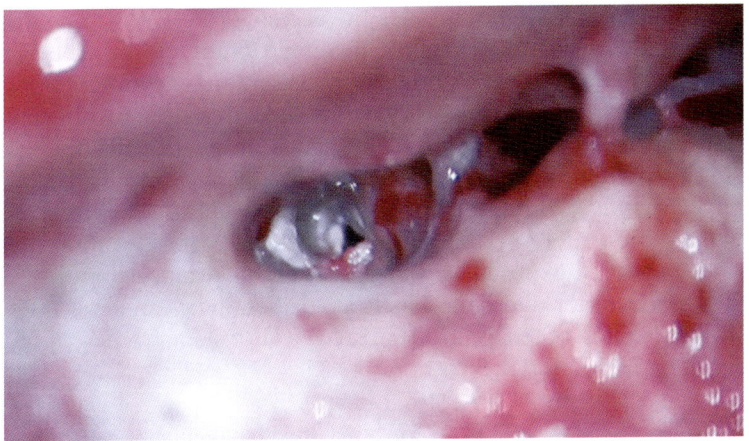

Fig. 5.5: Surgical view on a left ear demonstrating a cochleostomy with opened endosteum (arrowhead)

spiral lamina is avoided. Indeed, this was identified as one of the most frequent places at risk in temporal bone studies.[16] Initially, slim shaft 1.0 mm burrs are used; downscaling to 0.9 mm and 0.5 mm. The endosteum is exposed for 0.5 mm. Enlarging the exposure of the endosteum is done at a later stage. Care is taken not to use the aspiration near the endosteum site, as the suction pressure can make a small tear in the endosteum; aspirating perilymph, and exerting undue endocochlear pressure.

RW exposure (Fig. 5.6): First, the bone spur extending from the pyramidal process inferiorly to the facial recess posteriorly can limit the access to the RW region; this bony ridge is removed. In the majority of cases, the overhanging lip of the RW niche covering the RWM has to be shortened.

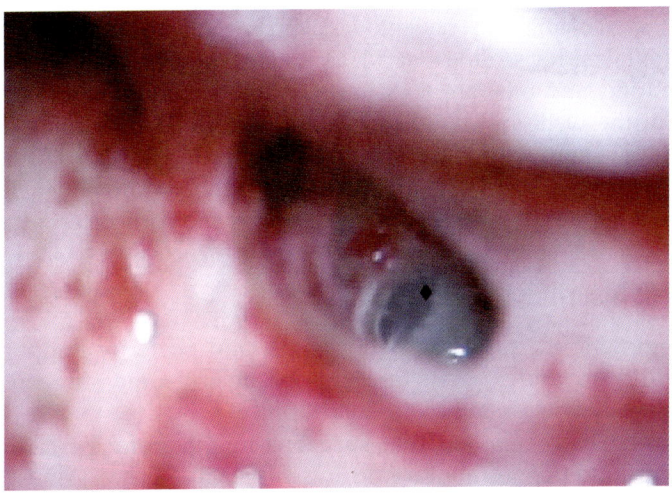

Fig. 5.6: Surgical view on a right ear demonstrating an exposed round window membrane after removing the overhanging promontory lip.

Also, a false membrane often hides the access to the RWM. The drilling is performed with a slim shaft; slow-drilling 0.9 mm diamond burr. Also, a skeeter burr can be used. A mucosal incision on the promontory at the superior edge of the RW niche is performed. With a slow turning 0.9 mm diamond burr, the lip is carefully trimmed from inferior to superoposterior. In case of mucosal fold, its insertion will separate from the bony overhang by carefully drilling the lip. The RW has a slightly convex structure with an anterior-inferior part and a more superior part. The anterior–inferior part has to be exposed without touching or desinserting the RWM. The superoposterior overhang has to be drilled away to some extend to allow the insertion of the electrode array at a later stage from a superoposterior to an anteroinferior direction.

Step 4: Topical Corticoid Application

First, the middle ear; RW and oval window region are cleaned of blood and debris. This region is submerged topically with a corticosteroid solution. Dexamethasone 1 mg/ml or triamcinolone 40 mg/ml solutions are recommended, as these solutions have shown to exhibit a broad safety profile. The solution is allowed for a minimum of 30 minutes to diffuse into the perilymph. After application of the corticoid application, the posterior tympanotomy and the attic are protected from blood and bone dust inflow.

Step 5: Placing the Implant

A subperiosteal pocket and the well for the implant are created. This part of the surgery is scheduled at this stage to allow the time for the corticosteroids to impregnate the retrotympanum. The entire middle ear, the incision site, and the surgical field are cleaned of bone dust and blood. The surgical team changes to new gloves. Three small subcutaneous fat autografts are taken for sealing—at a later stage—the perilymph leak around the electrode, and they are kept in an antibiotic solution. The implant is placed in the well, and fixed as usually performed in regular CI cases. During this stage, care is taken so that the electrode array is kept clean, and is prevented from coming into contact with the blood or dust. The electrode array is coated with a hyaluronic acid gel and corticosteroid solution.

Step 6: Inserting the Electrode Array

After removing the protection on the attic and posterior tympanotomy, the middle ear and mastoid are cleaned again; some surgeons prefer rinsing locally with an antibiotic solution.

It has to be mentioned that surgeons might prefer performing the drilling around the promontory during this stage.

In case of cochleostomy, the exposure to the endosteum is enlarged with a 0.5 mm or 0.6 mm burr until a size is achieved that is 0.1 mm larger than the diameter of the electrode array to be used; ranging from 0.6 mm to 1.0 mm. Sometimes, doing this enlargement is done under hyaluronic acid to prevent leaking out of perilymph. With a mini-knife or needle, the endosteum is incised along the inferior border of the bony cochleostomy. The incision should be broader than the diameter of the electrode array allowing flow-out of the perilymph volume as the electrode array is inserted. Before inserting the electrode, a new drop of topical corticoid solution is applied at the CS. A 4×7 mm thin silastic sheet can be placed between the facial ridge and the inferoposterior border of the CS as a temporary bridge, to facilitate directing the electrode array tip into the cochleostomy opening, and to prevent picking up bone dust, debris or blood. The electrode tip is placed in the opening, and is introduced into the ST. This introduction is done extremely slowly to prevent any buildup of intracochlear pressure. The insertion is stopped when the predefined depth is achieved, or when a first point of resistance is felt. The direction of insertion is parallel with the inferred ST direction going from superoposterior to anteroinferior. Touching of the tip against the inner ST modiolar wall has to be avoided. The silastic sheet is removed if used. The cochleostomy is closed with the pieces of fat autografts.

In case of RW approach, the view on the anterior-inferior part of the RWM is widened. Under the cover of hyaluronic acid, the membrane is punctured with a needle or a small paracentesis knife at the anteroinferior section, avoiding lifting of the insertion in the promontory. The posteroinferior region is to be avoided to avoid harming the semilunar process of the hook region. The opening is widened to an extent in order to accommodate the electrode to be inserted, allowing outflow of the perilymph volume as the electrode array is inserted. A drop of corticoid solution is applied. A 4×7 mm thin silastic sheet can be placed between the facial ridge and the RW as a temporary bridge, to facilitate directing the electrode array tip into the RW opening and to prevent picking up bone dust, debris or blood while introducing it in the ST. The electrode tip is placed in the opening of the RWM, and is inserted into the ST. The electrode introduction is done extremely slowly to prevent any buildup of intracochlear pressure. The insertion is stopped when the predefined insertion depth is achieved, or when a first point of resistance is felt. The direction of insertion is from superoposterior to anteroinferior. Touching of the tip against the inner ST modiolar wall has to be avoided. The silastic sheet is removed if used. The opening in the RWN around the electrode is closed with the pieces of fat autografts.

Step 7: Securing the Electrode and Closing the Retroauricular Incision in Three Layers

This is similar to the classical CI surgery. If bone pâté is used to secure and fix the electrode lead, care has to be taken so that the bone pâté is not touching the ossicular chain. For some electrodes, specific recommendations on fixation exist.

Although there is a growing consensus on the different aspects of HP surgery, the effect and necessity of many elements remain under debate,[22] and are subject to further improvement. The multicenter studies of Gstoettner et al.[5] and Helbig et al.[6] were closely monitored, and the surgical procedure described above with the cochleostomy approach was rigorously followed. James et al.[23] reported poorer outcome in the function of the number of surgical procedural violations.

COCHLEAR IMPLANT ELECTRODE DESIGN AND HEARING PRESERVATION

In order to be less traumatic to the intracochlear structures and thus avoid postimplantation hearing loss, particular care is taken in the design of electrode arrays for HP surgery. The improvement of HP surgery stimulated the development of electrode arrays specifically aiming at HP. The new HP electrodes are characterized by thinner calibers ranging from 0.25 at the tip to 0.8 mm at the cochleostomy or round window. The tip regions are more flexible than the traditional straight or "modiolar hugging" electrodes. This reduces the insertion force thereby reducing the risk of damaging the ST walls and the basilar membrane. The HP electrodes are are situated under the organ of corti (OC) near the lateral wall avoiding contact with the modiolar wall. Whereas, the initial standard electrodes provoked more damage with insertions over 360° in temporal bone studies;[16,24,25] this was less obvious with newer electrodes.[17,26] Figure 5.7 demonstrates the different electrodes: Flex soft, Flex28, Flex24 and Flex20 with respective lengths of 31 mm, 28 mm, 24 mm and 20 mm from Med-El GmbH, and Hybrid-L and Slim Half-Band Straight Array with lengths of 16 mm and 20–25 mm respectively from Cochlear Ltd. These specifically designed electrodes are appropriate for both RW and cochleostomy approaches.

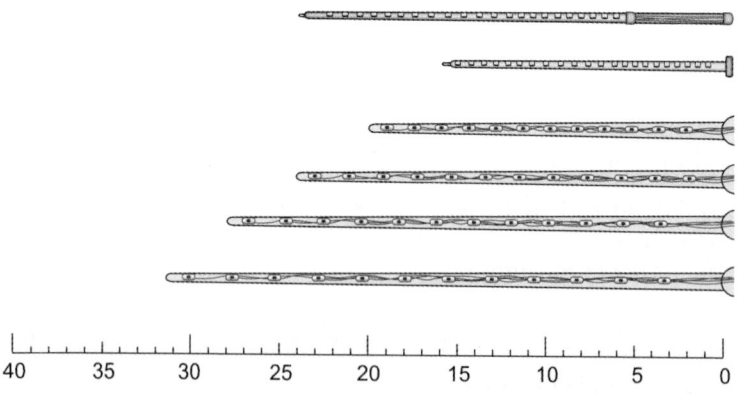

Fig. 5.7: Electrode arrays design for hearing preservation surgery. For each electrode design from top to bottom (name, length, "at the tip" and manufacturer): Hybrid-L, 16 mm, 0.25 mm, Cochlear; Slim straight array, 20 mm, 0.3 mm, Cochlear; EAS20, 20 mm, 0.3 mm, Medel; EAS24, 24 mm, 0.3 mm, Medel; EAS28, 28 mm, 0.3 mm, Medel; Flex soft, 31 mm, 0.5 mm, Medel

Lee et al.[27] showed a 3.6 mm average length difference to the helicotrema between RW and cochleostomy; the latter being nearest to the apex.

It remains unclear as to what extent electrode length influences the risk of hearing loss postimplantation, and how far the electrode array should be inserted into the cochlea remains under debate. An overview of studies reporting HP level, insertion depth and surgical cochleostomy or RW approach is given in Table 5.1. In Figure 5.8, the mean hearing loss at 125 Hz, 250 Hz, 500 Hz and 1,000 Hz is plotted as a function of insertion depth for the two surgical approaches—RW and CS. No statistical correlation between insertion depth and amount of hearing loss is found. This is in correspondence with the findings of Prentiss et al.[28] The graph and the table reveal that the publications of 2010 and 2011 using the more atraumatic electrodes report better HP levels.

Recent reports of HP with deeper insertions of Med-El FLEXsoft electrodes offer evidence that HP is also possible with longer electrodes.[17,28,29]

Table 5.1: Hearing preservation for various electrode insertion depths and both surgical approaches, and the mean hearing loss postoperatively

Hearing preservation surgery	Electrode insertion depth	Surgical approach	N	Post-op profound HL (N)	Mean hearing loss (dB)	Follow-up
Gantz et al. (2005)	10 mm	Cochleostomy	21	1	9.5	3 months
Skarzynski et al. (2007)	24 mm	Round window	10	1	28	12 months
Skarzynski et al. (2008)	24 mm	Round window	10	1	31	12 months
Gstoettner et al. (2008)	18–20 mm	Cochleostomy	18	3	23	15 months
Gantz et al. (2009)	10 mm	Cochleostomy	87	4	19.5	3–36 months
Kleine Punte et al. (2010)	30 mm	Cochleostomy	1	0	10	12 months
Woodson et al. (2010)	6–10 mm	Cochleostomy	87	9	15	1 month
Prentiss et al. (2010)	20–28 mm	Round window	18	0	15	18 months
Helbig et al. (2011)	18–24 mm	Cochleostomy and round window	18	0	20	15 months
Usami et al. (2011)	24–31 mm	Round window	5	0	5.5	7–16 months
Skarzynski et al. (2011)	28 mm	Round window	42	6	21.6	13 months

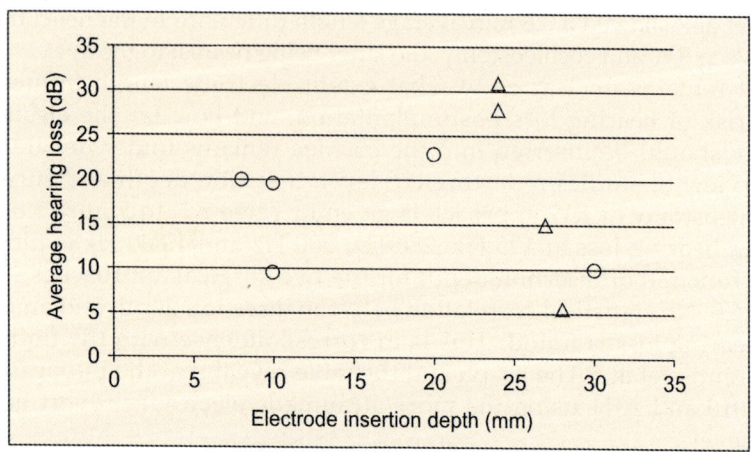

Fig. 5.8: Hearing loss outcomes of published EAS trials (Table 5.1) as a function of insertion depth. The mean average hearing loss at 125 Hz, 250 Hz, 500 Hz and 1000 Hz is plotted in the Y-axis. Cochleostomy approach is indicated by circles, and round window approach by triangles

Tailoring Insertion Depth

Many studies have shown a large intersubject variation in size of the cochlea, the scalae, and the cochlear duct length (CDL). The CDL may vary between 20–36 mm.[27] However, according to the Greenwood function,[30,31] the pitch-place relationship remains the same at constant angles. Because of this variation in cochlear size and CDL, the appropriate electrode length may also differ across patients. For example, as illustrated in Figure 5.9 with the cochleostomy approach; in order to reach the 1,000 Hz location, an insertion depth of 23 mm would be necessary in a large cochlea, and that for a small cochlea just 16 mm insertion depth would be sufficient. This has also as a consequence that for example, an electrode of 31 mm cannot be introduced entirely in a small cochlea; the ST just being too short. Hence, good estimates of the CDL appear essential to realize HP surgery and to choose the appropriate electrode length. Different experimental protocols have been presented using image processing of CT scans. Recently, Alexiades[32] presented a method to calculate the complete CDL based on a single radiographic basal turn dimension. On a standard cochlear view[33] or a Stenvers plane or reconstructed high resolution tomography in plane with the basal turn, the distance 'A' is measured which is the length of a straight line going from the RW to the maximum distance of the opposite lateral wall (Fig. 5.10). The CDL at the organ of Corti is given by the formula: CDL = (4.16×A)−3.98. This formula explains 80% of the variability of the actual CDL according to the author. When using an electrode array with a length of 31 mm, the dimension A should be greater than 8.4 mm when using a RW approach, and 8.9 mm when using a cochleostomy approach.

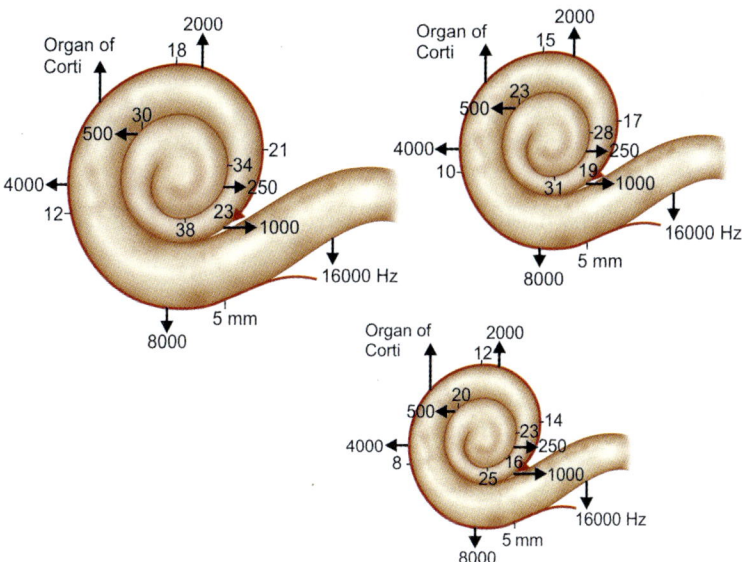

Fig. 5.9: Simulation of a large, average-sized, and small cochlea; demonstrating the respective insertion depths of 23 mm, 19 mm and 16 mm to reach the 1000 Hz point. Distances are considered from a cochleostomy approach

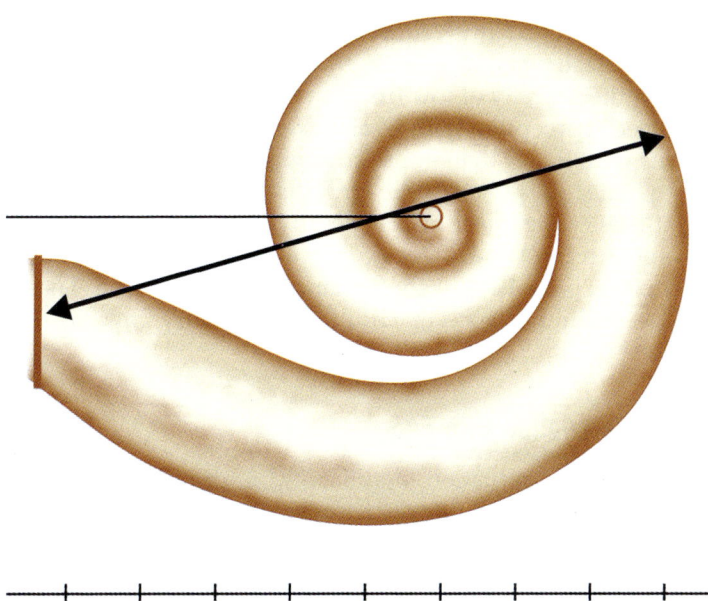

Fig. 5.10: On a cochlear view; measuring the distance A (double-arrow line) from the middle of the round window to the maximum distance of the opposite wall. Cochlear duct length (CDL) is calculated as: CDL = (4.16xA)−3.98 (after Alexiades 2011)

The decision for a certain electrode may depend on the amount RFLH and the CDL, and could be individualized per patient to reduce the risk of postoperative hearing loss and maximize the benefits of EAS. Future research needs to investigate whether taking this tailored insertion depth approach into account will result in better HP and speech perception.

OUTCOMES WITH COMBINED ELECTRIC ACOUSTIC STIMULATION

Hearing Preservation

The success of EAS depends on the preservation of RFLH. In the initial stage of EAS, straight and shorter electrodes were used. The Cochlear Hybrid implant using a 6 mm electrode and 10 mm electrode resulted in long-term HP in 75% of the subjects.[34] The first studies using Med-El Medium electrodes showed a successful HP in 12/18th subjects with a complete hearing loss, postimplantation in 3/18th subjects.[5,35] The long-term stability of preserved hearing up to 15 months after implantation with a FlexEAS electrode array has been demonstrated by a recent multi-center study by Helbig et al. with HP in all subjects.[6] This study shows an initial loss of low frequency hearing in the 125–500 Hz of on average 14.8 dB within the first month after implantation. However, after this period, RLFH remains relatively stable. Results of speech tests using HA only tend to drop initially after CI implantation. This is likely the result of the incurred partial low frequency hearing loss[6]. Also, after this initial reduction, speech perception with the HA only remains stable over time supporting the stability of low frequency hearing over time postimplantation. Speech perception with CI also seems to be better postoperatively in patients with RLFH than in patients with profound SNHL.[36] This may be due to better preserved nerve structures, e.g. spiral ganglion cells in these patients.[37] The effect of preoperative RFLH on speech perception is also reported by Woodson et al.[35]; together with duration of deafness, RLFH could explain 91% of the variance in performance. These results emphasize the importance of HP after CI surgery even in regular CI cases.

Speech Perception with EAS

Electric acoustic stimulation significantly improves speech perception in quiet and in noise compared to acoustic hearing only. Preoperatively, patients often use a HA, but do not have satisfactory speech perception due to the limitations of acoustic amplification in the high frequencies with HA and the poor acoustic thresholds at these frequencies of EAS candidates. The combination of electric and acoustic stimulation can significantly improve performance of patients with RLFH. The first study on EAS investigating the outcomes of EAS in patients with RLFH reported by Gstoettner el al.[5] showed significant improvements in speech perception performance with EAS compared to the best aided preoperative condition. EAS treatment yielded an improvement in speech perception in quiet from 24% preoperatively to 71% after 12 months of EAS experience. In noise, performance improved from 14% preoperatively in best aided condition to 60% after 12 months of EAS experience. Typical of EAS, is the synergistic effect of significantly better speech perception in noise with combined EAS compared to ES only or acoustic amplification only.[19] Also, often the combination of EAS yields higher scores than the scores with acoustic amplification only and ES only added together. This synergetic effect was also found in outcome studies with EAS published later on.[5,6] Recently, Helbig et al.[6] also reported a significant benefit of EAS for speech perception in quiet and in noise compared to acoustic hearing only or ES only (Fig. 5.11). Hybrid stimulation or EAS using shorter electrodes (6–10 mm) improves speech perception in both quiet and in noise in 48% of patients, however, 23% of subjects do not benefit from EAS when implanted with these shorter electrodes.[34] This may be due to a larger tonotopic mismatch[38] compared to longer electrodes, or due to insufficient stimulation of surviving auditory nerve fibers.

Music Appreciation and Subjective Benefit with EAS

Additional benefit of combined EAS are the higher sound quality and music appreciation with EAS compared to traditional CI. EAS users

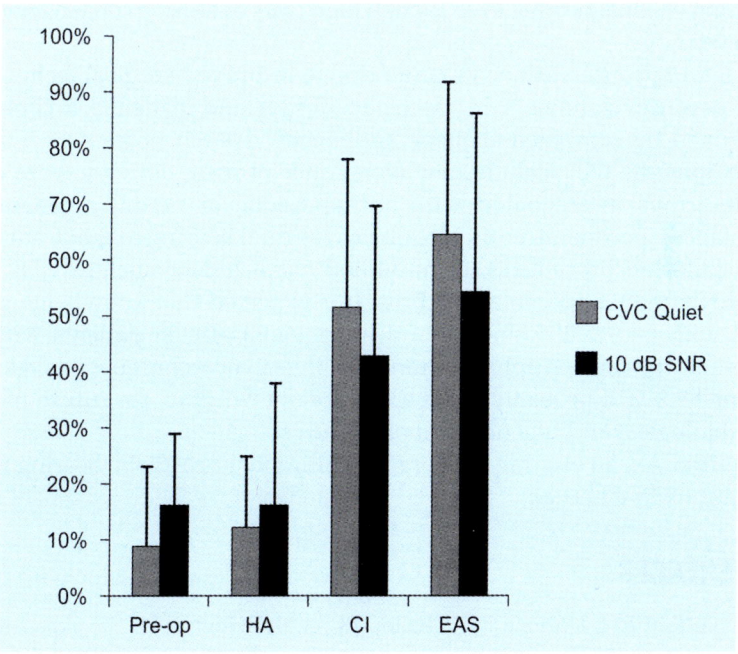

Fig. 5.11: Speech perception in quiet (gray bars) and in noise (black bars) preimplantation, and 12 months after first fitting in HA only, CI only, and EAS conditions (*Source:* Data derived from Helbig et al. 2011)

perform significantly better on melody recognition than CI users[40] and also, instrument identification tends to be better in EAS users than CI users.[39,40] The subjective benefit of EAS that was assessed with Abbreviated Profile of Hearing Aid Benefit (APHAB)[41] in multicenter studies[5,6] can already be observed after the first EAS fitting; improves further with more EAS experience.[42] This in contrast to objective measurements of speech perception where subjects need some experience with the device before improvement, is typically measured.

EAS: CONCLUSION ON COUNSELING AND FUTURE PERSPECTIVES

Inclusion criteria for ES of the auditory nerve via CI have significantly broadened over the years enabling patients with residual hearing to benefit from electrical stimulation as HP with EAS has increased considerably. Benefits of EAS are linked to providing full cochlear coverage with preservation of the specific acoustic benefits at low frequencies. Patients with severe sloping highfrequency hearing loss are partially deaf, experiencing great difficulties with speech perception especially in noisy conditions. Often, these patients have tried several HA with limited success. Nevertheless, many patients were afraid of losing their residual hearing through CI. Therefore of particular importance is also the evidence that speech perception improves considerably in CI mode only in case of loss of the acoustic hearing postoperatively or progressively over the years. Patients have indeed got to be aware of the risk of losing residual hearing even though high rates of hearing conservation are achieved.

Hearing conservation is mainly due to improved surgical techniques and new developments in electrode design and patient's acceptance improved by combined acoustic and electric speech processors. Future developments will include new techniques of drug delivery from electrode arrays impregnated with anti-apoptotic or neural regeneration substances, peroperative monitoring of residual hearing to guide surgical acts, tailoring procedures to individual characteristic such as CDL and improvement of speech algorithms. It is expected that knowledge gathered with EAS will influence and improve CI also in patients without residual hearing. Applying minimal invasive techniques developed under EAS will probably leave a therapeutic window for future molecular biological and regenerative procedures.

With EAS, an exciting new era in multimodal prosthetic hearing rehabilitation has emerged.

REFERENCES

1. Gifford RH, Dorman MF, Shallop JK, et al. Evidence for the expansion of adult cochlear implant candidacy. Ear Hear. 2010;31(2):186-94.
2. Papsin, BC, Gordon KA. Cochlear implants for children with severe-to-profound hearing loss. N Engl J Med. 2007;357:2380-7.

3. Van de Heyning P, Punte AK. Electric acoustic stimulation: a new era in prosthetic hearing rehabilitation. Adv Otorhinolaryngol. 2010;67:1-5.

4. von Ilberg C, Kiefer J, Tillein J, et al. Electric-acoustic stimulation of the auditory system. New technology for severe hearing loss. ORL J Otorhinolaryngol Relat Spec. 1999;61(6):334-40.

5. Gstoettner WK, Van de Heyning P, O'Connor AF, et al. Electric acoustic stimulation of the auditory system: results of a multi-centre investigation. Acta Otolaryngol. 2008;128(9):968-75.

6. Helbig S, Van de Heyning P, Kiefer J, et al. Combined electric acoustic stimulation with the PULSARCI(100) implant system using the FLEX(EAS) electrode array. Acta Otolaryngol. 2011;131(6):585-95.

7. Skarzynski H, Lorens A, Piotrowska A, et al. Partial deafness cochlear implantation in children. Int J Pediatr Otorhinolaryngol. 2007;71(9):1407-13.

8. Gantz BJ, Turner C, Gfeller KE, et al. Preservation of hearing in cochlear implant surgery: advantages of combined electrical and acoustical speech processing. Laryngoscope. 2005;115(5):796-802.

9. Vermeire K, Anderson I, Flynn M, et al. The influence of different speech processor and hearing aid settings on speech perception outcomes in electric acoustic stimulation patients. Ear Hear. 2008;29(1):76-86.

10. Helbig S, Baumann U. Acceptance and fitting of the DUET device—a combined speech processor for electric acoustic stimulation. Adv Otorhinolaryngol. 2010;67:81-7.

11. Moore BC, Glasberg B, Schlueter A. Detection of dead regions in the cochlea: relevance for combined electric and acoustic stimulation. Adv Otorhinolaryngol. 2010;67:43-50.

12. Skarzynski H, Lorens A, Piotrowska A, et al. Partial deafness cochlear implantation provides benefit to a new population of individuals with hearing loss. Acta Otolaryngol. 2006;126(9):934-40.

13. Skarzynski H, Lorens A, Piotrowska A, et al. Hearing preservation in partial deafness treatment. Med Sci Monit. 2010;16(11):CR555-62.

14. Skarzynski H, Lorens A, Skarzynski PH. Personal communication at the 28th Politzer Society, Athens 28/9-1/10/2011 and Hearring meeting Bradford 11-12/10/2012.

15. Wright CG, Roland PS. Temporal bone microdissection for anatomic study of cochlear implant electrodes. Cochlear Implants Int. 2005;6(4):159-68.

16. Adunka O, Kiefer J. Impact of electrode insertion depth on intracochlear trauma. Otolaryngol Head Neck Surg. 2006;135(3):374-82.

17. Helbig S, Settevendemie C, Mack M, et al. Evaluation of an electrode prototype for atraumatic cochlear implantation in hearing preservation candidates: preliminary results from a temporal bone study. Otol Neurotol. 2011;32(3):419-23.

18. Kiefer J, Gstoettner W, Baumgartner W, et al. Conservation of low-frequency hearing in cochlear implantation. Acta Otolaryngol. 2004;124(3):272-80.

19. Gstoettner WK, Helbig S, Maier N, et al. Ipsilateral electric acoustic stimulation of the auditory system: results of long-term hearing preservation. Audiol Neurootol. 2006;11 Suppl 1:49-56.

20. Skarzynski H, Lorens A, Piotrowska A, et al. Preservation of low frequency hearing in partial deafness cochlear implantation (PDCI) using the round window surgical approach. Acta Otolaryngol. 2007;127(1):41-8.
21. Van de Heyning P, Punte AK. Cochlear implants and hearing preservation. Preface. Adv Otorhinolaryngol. 2010;67:vii-viii.
22. Fitzgerald O'Connor E, O'Connor AF. Hearing preservation surgery: current opinions. Adv Otorhinolaryngol. 2010;67:108-15.
23. James C, Albegger K, Battmer R, et al. Preservation of residual hearing with cochlear implantation: how and why. Acta Otolaryngol. 2005;125(5):481-91.
24. Gstoettner W, Franz P, Hamzavi J, et al. Intracochlear position of cochlear implant electrodes. Acta Otolaryngol. 1999;119(2):229-33.
25. Adunka O, Kiefer J, Unkelbach MH, et al. Evaluating cochlear implant trauma to the scala vestibuli. Clin Otolaryngol. 2005;30(2):121-7.
26. Jolly C, Garnham C, Mirzadeh H, et al. Electrode features for hearing preservation and drug delivery strategies. Adv Otorhinolaryngol. 2010;67:28-42.
27. Lee J, Nadol JB Jr, Eddington DK. Depth of electrode insertion and postoperative performance in humans with cochlear implants: a histopathologic study. Audiol Neurootol. 2010;15(5):323-31.
28. Usami S, Moteki H, Suzuki N, et al. Achievement of hearing preservation in the presence of an electrode covering the residual hearing region. Acta Otolaryngol. 2011;131(4):405-12.
29. Punte AK, Vermeire K, Van de Heyning P. Bilateral electric acoustic stimulation: a comparison of partial and deep cochlear electrode insertion. A longitudinal case study. Adv Otorhinolaryngol. 2010;67:144-52.
30. Greenwood DD. A cochlear frequency-position function for several species—29 years later. J Acoust Soc Am. 1990;87(6):2592-605.
31. Greenwood DD. Critical bandwidth and consonance in relation to cochlear frequency-position coordinates. Hear Res. 1991;54(2):164-208.
32. Alexiades G, Bartels L, Jolly C. Method to estimate complete cochlear duct length using a single radiographic basal turn dimension, 2011.
33. Xu J, Xu SA, Cohen LT, et al. Cochlear view: postoperative radiography for cochlear implantation. Am J Otol. 2000;21(1):49-56.
34. Woodson EA, Reiss LA, Turner CW, et al. The Hybrid cochlear implant: a review. Adv Otorhinolaryngol. 2010;67:125-34.
35. Kiefer J, Pok M, Adunka O, et al. Combined electric and acoustic stimulation of the auditory system: results of a clinical study. Audiol Neurootol. 2005;10(3):134-44.
36. Rubinstein JT, Parkinson WS, Tyler RS, et al. Residual speech recognition and cochlear implant performance: effects of implantation criteria. Am J Otol. 1999;20(4):445-52.
37. Rask-Andersen H, Liu W, Linthicum F. Ganglion cell and 'dendrite' populations in electric acoustic stimulation ears. Adv Otorhinolaryngol. 2010;67:14-27.
38. Gantz BJ, Turner CW. Combining acoustic and electrical hearing. Laryngoscope. 2003;113(10):1726-30.
39. Gfeller KE, Olszewski C, Turner C, et al. Music perception with cochlear implants and residual hearing. Audiol Neurootol. 2006;11 Suppl 1:12-5.

40. Brockmeier SJ, Peterreins M, Lorens A, et al. Music perception in electric acoustic stimulation users as assessed by the Mu.S.I.C. test. Adv Otorhinolaryngol. 2010;67:70-80.

41. Cox RM, Alexander GC. The abbreviated profile of hearing aid benefit. Ear Hear. 1995;16(2):176-86.

42. Gstoettner WK, Van de Heyning P, Fitzgerald OA, et al. Assessment of the Subjective Benefit of Electric Acoustic Stimulation with the Abbreviated Profile of Hearing Aid Benefit. ORL J Otorhinolaryngol Relat Spec. 2011;73(6):321-9.

NOVEL APPROACHES TO THE DIAGNOSIS AND TREATMENT OF EUSTACHIAN TUBE DISORDERS

Dennis S Poe, Christian Pfeffer

INTRODUCTION

The auditory tube named after the anatomist Bartholomeus Eustachius who published a detailed anatomical and physiological description in 1562,[1] dynamically links the middle ear and the nasopharynx. The Eustachian tube function with its secretory, ciliary and dilatory components is critical for aeration and drainage of the middle ear, which is essential for the optimal conduction of sound through the tympanic cavity. Treatments for Eustachian tube disorders have met with little long-term success in the past. However, novel technologies and improved understanding of the anatomy, physiology and pathophysiology have led to improved diagnosis as well as strategies and advances in surgical intervention that will be discussed in this text.

CRITICAL ANATOMICAL AND PHYSIOLOGICAL ASPECTS

■ Overview

The anatomy and physiology of the Eustachian tube are tightly inter-linked.

The Eustachian tube, also called auditory tube or pharyngotympanic tube, measures approximately 31–38 mm in length in adults and about 21 mm in an infant. It connects the nasopharynx with the middle ear.[2,3] The pharyngotympanic tube is comprised of two portions, a proximal osseous portion about one-third in length contained within the temporal bone (petrosal part), and a distal cartilaginous portion of about two-third in length. The proximal and distal parts of the Eustachian tube are defined according to the mucociliary clearance flow within the Eustachian tube. It flows from the proximal middle ear cavity to the distal nasopharynx.[4]

The bony portion is lined with cuboidal respiratory epithelium[5] and becomes progressively narrow until reaching the isthmus, the narrowest diameter along the pharyngotympanic tube. This point marks the junction between the bony portion and the cartilaginous portion. The cartilaginous portion gradually flares out as it extends and opens into the nasopharynx. It is composed of a single segment of cartilage approximately 20 mm in length in adults and is anchored superiorly to the basisphenoid bone. The bony portion of the Eustachian tube is a fixed conduit and is always patent under normal conditions.

The cartilaginous portion is lined with pseudostratified columnar respiratory epithelium that is taller and more densely ciliated than in the bony portion. It contains abundant mucin secreting goblet cells, especially in the inferior aspect of the cross sectional area.[2,3,6] The lumen of the cartilaginous portion, particularly at the distal nasopharyngeal orifice, is closed at rest and opens through active muscular action against the curved cartilaginous skeleton that has a spring-like memory action to reclose the lumen after dilation.

PERITUBAL MUSCLES AND THEIR FUNCTION

There are four peritubal muscles, the tensor veli palatini (TVP), the levator veli palatini (LVP), the tensor tympani, and the salpingopharyngeus. The principal muscle for the opening action of the Eustachian tube is the TVP, which is innervated by the mandibular part of the trigeminal nerve.[7] The TVP muscle originates from the basisphenoid bone and the anterior-lateral lip of cartilaginous auditory tube. It is composed of two muscle fiber bundles. They course anteriorly and inferiorly, converging in a tendon that runs under, or at times inserts into the hamulus of the medial pterygoid processes before inserting into the soft palate and the palatine aponeurosis. The dilator tubae portion of the TVP originates directly along the antero-lateral membranous wall of the Eustachian tube and is important for active tubal dilation as well as tubal closure.[6]

The LVP is important for elevating and supporting the soft palate, as well as the torus tubarius throughout Eustachian tube dilation. The LVP originates from the petrous portion of the temporal bone. It runs along the floor of the Eustachian tube, inserts into the soft palate and is innervated by the vagus nerve.[8] The tensor tympani muscle arises from the cartilaginous portion of the Eustachian tube and attaches to the malleus in the middle ear cavity. The mandibular branch of the trigeminal nerve innervates this muscle.

The salpingopharyngeus muscle depresses the floor of the lumen in an action that appears to facilitate dilation and prevents backward displacement of the LVP muscle. It originates from the medial and inferior borders of the cartilaginous Eustachian tube and inserts into the musculature of the lateral pharynx wall. The pharyngeal plexus innervates this muscle.

The pediatric Eustachian tube shows critical anatomical differences compared to adults that may play a pivotal role in the pathogenesis of otitis media. In children the Eustachian tube is of considerably shorter length, has a narrower lumen, is more compliant, more horizontally oriented and contains more luminal mucosal folds.[6] These anatomical differences may predispose children to a different mucociliary clearance and reflux from the nasopharynx of pathogens, nasogastric contents, allergic or other inflammatory mediators.

VISUAL IDENTIFICATION AND LANDMARKS OF THE EUSTACHIAN TUBE

The Eustachian tube orifice can be readily identified just posterior to the inferior turbinate by the prominence of the torus tubarius, also known as the posterior cushion. It contains the mobile medial cartilaginous lamina. The lateral cartilaginous lamina is immobile, considerably smaller, and anchored to the basisphenoid bone shorter. The cartilaginous skeleton in its entirety resembles an inverted "J" hook. It is important to differentiate between the tubal orifice and the fossa of Rosenmüller, also called pharyngeal recess in the postero-lateral nasopharynx just posterior to the torus tubarius. At the base of this recess courses the internal carotid artery.[4] Within the mid-portion of the cartilaginous Eustachian tube, the mucosal surfaces of the anterolateral and posteromedial walls meet in apposition to close the lumen when in resting position. This approximately 8 mm long section is termed the "functional valve" and is comprised of the mucosa, submucosa, Ostmann fat pad, lateral cartilaginous lamina and the relaxed bulk of the tensor veli palatini muscle.

GENERAL PHYSIOLOGICAL ASPECTS

Intermittent brief tubal dilation is the main mechanism for equilibration of middle ear pressure to the ambient atmosphere.[9] Tubal dilation of the Eustachian tube occurs throughout the day through swallowing or yawning.

Muscular contractions of the TVP, LVP and salpingopharyngeus muscles initiate rotational movements of the cartilaginous framework, thereby creating tension with effacement and lateral rounding of the anterolateral wall that leads to active dilation of the lumen and transient opening of the Eustachian tube. Surfactants are produced within the tubal mucosa, and aid in reducing the surface tension of the lumen thus reducing the work required to dilate the tube.[10]

Middle ear and mastoid gas exchange through the mucous membranes and vasculature is a continuous process, and generates a net absorption of gases resulting in an increasingly negative pressure relieved by intermittent tubal dilations.

Fluid and secretions in the middle ear are cleared by mucociliary activity,[11] combined with the muscular pumping action and the tubal closing. Reflux of nasopharyngeal secretions as well as breathing sounds and vocalizations into the middle ear are prevented by the closed position of the pharyngeal Eustachian tube, and by the remaining gas volume in the middle ear and mastoid bone.

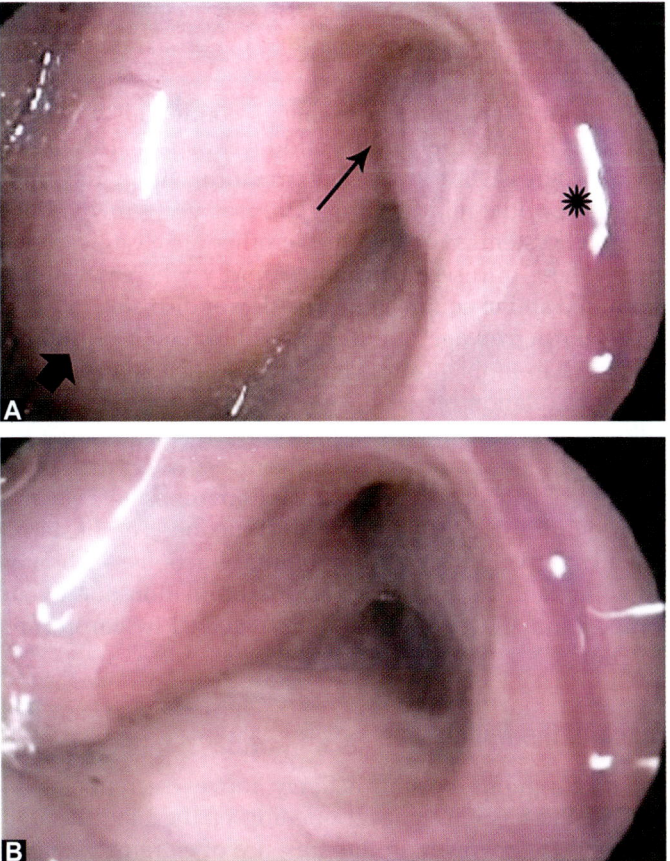

NEW CONSIDERATIONS IN PHYSIOLOGY

█ Eustachian Tube Dilation and Closure

The cartilaginous portion of the pharyngotympanic tube is closed in the resting state as the mucosal walls are in apposition. The closure occurs over a variable length, about a 5–10 mm stretch, and just a few millimeters distal from the bony isthmus where the cartilaginous skeleton becomes flexible. This portion of the cartilaginous Eustachian tube that intermittently dilates actively and closes is termed "valve." Tubal dilation with opening of the valve occurs in two distinct phases (Figs 6.1A and B). Tubal dilation is initiated through palatal elevation as the LVP muscle contracts. This also results in medial rotation of the torus tubarius and the posteromedial wall of the cartilaginous Eustachian tube. The LVP contraction is maintained throughout the tubal dilation cycle. It serves as

Figs 6.1A and B: Normal left Eustachian tube depicting the torus tubarius (arrowhead), orifice (arrow), anterolateral wall (asterisk). A 30° Hopkins rod endoscope in the ipsilateral nasal cavity was used to capture the images. (A) Closed resting position; (B) Open dilated position

a scaffold against which the TVP subsequently acts. The second phase of tubal dilation follows the contraction of the TVP, which actively dilates the Eustachian tube's functional valve thereby exerting a lateral traction force on the anterolateral membranous wall. Full contraction of the TVP results in maximal opening of the valve and creates a rounded Eustachian tube lumen. Tubal dilation propagates from the nasopharyngeal orifice toward the isthmus of the Eustachian tube. The closing of the auditory tube proceeds in the opposite direction, from the isthmus to the nasopharynx. When closed, the functional valve creates an air- and water-tight seal. To adequately ventilate the middle ear space, the functional valve dilation of the Eustachian tube has to be sufficiently wide and frequent to allow gas exchange with the middle ear and to maintain air pressure at near ambient levels. Under normal conditions, the Eustachian tube dilates approximately 1.4 times per minute throughout waking hours, lasts approximately 400 milliseconds, and is substantially decreased during sleep.[12,13]

Middle Ear Gas Exchange

Gases (air) within the middle ear exchange continuously with the gases from the venous blood supply of the middle ear space. This gas exchange results in a progressively lower net pressure within the middle ear. Nitrogen as part of the middle ear air diffuses very slowly, but steadily into the venous system compared to the other air gases, carbon dioxide and oxygen. These diffuse much more rapidly whereas water vapor is always saturated and in equilibrium. The slower diffusion rate of nitrogen creates a greater percentage of nitrogen within the air of the middle ear space compared to ambient air. Thus, at insufficiently wide or insufficiently frequent dilation of the Eustachian tube to adequately ventilate the middle ear gases, the middle ear pressure remains negative and with a higher ratio of nitrogen compared to ambient air. The gradient of nitrogen relative to the ambient air is believed to play an important role in the regulation of pressure in Eustachian tube dysfunction. The Eustachian tube actively dilates by voluntary and involuntary actions, such as yawning and swallowing, and by autonomic reflex stimulation due to alterations in gas composition and pressure that are detected by baroreceptors and chemoreceptors.[9,14]

Clearance of the Middle Ear

The distal cartilaginous portion actively moves secretions, fluids and debris toward the nasopharyngeal opening of the tube through mucociliary transport.[1,15] However, in the presence of extremely viscous secretions, mucociliary clearance can be hindered. Surfactants have been found in the Eustachian tube and may serve to help reduce surface tension within the lumen, effectively aiding mucociliary clearance, tubal dilation, and exchange of gases across the mucosal barrier.[16,17]

There is a muscular pumping action during the tubal closing process that additionally facilitates tubal clearance. In the closing process after dilation as the Eustachian tube progressively closes in a proximal-to-distal direction, it creates an expelling force from the relaxing cartilage and peritubal muscles.[15]

Protection of the Middle Ear

The functional valve of the Eustachian tube protects the middle ear against the reflux of sounds and material from the nasopharynx.[1] During the brief periods of intermittent tubal patency, the existing air pressure within the middle ear and mastoid cavity provides a gas cushion that further inhibits the reflux of material from reaching the middle ear.[13]

EVALUATION OF THE EUSTACHIAN TUBE

History and Physical Examination

A comprehensive history and physical examination are the most important means for evaluation of the Eustachian tube. In patients with dilatory Eustachian tube dysfunction, inflammation of the cartilaginous portion of the Eustachian tube is the most common pathological finding. Patients should therefore be questioned about inflammatory disorders, such as allergies, chronic rhinosinusitis, laryngopharyngeal reflux, vasomotor rhinitis and other less common causes such as Samter's triad. In the pediatric patients, it is important to additionally inquire about recurrent or persistent otitis media, respiratory infections, smoke or wood stove exposure, daycare attendance and immune deficiency.[18] Eustachian tube disorders may also have a familial genesis. Therefore, refractory cases should be evaluated for ciliary motility disorders such as Kartagener's syndrome or cystic fibrosis. Tobacco use or smoke exposure negatively affects mucociliary clearance.

Patients with dilatory dysfunction typically complain of aural fullness and varying degrees of conductive hearing loss. Typically, the tympanic membrane appears abnormal as well. Less common symptoms may include otalgia, otorrhea and fever. Patients with chronic aural fullness, but without tympanic membrane retractions, effusion, or abnormalities are unlikely to have Eustachian tube dilatory dysfunction. For these patients, other causes should be investigated.

Endoscopic Examination of the Eustachian Tube

A flexible or Hopkins rod endoscope is used to evaluate the Eustachian tube. A thorough examination assessing the nasal mucosa, nasopharynx, pharynx, larynx, hypopharynx and subglottic space for signs of inflammation or underlying allergy, granulomatous, laryngopharyngeal reflux, or other diseases should be performed prior to evaluating the Eustachian tube in detail.[19]

When examining the Eustachian tube with a flexible endoscope, the optimal view into the depths of the tubal lumen may be obtained by either advancing the instrument through the ipsilateral nostril or via the contralateral nostril, passing it behind the vomer and positioning it close to the nasopharyngeal orifice of the auditory tube. To best inspect the tubal valve during swallowing and yawning, the endoscope should be directed down the longitudinal axis of the lumen which courses approximately 45° laterally and 45° superiorly from the floor of the nasal cavity. When examining with a rigid endoscope, 4 mm scopes with a 30° or 45° viewing angle are ideal. As the instrument is introduced into the nasal cavity, the scope should be initially directed laterally or superiorly to watch the turbinates. Then it can be rotated to bring the auditory tube orifice into view when entering the nasopharynx.[20] When the healthy and intact Eustachian tube is closed, the tissues of the anterolateral wall create a convex bulge and create an S-shaped appearance from the opposed mucosal walls.

The most common findings in Eustachian tube dilatory dysfunction are mucosal inflammation with edema, hypertrophy, excessive mucus secretion, hyperemia and cobblestone appearance from lymphoid hyperplasia.[21] These changes are frequently most pronounced in the mucosa of the torus tubarius (Fig. 6.2).

Evaluation with slow-motion endoscopy aids to differentiate between obstructive and dynamic causes of Eustachian tube dilatory dysfunction. To assess the principal peritubal muscle function, the patient is asked to phonate the letter "K" repeatedly. This causes isolated contraction of the LVP muscle and medial rotation of the torus tubarius without tubal dilation. Normal tubal dilation is then assessed during repeated swallows and lastly, the patient is asked to forcefully yawn to produce a maximal

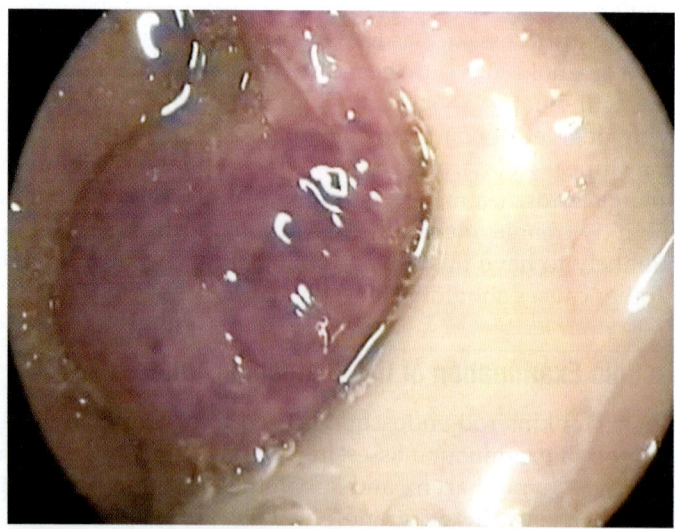

Fig. 6.2: Left Eustachian tube with inflamed torus tubarius and lymphoid hyperplasia. In addition, the patient shows otitis media with effusion

voluntary dilatory effort. Video endoscopy recorded with either analog or digital media can be reviewed in slow motion. This allows a detailed assessment of the tubal dilatory phases, with the orifice seen changing from its resting S-shaped convexity into a rounded opening.

PATHOLOGY OF EUSTACHIAN TUBE DYSFUNCTION

Overview, Etiology and Pathophysiology

Endoscopy of the Eustachian tube has revealed that most patients with Eustachian tube dysfunction have identifiable pathology within the cartilaginous portion.[5,22] Insufficient dilation of the Eustachian tube (dilatory dysfunction) is the most common type of tubal dysfunction. Second most is the patulous Eustachian tube, the failure of proper closure of the tubal valve.

Dilatory dysfunction is most commonly due to functional obstruction or insufficient dilation rather than true blockage of the lumen. The most common finding in dilatory dysfunction is mucosal inflammation within the cartilaginous Eustachian tube. The inflammation appears to involve the lymphoid tissues in the torus tubarius and the glandular mucosal surfaces of the nasopharyngeal orifice. The mucosa deeper within the lumen, i.e. closer to the isthmus is typically much less inflamed. In one study of dilatory obstructive dysfunction, mucosal edema near the orifice was found in 83% of the subjects and 74% had reduced anterolateral wall movement of the Eustachian tube, most likely due to the thickness of the inflamed mucosa.[23] Adjacent inflammation in the adenoid is common. Inflammation has correlated significantly with the presence of laryngopharyngeal reflux and allergies in adults, raising suspicions that these factors may be important contributors to dilatory dysfunction.[22,23] Inflammation due to infection can result from diseases in the respiratory tract including those affecting the nasal cavity, sinuses, nasopharynx and the remainder of the upper and lower airway. Primary disorders of the mucosa or submucosa such as Wegener's disease, Samter's triad and granulomatous diseases are less common etiologies. Children are additionally affected by frequent upper respiratory infections that are increased with day care, reflux disease in younger children and exposure to tobacco smoke or wood-burning stoves.[18] Smoke impairs the mucociliary function. Increased viscosity of secretions and primary ciliary disorders are other causes for compromised mucociliary clearance function. Hormone level changes, in particular, progesterone that are increased during pregnancy or oral contraceptive intake can induce mucosal hypertrophy.

Anatomical obstruction of the Eustachian tube from neoplasms is less common. However, adenoid hypertrophy that encroaches on the torus tubarius can interfere with the dilatory process thereby causing a functional obstruction. The contraction of pharyngeal constrictors during swallowing can press an enlarged adenoid into the torus tubarius and force it anteriorly to close the tubal orifice instead of dilating it open[23,24] (Figs 6.3A and B).

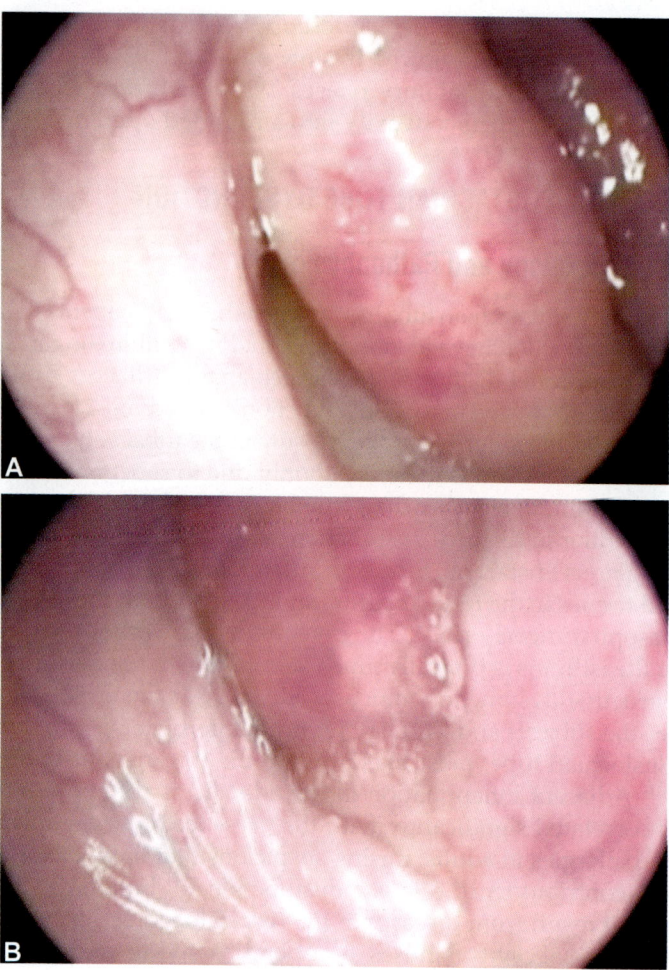

Figs 6.3A and B: Right Eustachian tube with inflamed adenoid in upper right corner. The adenoid reaches and contacts the inflamed torus tubarius. Otitis media with effusion is seen. (A) Closed resting position; (B) Swallow with attempt to open the Eustachian tube. The swollen torus tubarius is compressed against the adenoid thus forcing the torus anteriorly and preventing opening of the orifice

Dynamic causes of Eustachian tube dilatory dysfunction may be due to hypoactive, hyperactive or uncoordinated contraction of TVP or LVP muscles. Muscular dysfunction and weakness of the TVP muscle is the most common dynamic cause of decrease in anterolateral wall dilatory movement. Diminished or disorganized TVP contractions may reduce the lateral excursion of the anterolateral wall in the final step of dilation. Excessive contractions have been observed in both TVP and LVP muscles. This leads to a bulky mass effect thereby paradoxically impairing the valve dilation at the moment it should be opening (Figs 6.4A and B). Uncoordinated contractions can result in inadequate dilation when the LVP relaxes prematurely prior to the contraction of the TVP. This provides additional

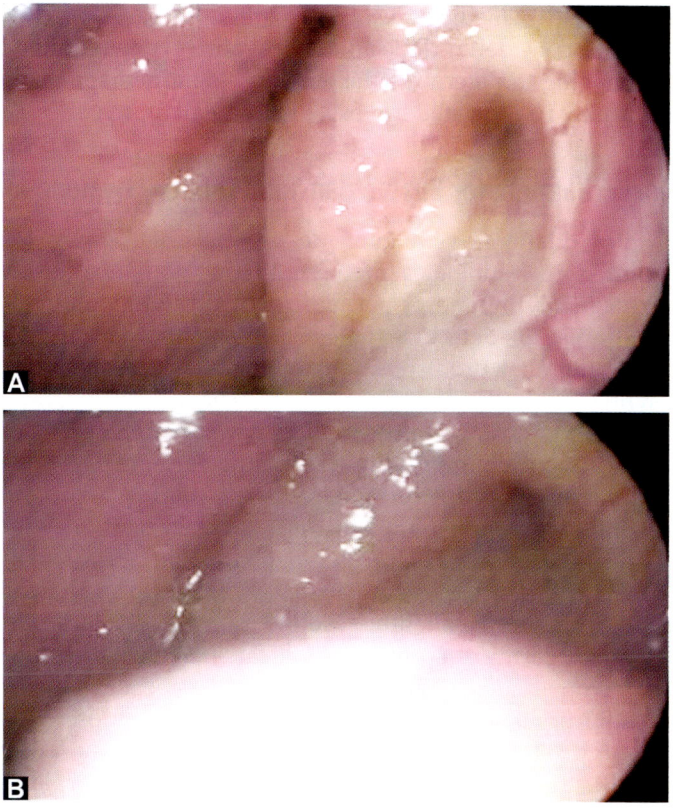

Figs 6.4A and B: Left Eustachian tube demonstrating dynamic dysfunction of the LVP muscle. The muscle contracts excessively high during swallows, thus blocking the lumen during the dilatory effort. Otitis media with effusion is present. (A) Resting closed position; (B) Swallow with high elevation of the palate; LVP muscle blocks the tubal lumen

evidence that the LVP serves a scaffold-function against which the weak action of the TVP is dependent for adequate dilation function.

Medical Treatment for Eustachian Tube Dilatory Dysfunction

Mucosal disease is the most common cause of dilatory dysfunction. Identifying the underlying etiology of the disease and treating it appropriately is advised. Allergies are a common cause of dilatory dysfunction. These persist or start after the age of six and evaluation is often indicated. Allergen avoidance, oral antihistamines, nasal topical steroid drops (available in Europe, but not in the USA) or sprays (less effective than drops), saline irrigations, nasal antihistamine, mast cell stabilizer sprays, leukotriene inhibitors, combination therapy and immunotherapy may all be considered. Recurrent nasal or sinus infections should be maximally treated as indicated. Granulomatous diseases usually require immunosuppressant therapy, but some topical treatments may be indicated. Laryngopharyngeal reflux should be treated with behavioral and dietary modifications as well as anti-reflux medications. For severe reflux cases, fundoplication surgery may be considered. True anatomical obstruction requires contrast enhanced imaging to determine the etiology. Identified benign or malignant lesions may be indicated for excision as the definitive therapy.

Surgical Treatment for Eustachian Tube Dilatory Dysfunction

Persistence of dilatory dysfunction despite maximal efforts to control various underlying etiologies may imply that the tubal mucosa has become irreversibly injured or perhaps involved with biofilms. A structural compromise or defect of the Eustachian tube may be present in patients with familial predisposition for tubal dysfunction, cleft lip or palates, syndromic and other craniofacial anomalies.

Inserting tympanostomy tubes into the tympanic membrane may alleviate the negative pressure within the middle ear and relieve tympanic membrane retraction, effusion and atelectasis. Effusion or inflammation that continues despite tympanostomy tubes in place may indicate a primary mucosal disorder. Thick glue-like effusions are associated with up regulation of the MUC genes causing increased protein production. These conditions will frequently respond to oral or topical corticosteroids.[25] Adenoidectomy can provide significant relief to patients with otitis media and demonstrated adenoid hypertrophy, especially if the hypertrophied adenoid tissue reaches the torus tubarius.[26,27] Endoscopic-assisted adenoidectomy permits more complete removal of the tissue encroaching the torus. It further allows for some debulking of the hyperplastic tissue of the torus, if considered necessary.

In recent years, Eustachian tuboplasty has received increased attention as a safe and possibly effective surgical option for patients with dilatory dysfunction. Candidates for Eustachian tuboplasty are patients with chronic tubal dilatory dysfunction after receiving maximal yet ineffectual medical therapy. They experience improvement with tympanostomy tube placement, but their dilatory dysfunction recurs upon extrusion of the tympanostomy tubes. Eustachian tuboplasty can be accomplished by removing inflamed soft tissue and cartilage as indicated from the luminal side of the posteromedial wall, beginning from the leading edge of the torus tubarius and extending up to or into the valve. This is accomplished using either a laser or microdebrider (Figs 6.5A to D). This procedure is based on the following hypothesis. Dilation of the lumen by surgical debulking facilitates the dilatory action of the TVP muscle and removes irreversibly diseased mucosal tissue allowing for regrowth of healthy mucosa. Submucosal tissue and cartilage within the valve region may be removed, but the mucosa is conserved to prevent synechiae. Similarly, care is taken to avoid injury to the contralateral anterolateral wall.[28] Great care should always be taken to protect and avoid contact with the internal carotid artery. The artery lies in increasingly close proximity to the Eustachian tube as it courses superiorly. In some cases the artery becomes even dehiscent within the bony portion.

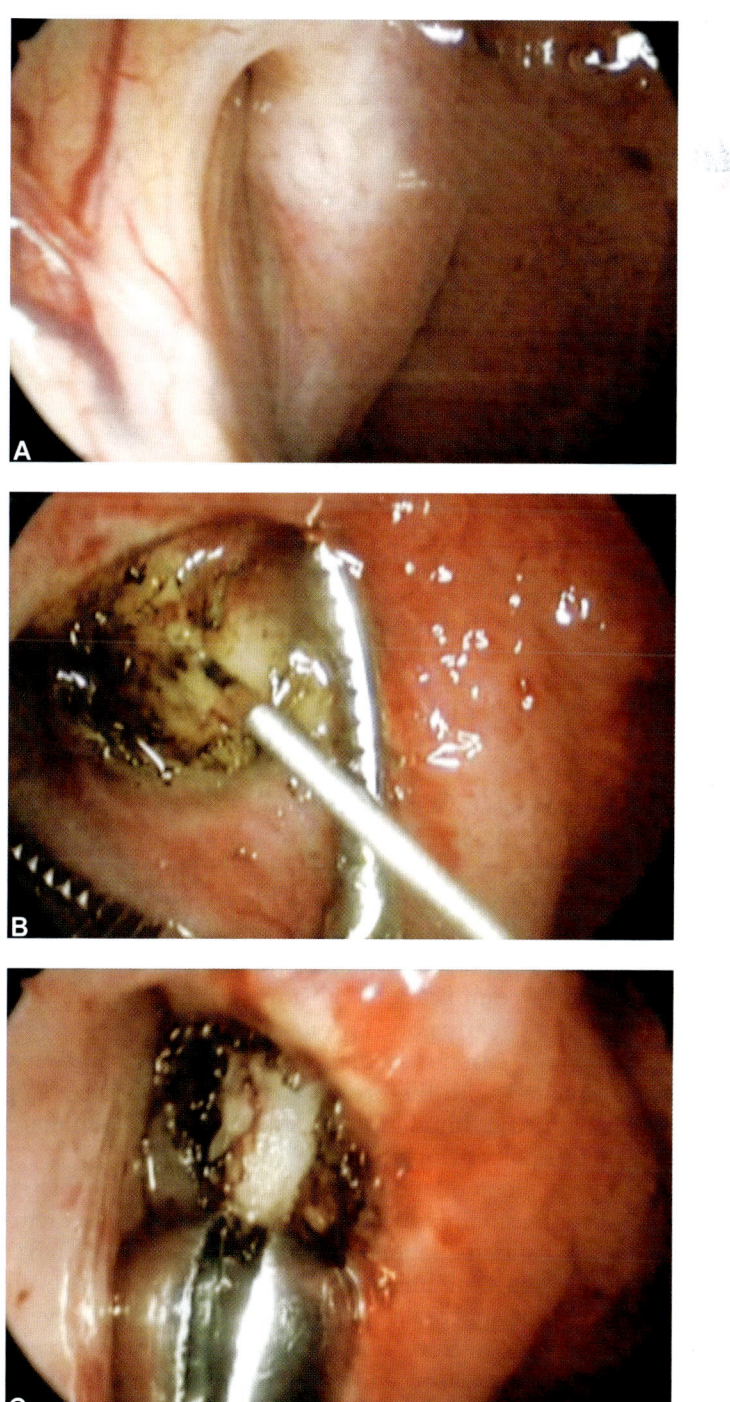

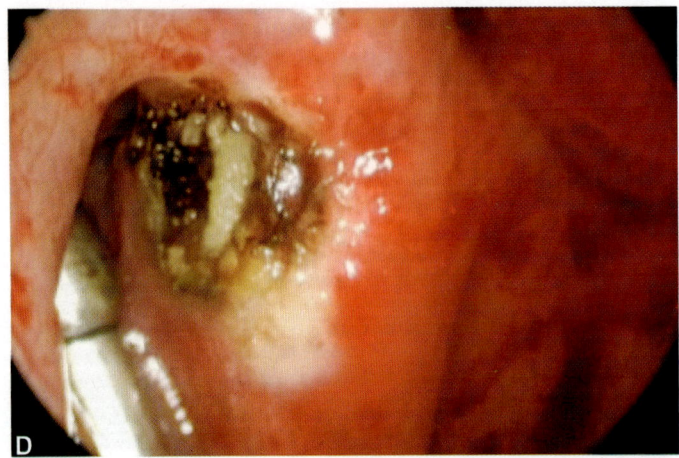

Figs 6.5A to D: Laser tuboplasty on the right Eustachian tube; patient has refractory otitis media with effusion. (A) Intraoperative view of orifice prior the procedure. The mucosa of the torus tubarius is edematous; (B) An optional retractor is in place; with a KTP laser, fiber mucosa and soft tissue is removed down to the level of the medial cartilaginous lamina; (C) A portion of cartilage that protruded into the lumen has been divided with scissors, and cup forceps are used for removal; (D) The completed operative field with the exposed tubal cartilage showing the mucosal and submucosal defect. An olive tipped curved suction is retracting the torus tubarius medially for exposure

In the senior author's two-year follow-up study of Eustachian tuboplasty using an otologic Argon or KTP laser for tissue ablation, 38% of 13 adults with refractory, very long-term otitis media with effusion and multiple prior tympanostomy tubes had remission of their effusion. Three other patients developed intermittent effusions and considered themselves substantially improved for an overall improvement rate of 68%.[29] There were no significant complications. Postoperatively there is a scaphoid defect in the torus tubarius and in most cases a deeper view into the valve (Figs 6.6A to D). In our studies, failures of laser based Eustachian tuboplasty correlated with the presence of allergies or laryngopharyngeal reflux. This further highlights the need to continue to manage any underlying conditions postoperatively.[29,30]

Most recently balloon dilation of the cartilaginous Eustachian tube has been assessed for feasibility, safety and early clinical application. Cadaveric studies using balloon dilation catheters for tubal dilation have proven to be effective and show minimal complication risks. Adverse events, such as minor tears in the mucosal lumen were observed. However, neither osseous cartilaginous fracture nor trauma to the internal carotid did occur.[31] A clinical study was recently performed on 11 patients presenting with Eustachian tube dilation dysfunction showing refractory otitis media with effusion for over five years duration, interrupted only with a tympanostomy tube placement.[32] Endoscopic-assisted dilation with a 6 or 7 mm diameter × 16 mm long sinuplasty balloon for one minute was done under

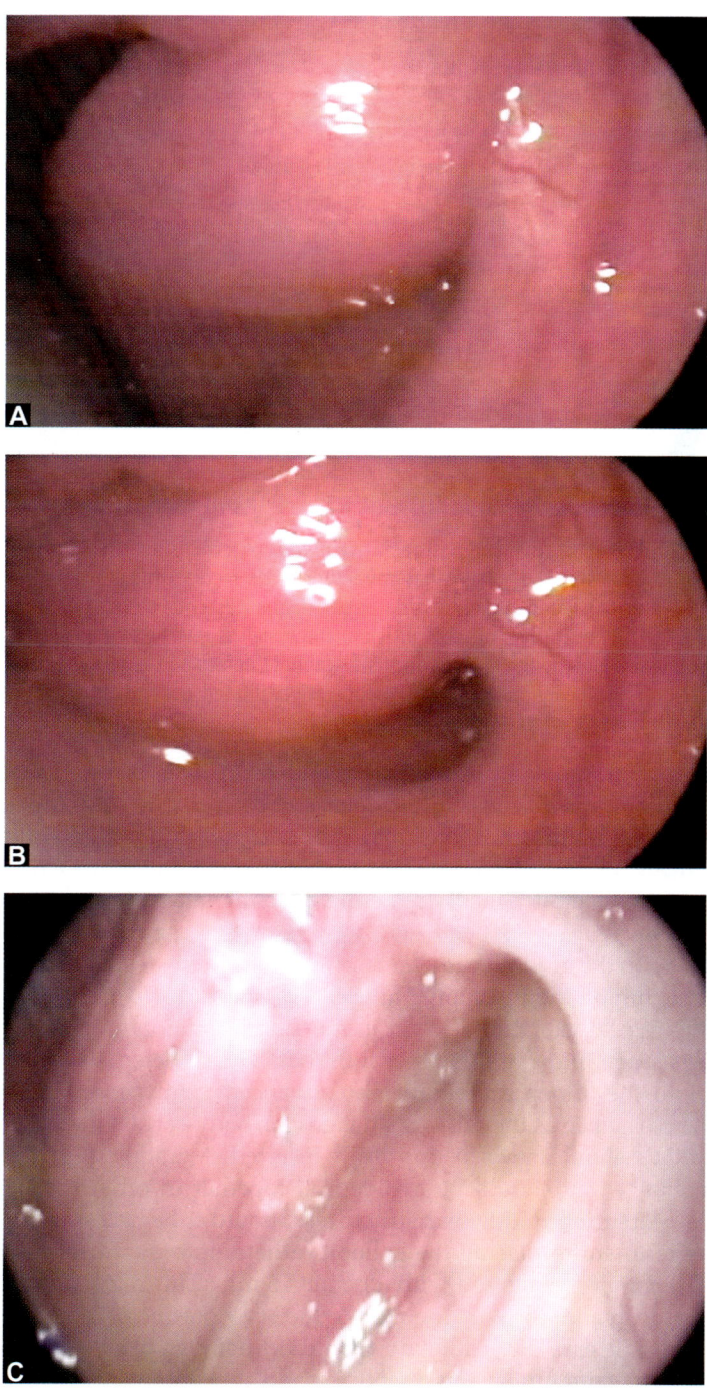

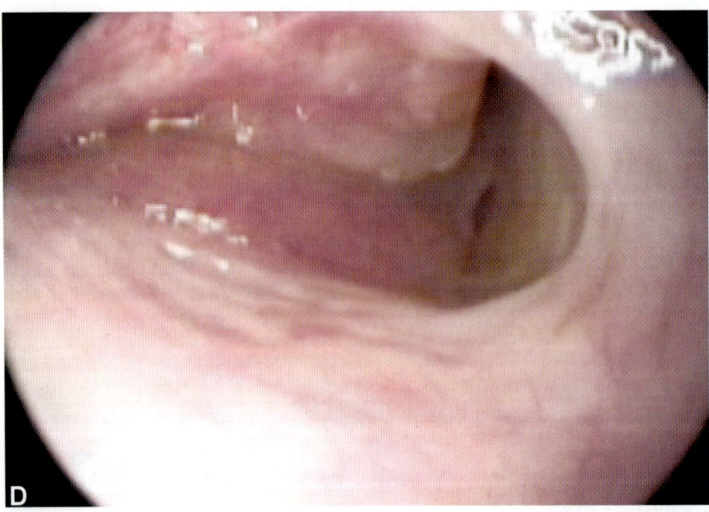

Figs 6.6A to D: Preoperative and postoperative photos of left Eustachian tube orifice laser Eustachian tuboplasty. The patient has refractory otitis media with effusion and severe allergic disease. (A) Preoperative, resting position; the posterior cushion is bulbous and edematous; (B) Preoperative, dilated position; the lumen is revealed minimally; (C) Postoperative, resting position; the torus shows a scaphoid defect on the luminal surface; the inflammation is markedly reduced; (D) Postoperative, dilated position; the lumen is now exposed with dilatory effort

general anesthesia. A 4 mm, 45° rigid endoscope was placed in the ipsilateral or contralateral nostril for viewing. The balloons were introduced through a 70° guiding catheter that was designed for frontal sinus dilation. During surgery it is important to recognize that the Eustachian tube initially curves slightly medially before coursing laterally toward the ear. The lumen should be opened gently by retracting medially on the torus tubarius with the guiding catheter allowing for a view deep into the lumen before beginning the insertion. Failure to rotate the torus medially before inserting the catheter could result in mucosal laceration with bleeding or a false passage into the submucosal tissues. The catheter is passed superiorly into the lumen atraumatically, advanced gently and slowly until meeting resistance as the catheter engages the bony-cartilaginous isthmus. The catheter should never be forcefully inserted. A guidewire is generally not necessary and should be avoided all together in order to minimize the risk of injuring middle ear structures. Should it be necessary to use a guidewire to aid in placing the balloon catheter into the Eustachian tube lumen, it should be marked with a pen at 16 mm. This mark prevents the surgeon to advance the wire too far into the bony portion of the Eustachian tube or middle ear. The guidewire should be removed prior to inflation so that the catheter's lumen can open fully and prevent over pressurization from a trapped air pocket. The balloon catheter shows a yellow mark at 16 mm from its tip. It should be inserted into the tubal lumen no further than to this marker and the yellow marker should just be visible at the tubal orifice. This assures that the balloon catheter is inserted at the proper depth into the tubal lumen. The inflation is currently performed at 12 atm for two minutes as opposed to one minute used in the pilot study. After this procedure the balloon is deflated and removed (Figs 6.7A to D). The procedure may be done bilaterally. The sinuplasty balloon system (Acclarent corp., Palo Alto, CA, USA) is not FDA approved for Eustachian tube dilation.

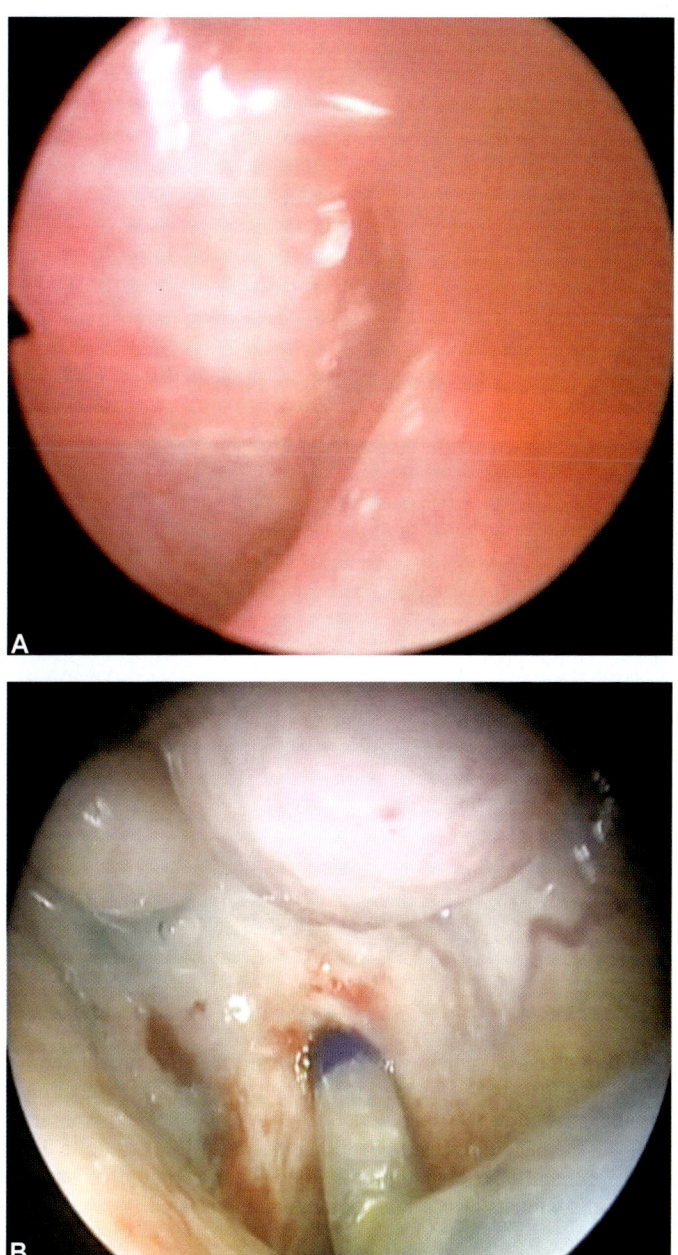

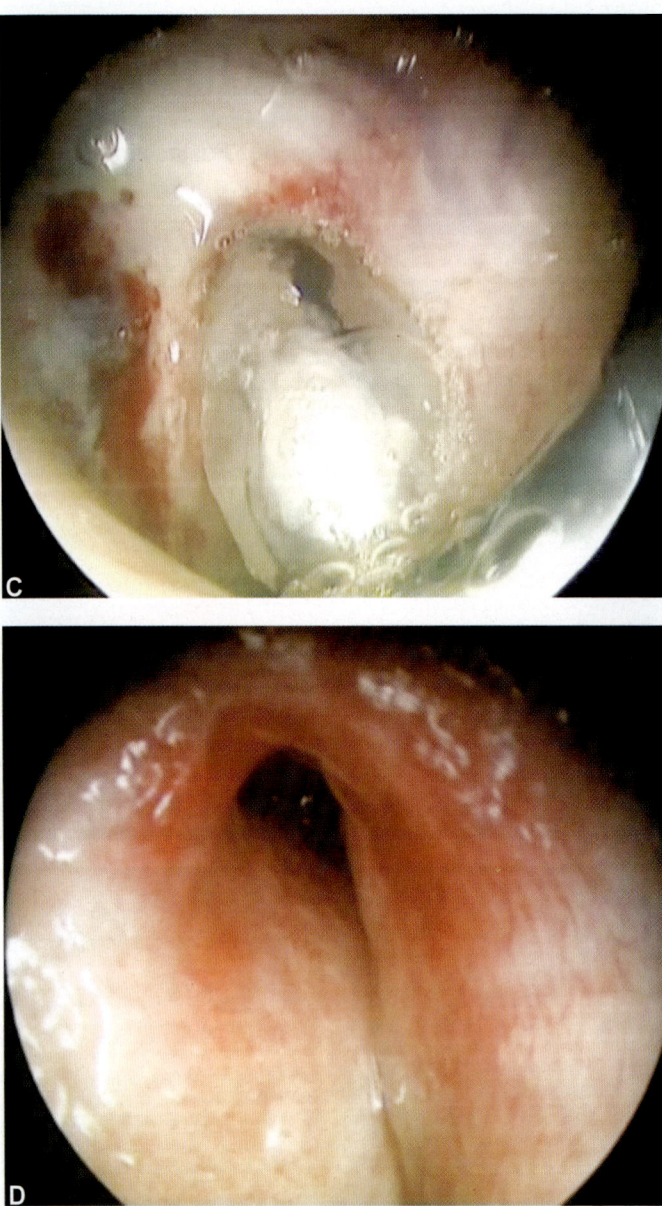

Figs 6.7A to D: Balloon dilation of a left Eustachian tube. The patient shows refractory otitis media with effusion. (A) Preoperative resting position of the auditory tube with edema and inflammation of the torus tubarius; (B) A guide catheter is inserted into the tubal lumen; (C) The balloon catheter; 7x16 mm has been inserted up to 16 mm depth, and inflated to 12 atm for two minutes; (D) The balloon catheter has been removed. A widened lumen and minimal mucosal lacerations are appreciated

Eleven out of eleven (100%) patients were able to perform a Valsalva maneuver postoperatively which they could not perform before this procedure. This result declined to 63.6% after a 6–14 months follow-up period. Resolution of OME occurred in five out of eleven (45.4%) patients with an intact tympanic membrane (no perforation or tube). There was significant reduction in inflammatory rating scores of the mucosa of the Eustachian tube. Additional controlled clinical studies of balloon dilation and Eustachian tuboplasty are needed to determine the value and long-term results of these novel procedures. Additional basic research is required to investigate and understand the apparent potential benefits in reducing mucosal inflammation.

PATULOUS EUSTACHIAN TUBE DYSFUNCTION

Overview, Etiology and Pathophysiology

Patulous Eustachian tube dysfunction refers to persistent patency of the tubal lumen. Air and sound pass unrestricted between the nasopharynx and the middle ear space. Patients with this disorder complain of a disturbing amplified perception of one's own voice and nasal breathing sounds (autophony), an accompanying sensation of aural fullness, and in few cases otalgia. Although benign, patulous dysfunction and the resulting autophony cause a wide range of symptom severity ranging from asymptomatic to severe psychological impairment. Symptoms are often intermittent and can last from seconds to hours. In extreme cases they persist continuously throughout the day. Symptoms may be worsened with nasal steroids or decongestants and improved with upper respiratory tract infections. Etiologically, symptoms occur after a dramatic and substantial weight loss such as during post-pregnancy, cachectic diseases, dietary weight loss, or bariatric surgery. In the author's experience, one-third of cases of patulous Eustachian tube have a history of substantial weight loss, one-third have an associated systemic rheumatologic disorder, and the remaining third are idiopathic. Oral contraceptives may also contribute to the disorder. Loss of tubal tissue volume within the valve is the likely etiology for many patients. Endoscopic examination reveals a longitudinal concavity in the anterolateral wall in the resting position of the auditory tube resulting in inadequate closing of the tubal lumen (Fig. 6.8).[33] The anterolateral wall normally contains a convex bulge into the lumen that contributes to the valve function. This bulge is diminished or absent in these patients. A majority of cases have an underdeveloped lateral cartilaginous lamina constituting a potential risk for patulous Eustachian tube. Patients with a thin build may have less Ostmann's fat and if combined with a lack of cartilage in the bulge of the valve, may lead to patulous Eustachian tube. Exercise frequently initiates or exacerbates symptoms. They tend to abate in the supine or head dependent positions. Recently, CT scans revealed smaller Ostmann's fat pad and glandular tissues in patulous patients compared to normal control subjects.[34]

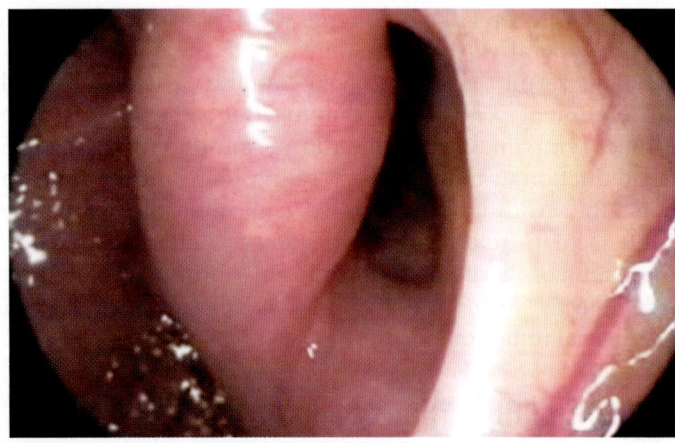

Fig. 6.8: Left patulous Eustachian tube. It shows a marked scaphoid anterolateral wall. No visible lateral cartilaginous lamina or evidence of a significant Ostmann's fat pad

The symptoms of patulous Eustachian tube can overlap with other conditions making the differential diagnosis more challenging. Patients should be examined while they are experiencing active autophony symptoms. Otoscopy or micro-otoscopy in the sitting position will usually reveal the pathognomonic sign of a patulous tube with medial and lateral excursions of the tympanic membrane during nasal breathing while the opposite nostril is held shut. If the symptoms are not initially active, they can usually be triggered by a few minutes of physical activity prior to otoscopy.

Impedance tympanometry is the most sensitive test to aid in the diagnosis of patulous Eustachian tube dysfunction. It shows ventilatory fluctuations in the compliance of the tympanic membrane while a 15 second run is performed with the instrument set for reflex decay testing. Irregular inspirations and expirations through the ipsilateral nostril with the opposite nostril occluded should show sawtooth-like perturbations of the baseline tympanogram tracing. The breathing is performed irregularly to not confuse the tracing with the regular sawtooth waveforms that can occur from intracranial pulsations.

If the tympanogram test is negative despite the patient having active autophony, other pathologies should be considered, such as semicircular canal dehiscence syndrome. Vestibular evoked myogenic potential (VEMP) and electrocochleography (ECoG) testing can aid in differentiating patulous dysfunction from Minor's semicircular canal dehiscence syndrome. Although less common, endolymphatic hydrops can cause recruitment with hyperacusis and autophony. Patients with Minor's syndrome generally lack autophony of their nasal breathing sounds as opposed to the bone-conducted autophony of their voice. These patients will show an abnormally low threshold VEMP. If the patient has tympanostomy tubes still in place, ventilatory excursions can still be observed. To achieve this, a drop of clear topical otologic medication is placed on top of the tympanostomy tube and movements of the fluid meniscus forming on top of the tube can be observed.

Additionally, sonotubometry research with recent improvements in detecting tubal patency status have demonstrated a correlation between the severity of autophony and measured tubal function.[35]

Medical Treatment for Patulous Eustachian Tube Dysfunction

The therapeutic goals for patulous Eustachian tube are the restoration of the healthy humidified mucosa and competence of the tubal valve. Patients should be treated in a stepwise fashion. The initial step is to reassure the patients that the condition is entirely benign. Next steps are the discontinuation of decongestants and topical nasal corticosteroid, encouraging patients to increase their fluid intake particularly during exercise, adding nasal saline drops or irrigations to improve hydration of the mucosa.

Although approximately one-third of patulous patients have a history of significant weight loss, weight gain is generally not advised unless medically indicated. The following medications have been used, but with mixed results. The concept behind these medications is to stimulate a temporary closure of the Eustachian tube. Among them, saturated solution of potassium iodide (SSKI), eight to ten drops diluted in water or juice taken three times daily, enhances the viscosity of the mucus. Application of irritants, such as boric and salicylic acid powder, silver nitrate, nitrate acid and phenol cause tissue inflammation and thus increased mucus production. Chlorine based drops are available but have only variable success as well. The off-label use of Premarin (25 mg in 30 ml normal saline topical nasal drops, three drops three times daily for a 6 weeks trial) or depo-estradiol estrogens (5 mg in 30 ml normal saline) may provide some temporary relief by causing localized mucosal hypertrophy and thus temporary closure of the open Eustachian tube.

Drops are most effectively applied with the nose pointed straight upward and the head turned 45° to the ipsilateral side as the drops pass through the nasal cavity. A tickle or sensation of irritation should radiate toward the ear when the drops come in contact with the tubal orifice.

Surgical Treatment of Patulous Eustachian Tube Dysfunction

When medical treatments lead to insufficient relief only, surgical options may be considered. The following strategies are considered. Myringotomy with tympanostomy tube placement is commonly tried as an initial procedure.[36] This procedure is effective for aural fullness and tympanic membrane excursions. However, it is generally not effective for treating autophony. To alleviate autophony, complete occlusion of the Eustachian tube lumen can be considered. However, tubal function is not preserved and makes long-term tympanostomy tube ventilation necessary.

Occlusion can be accomplished through the ear by placing one or more catheters into the osseous portion of the Eustachian tube lumen, filling them with bone wax if desired and even packing around the catheters with bone wax for a complete seal. Alternatively, circumferential monopolar cauterization of the lumen within the nasopharyngeal orifice lumen can be performed, obliterating the lumen and occluding it with a fat graft.[37] These procedures can lead to a complete relief of the patulous symptoms. Occasionally, however, thick mucus secretions can develop, and cause repeated occlusion of the tympanostomy tube. Therefore, occlusion options that do not reconstruct or preserve tubal function should only be considered as a last resort.

In an effort to correct the patulous symptoms while preserving tubal function, a shim can be inserted into the lumen. Alternatively, autologous cartilage can be placed into the submucosal pockets within the lumen. A shim can be introduced into the nasopharyngeal orifice, wedging it into position within the isthmus. Being long and thin, the shim can be positioned into the length of the longitudinal concave defect of the valve to effectively restore some valve function and thus relieve the symptoms. An intravenous catheter filled with bone wax can be employed in this off-label application. A 14 gauge (2.1 mm diameter) catheter will appropriately fit most adult patients. A CT scan is necessary for all patients preoperatively to assure that there is bony coverage of the internal carotid artery. Dehiscence of the artery into the tubal lumen is a contraindication for catheter insertion into the pharyngeal opening of the auditory tube.

The placement of the catheter is performed under general anesthesia. Bone wax is heated until molten, then aspirated through the catheter using a syringe. The wax then quickly cools and solidifies. The catheter is cut to 36–38 mm length for most females and 38–40 mm for most males. It is inserted under endoscopic guidance using an insertion tool. It consists of a hollow tube that is passed through the oral cavity and an internal piston that pushes the catheter forward and outward towards the distal end. The insertion tool is also utilized to push the torus medially. This maneuver reveals the curvature of the Eustachian tube. To visualize this anatomy is essential prior to introducing the catheter in the same fashion discussed with the insertion of the balloon catheter. The catheter should pass smoothly and atraumatically at all times. The insertion should be bloodless. The catheter will begin to meet some resistance at the isthmus and is allowed to straighten itself out. It can then be advanced with some firmer pressure to wedge it into position within the isthmus. Proper catheter placement is achieved when the distal catheter end is at the level with the margin of the free torus tubarius (Figs 6.9A to D). A 16 gauge catheter may be used if the 14 gauge one is too large to pass smoothly. A 12 gauge catheter is rarely used. In most patients, the catheters stay in place nicely and are not felt by the patients at all.

In the event that the catheter extrudes prematurely, patulous Eustachian tube reconstruction may be done with autologous cartilage grafts taken from the conchal or septal cartilage. Under endoscopic guidance, a submucosal pocket is created in the superior and anterolateral wall of the pharyngeal opening of the auditory tube. The harvested cartilage grafts are cut into

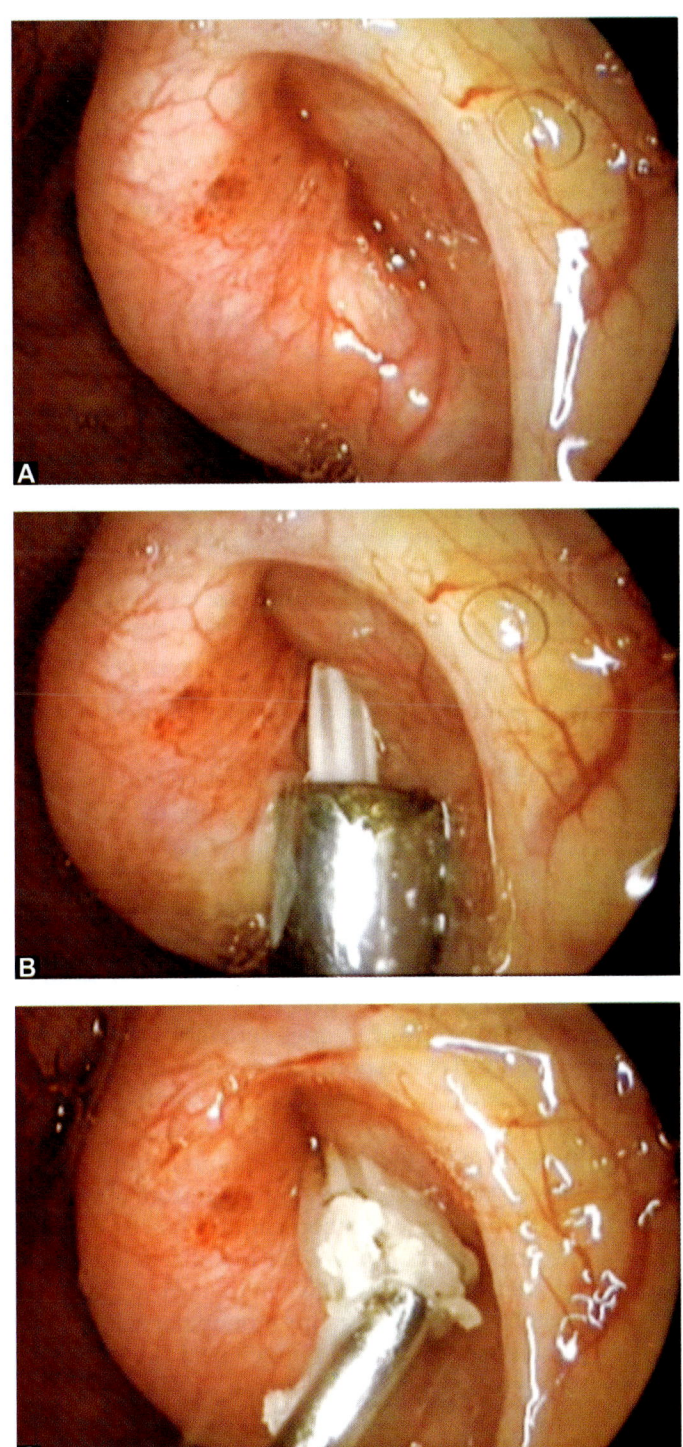

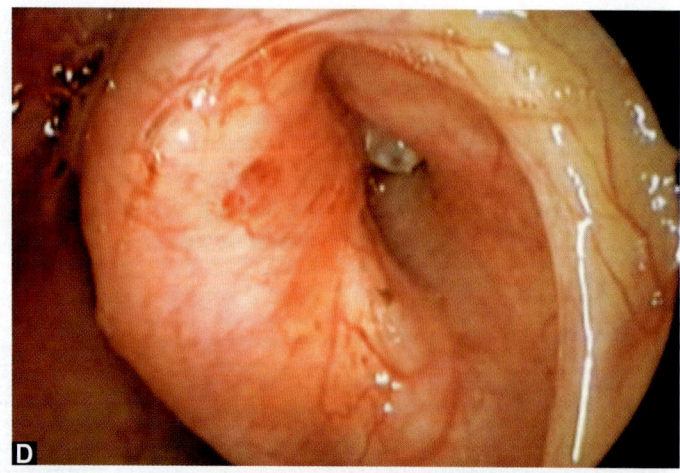

Figs 6.9A to D: Left patulous Eustachian tube showing insertion of an intravenous catheter filled with bone wax. (A) The left tubal orifice before intervention; (B) The catheter is housed in an introducer tool. It is being positioned into the tubal orifice. The torus is rotated medially to open the lumen, and view the direction of the lumen. The lumen usually curves slightly medially before subsequently coursing laterally toward the temporal bone. Failure to recognize this curve can result in mucosal lacerations or false passages during catheter advancement; (C) The catheter is firmly wedged into the bony-cartilaginous isthmus; (D) The catheter is in the final position at the level of the torus tubarius

small wedges of about 8 mm lengths and are inserted into the pocket. After confirming proper placement of the cartilage graft, the incision is closed with sutures. A curved needle driver that can be passed through the oral cavity is used and the knot is cinched down into place by passing one end of the suture through a curved olive antral suction tip. While the suction is engaged, the suture is passed into the lumen of the suction catheter. The suction tubing is then removed, allowing the surgeon to grasp the now threaded suction and to advance the suction catheter up to cinch down the throws of the knot. A pilot study of 14 cases demonstrated to be 100% effective for this procedure in all cases shortly post procedure. The effectiveness decreased to 43% after a follow-up period of 15.8 months.[33]

The Eustachian tube lumen can be further narrowed by longitudinally cutting through the base of the medial cartilaginous lamina using a curved scissors, sickle knife or laser, thereby separating it from the basisphenoid. At the posterior extent of the dissection caution has to be exercised as the internal carotid artery approaches. Once mobilized, the cartilage loses much of its spring like effect and will give in to narrow the lumen. Additional narrowing can be achieved with fine monopolar cauterization of the inferior cross sectional half of the tubal lumen near the orifice supported by placing a suture across the orifice to lateralize the now mobile medial cartilaginous lamina.

Injection of materials into the submucosal space within the lumen of the Eustachian tube can be done exercising caution. However, it should be considered that the material may migrate within the loose tissue planes in the anterolateral wall. Non-FDA approved use of calcium hydroxyapatite paste has been done anecdotally, but the symptom relief is usually temporary, lasting weeks to months only.

Most patients will not require a tympanostomy tube following patulous Eustachian tube repairs as discussed above through either catheter placement or autologous cartilage grafts. If an effusion occurs, it will usually subside within 3 weeks. A tympanostomy tube could be considered for effusions lasting beyond that time.

CONCLUSION

Proper function of the Eustachian tube is essential for aeration, clearance and protection of the middle ear space. Disorders of the Eustachian tube most commonly have identifiable pathology within the cartilaginous portion of the tube. In the majority of cases, these can be managed conservatively. In selected cases, surgical intervention for Eustachian tube disorders is now possible. However, more data from controlled clinical trials are needed to determine the long-term benefit of the procedures. Additionally, basic science investigations are required to better understand the etiology of Eustachian tube dysfunction as well as the impact of the surgical therapies.

REFERENCES

1. Bluestone CD. Introduction. In: Bluestone MB (Ed). Eustachian tube : structure, function, role in otitis media. Ontario: BC Decker; 2005. pp. 1-9.
2. Proctor B. Anatomy of the eustachian tube. Arch Otolaryngol. 1973;97(1):2-8.
3. Sando I, Takahashi H, Matsune S, et al. Localization of function in the eustachian tube: a hypothesis. Ann Otol Rhinol Laryngol. 1994;103(4 Pt 1):311-4.
4. Poe DS, Gopen Q. Endoscopic diagnosis and surgery of eustachian tube dysfunction. In: Gulya AJ, Minor LB, Poe D (Eds). Glasscock-Shambaugh surgery of the ear. Connecticut: People's Medical Publishing House-USA; 2010. pp. 245-253.
5. Hopf J, Linnarz M, Gundlach P, et al. [Microendoscopy of the Eustachian tube and the middle ear. Indications and clinical application]. Laryngorhinootologie. 1991;70(8):391-4.
6. Bluestone CD. Anatomy. In: Bluestone MB (Ed). Eustachian tube: structure, function, role in otitis media. Ontario: BC Decker; 2005. pp. 25-50.
7. Cantekin EI, Doyle WJ, Reichert TJ, et al. Dilation of the eustachian tube by electrical stimulation of the mandibular nerve. Ann Otol Rhinol Laryngol. 1979;88(1 Pt 1):40-51.
8. King PF. The Eustachian tube and its significance in flight. J Laryngol Otol. 1979;93(7):659-78.
9. Sadé J, Ar A. Middle ear and auditory tube: middle ear clearance, gas exchange, and pressure regulation. Otolaryngol Head Neck Surg. 1997;116(4):499-524.

10. Chandrasekhar SS, Mautone AJ. Otitis media: treatment with intranasal aerosolized surfactants. Laryngoscope. 2004;114(3):472-85.

11. Bluestone CD, Klein JO. Otitis media, atelectatis, and eustachian tube dysfunction. In: Bluestone CD, Stool SE, Kenna MA (Eds). Pediatric Otolaryngology, 3rd edition. Philadelphia: WB Saunders; 1996.

12. Mondain M, Vidal D, Bouhanna S, et al. Monitoring eustachian tube opening: preliminary results in normal subjects. Laryngoscope. 1997;107(10):1414-9.

13. Bluestone CD. Physiology. In: Bluestone MB (Ed). Eustachian tube : structure, function, role in otitis media. Ontario: BC Decker; 2005. pp. 51-63.

14. Rockley TJ, Hawke WM. The middle ear as a baroreceptor. Acta Otolaryngol. 1992;112(5):816-23.

15. Honjo I, Hayashi M, Ito S, et al. Pumping and clearance function of the eustachian tube. Am J Otolaryngol. 1985;6(3):241-4.

16. McGuire JF. Surfactant in the middle ear and eustachian tube: a review. Int J Pediatr Otorhinolaryngol. 2002;66(1):1-15.

17. Grace A, Kwok P, Hawke M. Surfactant in middle ear effusions. Otolaryngol Head Neck Surg. 1987;96(4):336-40.

18. Bluestone CD. Epidemiology. In: Bluestone MB (Ed). Eustachian tube : structure, function, role in otitis media. Ontario: BC Decker; 2005. pp. 11-24.

19. Poe DS, Gopen Q. Eustachian tube dysfunction. In: Snow JB, Wackym PA, Ballenger JJ, (Eds). Ballenger's Otorhinolaryngology: Head and Neck Surgery. New York: BC Decker; 2009. pp. 201-8.

20. Poe DS, Pyykkö I, Valtonen H, et al. Analysis of eustachian tube function by video endoscopy. Am J Otol. 2000;21(5):602-7.

21. Takahashi H, Honjo I, Fujita A. Endoscopic findings at the pharyngeal orifice of the eustachian tube in otitis media with effusion. Eur Arch Otorhinolaryngol. 1996;253(1-2):42-4.

22. Edelstein DR, Magnan J, Parisier SC, et al. Microfiberoptic evaluation of the middle ear cavity. Am J Otol. 1994;15(1):50-5.

23. Poe DS, Abou-Halawa A, Abdel-Razek O. Analysis of the dysfunctional eustachian tube by video endoscopy. Otol Neurotol. 2001;22(5):590-5.

24. Kindermann CA, Roithmann R, Lubianca Neto JF. Obstruction of the eustachian tube orifice and pressure changes in the middle ear: are they correlated? Ann Otol Rhinol Laryngol. 2008;117(6):425-9.

25. Elsheikh MN, Mahfouz ME. Up-regulation of MUC5AC and MUC5B mucin genes in nasopharyngeal respiratory mucosa and selective up-regulation of MUC5B in middle ear in pediatric otitis media with effusion. Laryngoscope. 2006;116(3):365-9.

26. Gates GA. Adenoidectomy for otitis media with effusion. Ann Otol Rhinol Laryngol Suppl. 1994;163:54-8.

27. Nguyen LH, Manoukian JJ, Yoskovitch A, et al. Adenoidectomy: selection criteria for surgical cases of otitis media. Laryngoscope. 2004;114(5):863-6.

28. Poe DS, Metson RB, Kujawski O. Laser eustachian tuboplasty: a preliminary report. Laryngoscope. 2003;113(4):583-91.

29. Poe DS, Grimmer JF, Metson R. Laser eustachian tuboplasty: two-year results. Laryngoscope. 2007;117(2):231-7.

30. Kujawski OB, Poe DS. Laser eustachian tuboplasty. Otol Neurotol. 2004;25(1):1-8.
31. Poe DS, Hanna BM. Balloon dilation of the cartilaginous portion of the eustachian tube: initial safety and feasibility analysis in a cadaver model. Am J Otolaryngol. 2011;32(2):115-23.
32. Poe DS, Silvola J, Pyykkö I. Balloon dilation of the cartilaginous eustachian tube. Otolaryngol Head Neck Surg. 2011;144(4):563-9.
33. Poe DS. Diagnosis and management of the patulous eustachian tube. Otol Neurotol. 2007;28(5):668-77.
34. Kikuchi T, Oshima T, Ogura M, et al. Three-dimensional computed tomography imaging in the sitting position for the diagnosis of patulous eustachian tube. Otol Neurotol. 2007;28(2):199-203.
35. Hori Y, Kawase T, Oshima T, Sakamoto S, et al. Objective assessment of autophony in patients with patulous Eustachian tube. Eur Arch Otorhinolaryngol. 2007;264(12):1387-91.
36. Dyer RK Jr, McElveen JT Jr. The patulous eustachian tube: management options. Otolaryngol Head Neck Surg. 1991;105(6):832-5.
37. Doherty JK, Slattery WH 3rd. Autologous fat grafting for the refractory patulous eustachian tube. Otolaryngol Head Neck Surg. 2003;128(1):88-91.

Chapter

7

VESTIBULAR-EVOKED MYOGENIC POTENTIAL TESTING IN OTOLOGY

Yi-Ho Young

ABSTRACT

By stimulating the ear with air-conducted sound (ACS) or bone-conducted vibration (BCV) stimuli, vestibular-evoked myogenic potential (VEMP) can be recorded on the contracted neck muscles, so-called cervical VEMP (cVEMP), and on the extraocular muscles termed ocular VEMP (oVEMP). These two newly developed electrophysiological tests expand the test battery available to clinicians for exploring dynamic otolithic function, and create a potential use for the sacculocollic reflex and vestibulo-ocular reflex (VOR) respectively. Animal models for cVEMP and oVEMP have been established in guinea pigs, which set the stage for evaluating the mechanism of saccular and utricular disorders in humans.

INTRODUCTION

Vestibular end organs comprise three semicircular canals for sensing angular acceleration, and two otolithic organs, the utricle and saccule for perceiving linear acceleration. In 1964, Bickford et al.[1] demonstrated that loud sound stimuli could cause myogenic "inion response" indicative of the activation of vestibular organs. However, only with the revision of the recording setting by Colebatch et al.[2] did VEMP become a practical clinical tool posited to be generated via a disynaptic pathway, beginning in the saccular macula, then via the inferior vestibular nerve, lateral vestibular nucleus, and medial vestibulospinal tract, terminating on the motor neurons of the sternocleidomastoid (SCM) muscle.[3]

Subsequently, Rosengren et al.[4] reported that VEMP can also be recorded from extraocular muscles. This form of VEMP is known as oVEMP, and is elicited via the superior vestibular nerve along the crossed VOR, and recorded on the extraocular muscles.[5] For discrimination, VEMPs recorded from the neck muscles thus, subsequently came to be termed cVEMP.[6] Figure 7.1 illustrates the pathways responsible for the VEMPs.

Recently, both oVEMP and cVEMP tests have been introduced into clinical practice for detecting dynamic otolithic function (Table 7.1). Additionally, both tests are used to differentiate lesions between the superior and inferior vestibular nerves. The cVEMP can be elicited by either ACS stimuli or tapping the head to assess the saccular function,[2,7] whereas oVEMP is induced by ACS or BCV stimuli and is thought to arise from stimulation of the otolithic macula.[8] Notably, these stimulation modes work differently. BCV stimulation applied to the head causes waves to travel around and through the head, resulting in linear accelerations at mastoids.[9] In contrast, ACS stimulation cannot induce acceleration, but moves stapes and then causes endolymph flow.[10]

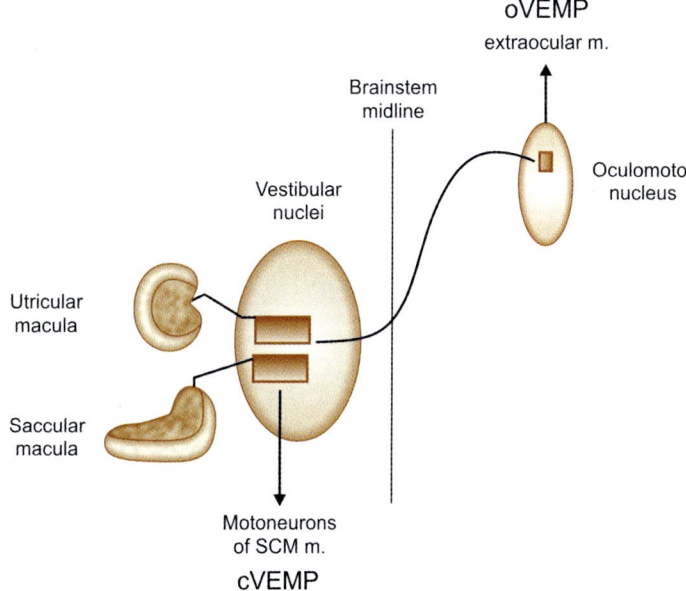

Fig. 7.1: Illustration of the pathways responsible for the cVEMP and oVEMP; (SCM: sternocleidomastoid)

Table 7.1: Characteristics of cervical vs. ocular vestibular-evoked myogenic potentials			
	Optimal stimulation mode	Afferent	Pathway	Recording site
cVEMP	Air-conducted sound	Inferior vestibular nerve	Ipsilateral sacculo-collic reflex	Sternocleido-mastoid muscle
oVEMP	Bone-conducted vibration	Superior vestibular nerve	Crossed vestibulo-ocular reflex	Extraocular muscle

In experimental animals, the ACS mode primarily activates the saccule[11] whereas the BCV mode stimulates primary vestibular neurons of both utricular and saccular macula.[8] Animal models of cVEMP and oVEMP have been established in guinea pigs, which set the stage for evaluating the mechanism of saccular and utricular disorders in humans.[12,13]

MODES OF STIMULATION AND RECORDING

Figure 7.2 illustrates the equipment of VEMP machine (Smart EP 3.95, Intelligent Hearing Systems, Miami, FL, USA) which can be used for recording both oVEMPs and cVEMPs.

▋ Air-Conducted Sound Mode

Constant short-tone burst (95 dBnHL, 500 Hz, ramp = 2 ms, plateau = 2 ms) with rarefaction polarity was given through an insert earphone (Fig. 7.3A). EMG signals were amplified and bandpass filtered between 30 Hz and 3,000 Hz at a repetition rate of 5 Hz. The analysis time for each stimulus was 50 ms, and responses up to 100 stimuli were averaged for each run. Two consecutive runs were averaged to obtain the final response.

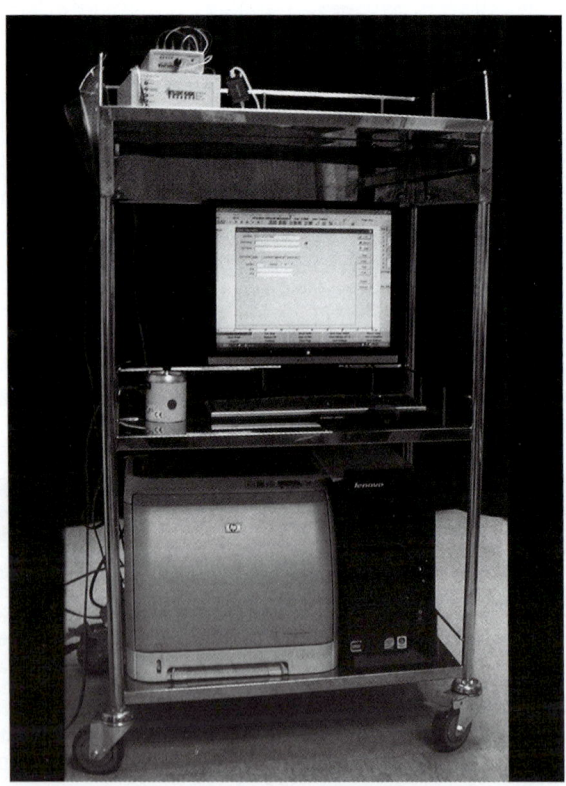

Fig. 7.2: Equipment for recording both cervical and ocular VEMPs

Bone-Conducted Vibration Mode

Halmagyi et al.[7] reported that cVEMPs are typically absent in cases of conductive hearing loss with air-bone gap measuring greater than or equal to 20 dB and hence, the tapping method exhibits higher provocation rate of cVEMPs in patients with conductive hearing loss.[14] However, the pitfall of the tapping method is non-uniform stimulation, leading to this method being replaced by BCV stimulation via a minishaker.

The BCV mode utilized a hand-held electro-mechanical vibrator fitted with a short M4 bolt (2 cm in length) terminated in a bakelite cap (1.6 cm in diameter; V201 shaker, Ling Dynamic Systems, Royston, England). The input signal was one half cycle of 500 Hz sine wave driven by a custom amplifier. The maximal peak driving voltage was approximately 8V, equivalent to 128 dB force level (FL); 0 dBFL = 1 μN. The operator held the vibrator by hand, and supported most of its weight such that the axis of the connected bakelite cap perpendicularly delivered a repeatable tap on the subject's head at Fz (midline forehead at the hairline; Fig. 7.3B). A total of 50 responses were averaged for each run.[15]

Galvanic Vestibular Stimulation Mode

Watson and Colebatch[16] suggested that galvanic stimulation would stimulate the most distal portion of the vestibular nerve while the clicks act at the receptor level.

To deliver galvanic stimuli, electrodes were placed on both sides of the mastoid process (cathode) and the forehead (anode). A direct 5 mA current was applied for 1.0 ms (Fig. 7.3C). Responses to 100 galvanic stimuli were averaged for each run and the results of two duplicate runs were averaged. Since the original waveform contained large electrical artifacts, the cVEMP responses obtained without muscle contraction were subsequently subtracted from those obtained with SCM muscle contraction to provide the final galvanic cVEMPs (Fig. 7.4).[17] Likewise, the oVEMPs obtained with subjects gazing downward were subtracted from those upon gazing upward to provide the final galvanic oVEMPs.[18]

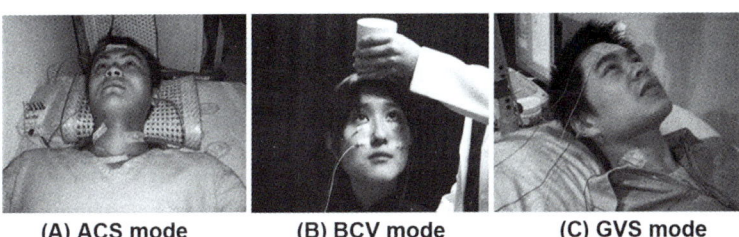

| (A) ACS mode | (B) BCV mode | (C) GVS mode |

Figs 7.3A to C: Three modes for VEMP test; (A) ACS: air-conducted sound; (B) BCV: bone-conducted vibration; (C) GVS: galvanic vestibular stimulation

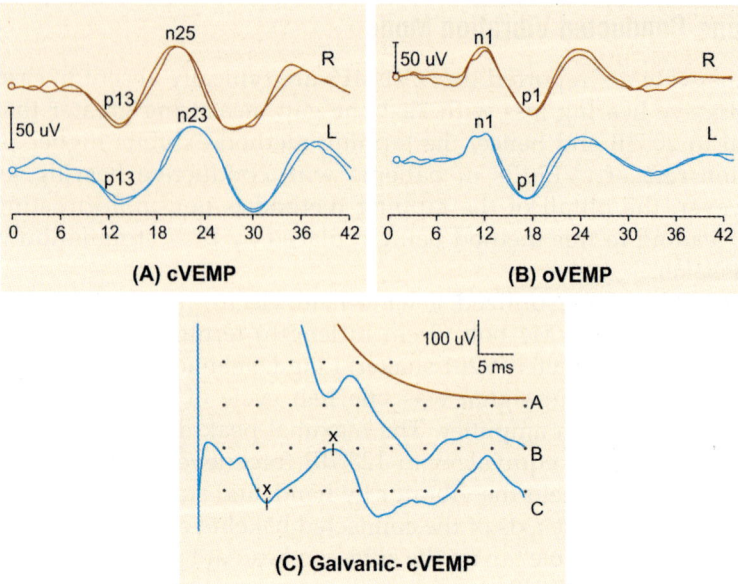

Figs 7.4A to C: Illustration of three kinds of VEMPs. (R: right; L: left; A: without muscle contraction; B: with muscle contraction; C: subtraction wave A from wave B)

Recording of cVEMPs

The subject was in a supine position. Two active electrodes were placed on the upper half of the SCM muscles; one reference electrode was positioned on the suprasternal notch, and a ground electrode was situated on the forehead. The SCM muscles were activated bilaterally by maintaining an elevated head in the supine position during examination (Fig. 7.3A). For those unable to sustain SCM muscle contraction, an alternative was to rotate the head sideways towards one shoulder head down in the yaw plane.[19] To measure background muscle activity, subjects were given feedback on the level of EMG activity in their SCM muscles, and were required to maintain a background muscle activity of at least greater than 50 µV.[20]

The peak latencies of waves p13 and n23, and amplitude p13–n23 were measured (Fig. 7.4). Delayed cVEMP indicates the mean latency of p13 exceeds the value (mean + 2SD), suggesting lesion in the retrolabyrinthine especially the brainstem.[21] Asymmetry ratio is defined as interaural peak-to-peak amplitude difference over the sum of amplitudes of both ears.[22]

Recording of oVEMPs

The subject was in a sitting position for recording oVEMPs. A pair of active electrodes was placed on the face inferior to each eye, around 1 cm below the center of the lower eyelid. The reference electrodes were positioned 1–2 cm below the corresponding active ones. One ground electrode was placed over the sternum. During recording, the subject was instructed to look upwards at a small fixed target greater than 2 m from the eyes, with a vertical visual angle of approximately 30–35° above the horizontal (Fig. 7.3B).[15]

The initial negative-positive biphasic waveform comprised the nI and pI peaks (Fig. 7.4). Consecutive runs were performed to confirm the reproducibility. The latencies of the nI and pI peaks, and the amplitude of nI–pI were then measured.

ANIMAL MODEL

Animal Model of cVEMP

A pair of needle electrodes was placed on both neck extensors, while a reference electrode was placed on the occipital area at the midline. During recording, the animal was fixed with its head elevated and neck hyperextended (Fig. 7.5). Click stimuli were delivered via a short tube inserted into the ear canal. Each animal was evoked by monaural acoustic stimulation with unilateral recording. The stimulation rate was 5 Hz and the analysis time for each response was 24 ms, with 200 responses being averaged for each run.[12] Absence of cVEMPs in guinea pigs treated with gentamicin is likely due to saccular toxicity,[23] and histological analyses have demonstrated that cVEMPs are heavily dependent on type I hair cell activities of the saccular macula.[24]

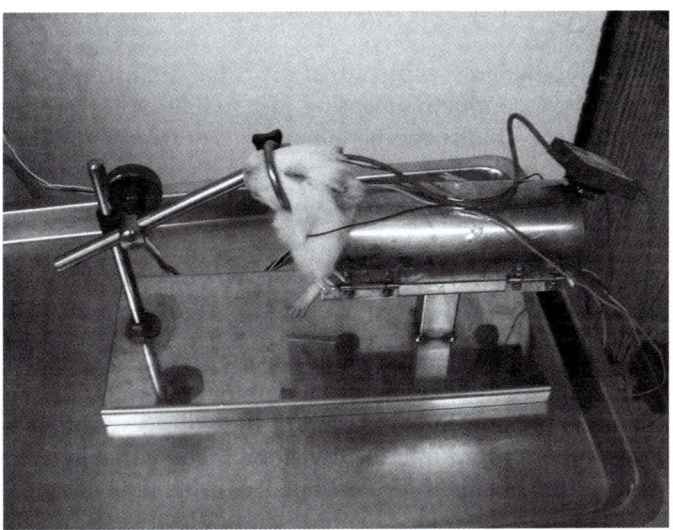

Fig. 7.5: Illustration of the cVEMP test in a guinea pig. The animal was fixed with its head elevated and neck hyperextended. A pair of needle electrodes was placed on both neck extensors while a reference electrode was placed on the occipital area at the midline

Animal Model of oVEMP

Five needle-electrodes were employed. On each side, one active electrode was inserted vertically on the skin 5 mm above the inferior orbital rim in or near the inferior extraocular muscle. Another (reference) electrode was inserted approximately 15 mm below the respective active electrode. The ground electrode was placed on the parietal area at the midline. Single square wave stimuli with duration 0.6 ms were transmitted to a hand-held vibrator. The drive voltage was adjusted and fixed to produce a peak of 128 dBFL (re 1 μN) from the vibrator. The operator held the vibrator by hand, and the device delivered a repeatable tap on the midline frontal bone of a guinea pig. The stimulation rate was 5 Hz; the analysis time for each response was 24 ms, and 30 responses were averaged for each run.[13] The cVEMP test via ACS mode is specific for investigating the saccular disorders, whereas the oVEMP test via BCV mode is preferable for investigating the utricular disorders in humans. The guinea pig model is consistent with the findings of humans.[25,26]

CLINICAL APPLICATION

Conductive Hearing Loss

When the stimulated sound is attenuated by middle ear pathology such as chronic otitis media or otosclerosis, the cVEMP can be expected to be poorly elicited. Subsequent cVEMP test performed through tapping evocation or bone-conducted stimulation should be conducted to elucidate the absent cVEMPs originating from middle ear or inner ear pathology.[14,27]

Additionally, patients with superior canal dehiscence syndrome can have apparent conductive hearing loss, while cVEMP responses to tones remain intact. This phenomenon may result from a mobile window created by the superior canal dehiscence enhancing the transmission of sound pressure through the vestibule required for activation of the sacculus.[6]

Vestibular Neuritis

Halmagyi et al. proposed three clinical patterns of vestibular neuritis, namely superior vestibular nerve inflammation, inferior vestibular nerve inflammation, and inflammation of the entire vestibular ganglion including its superior and inferior divisions.[28] The variable oVEMP and cVEMP test results obtained for vestibular neuritis patients thus are not surprising.[5] Through the caloric, oVEMP and cVEMP tests, this inner ear monitoring system is useful for identifying the affected branches of the vestibular nerve in cases of vestibular neuritis providing insight into the interval for the relief of vertigo.[29]

Meniere's Disease

Since the saccule, next to the cochlea, is the second most frequent site for hydrops formation, cVEMP is supposed to reflect the stage of Meniere's disease. Asymmetry ratio and Meniere's stage are significantly related, indicating that the asymmetry ratio of cVEMPs can be used to assess Meniere's stage.[22] The abnormal rates for hearing, ACS-cVEMP, BCV-oVEMP, and caloric tests in Meniere's ears were 65%, 45%, 25%, and 20%, respectively. This decreasing order of abnormal percentages in the function of the cochlea, saccule, utricle and semicircular canals mimics the declining sequence of hydrops formation in temporal bone studies.[30] Thus, an inner ear test battery may provide further insight into the localization and prevalence of hydrops formation in Meniere's disease.[31]

Most patients (67%) suffering Meniere attacks revealed abnormal cVEMPs, indicating that the saccule participates in the event of Meniere attack, an important idea that stimulates consideration of the mechanism of Meniere attack.[32] Recently, Manzari et al. observed dissociation between cVEMPs and oVEMPs during Meniere's attack.[33]

Posterior Fossa Stroke

The cVEMP test can discriminate lower from upper brainstem lesions. Some patients with lower brainstem stroke but normal VOR can have abnormal cVEMPs, presumably because the VOR ascends via the upper brainstem while the cVEMP descends through the lower brainstem.[34]

The oVEMP test can differentiate between cerebellar and brainstem lesions. Abnormal oVEMPs in patients with cerebellar disorder may indicate adjacent brainstem involvement. Although the cerebellum affects VOR, it does not affect the presence of oVEMPs, probably because caloric nystagmus is a slow response lasting minutes, while oVEMPs are very short responses lasting milliseconds.[35]

Acoustic Neuroma

For cases with acoustic neuroma (AN), caloric test results correlate significantly with oVEMP test results as both tests transit along the superior vestibular nerve.[36] Conversely, no correlation exists between oVEMP and cVEMP test results, primarily because the cVEMP test runs via the inferior vestibular nerve. Thus, the oVEMP test combined with the cVEMP test can determine whether AN originates from the superior or inferior vestibular nerve.[37] The tumor size of AN correlates with cochleovestibular deficits, with the estimated tumor size for those with abnormal caloric or cVEMP responses increased by 1.43 cm or 1.35 cm respectively.[38]

Table 7.2 summarizes the clinical application of cVEMP and oVEMP tests.

Table 7.2: Clinical application of cVEMP and oVEMP testing		
	cVEMP test	*oVEMP test*
Superior canal dehiscence syndrome	Augmented	Augmented
Superior vestibular neuritis	Present	Absent
Inferior vestibular neuritis	Absent	Present
Meniere's disease	Present (55%)	Present (75%)
Upper brainstem stroke	Present	Absent
Lower brainstem stroke	Absent	Present
Superior vestibular schwannoma	Present	Absent
Inferior vestibular schwannoma	Absent	Present

FUTURE

Based on the hypothesis of "efferent specificity" proposed by Curthoys,[8] there is now a lot of evidence that the ACS- and BCV-oVEMPs show dependence on the integrity of the superior division of the vestibular nerve, and the ACS-cVEMPs on the integrity of the inferior division. On the other hand, the behavior of the BCV-cVEMPs show stimulus site and direction dependence that is compatible—at least in part—with some influence of the utricle.[39,40]

REFERENCES

1. Bickford RG, Jacobson JL, Cody DT. Nature of averaged evoked potentials to sound and other stimuli in man. Ann N Y Acad Sci. 1964;112:204-23.
2. Colebatch JG, Halmagyi GM, Skuse NF. Myogenic potentials generated by a click-evoked vestibulocollic reflex. J Neurol Neurosurg Psychiatry. 1994;57(2):190-7.
3. Uchino Y, Sato H, Sasaki M, et al. Sacculocollic reflex arcs in cats. J Neurophysiol. 1997;77(6):3003-12.
4. Rosengren SM, McAngus Todd NP, Colebatch JG. Vestibular-evoked extraocular potentials produced by stimulation with bone-conducted sound. Clin Neurophysiol. 2005;116(8): 1938-48.
5. Iwasaki S, McGarvie LA, Halmagyi GM, et al. Head taps evoke a crossed vestibulo-ocular reflex. Neurology. 2007;68(15):1227-9.
6. Welgampola MS, Myrie OA, Minor LB, et al. Vestibular-evoked myogenic potential thresholds normalize on plugging superior canal dehiscence. Neurology. 2008;70(6):464-72.
7. Halmagyi GM, Yavor RA, Colebatch JG. Tapping the head activates the vestibular system: a new use for the clinical reflex hammer. Neurology. 1995;45(10): 1927-9.
8. Curthoys IS. A critical review of the neurophysiological evidence underlying clinical vestibular testing using sound, vibration and galvanic stimuli. Clin Neurophysiol. 2010;121(2):132-44.
9. Iwasaki S, Smulders YE, Burgess AM, et al. Ocular vestibular evoked myogenic potentials in response to bone-conducted vibration of the midline

forehead at Fz. A new indicator of unilateral otolithic loss. Audiol Neurootol. 2008;13(6):396-404.

10. Curthoys IS, Vulovic V. Vestibular primary afferent responses to sound and vibration in the guinea pig. Exp Brain Res. 2011;210(3-4):347-52.

11. Murofushi T, Curthoys IS, Topple AN, et al. Responses of guinea pig primary vestibular neurons to clicks. Exp Brain Res. 1995;103(1):174-8.

12. Yang TH, Young YH. Click-evoked myogenic potentials recorded on alert guinea pigs. Hear Res. 2005;205(1-2):277-83.

13. Yang TH, Liu SH, Wang SJ, et al. An animal model of ocular vestibular-evoked myogenic potential in guinea pig. Exp Brain Res. 2010;205(2):145-52.

14. Yang TL, Young YH. Vestibular evoked myogenic potentials in otosclerosis patients using air- and bone-conducted tone-burst stimulation. Otol Neurotol. 2007;28(1):1-6.

15. Wang SJ, Weng WJ, Jaw FS, et al. Ocular and cervical vestibular-evoked myogenic potentials: a study to determine whether air- or bone-conducted stimuli are optimal. Ear Hear. 2010;31(2):283-8.

16. Watson SR, Colebatch JG. Vestibulocollic reflexes evoked by short-duration galvanic stimulation in man. J Physiol. 1998;513(Pt 2):587-97.

17. Cheng PW, Yang CS, Huang TW, et al. Optimal stimulation mode for galvanic-evoked myogenic potentials. Ear Hear. 2008;29(6):942-6.

18. Cheng PW, Chen CC, Wang SJ, et al. Acoustic, mechanical and galvanic stimulation modes elicit ocular vestibular-evoked myogenic potentials. Clin Neurophysiol. 2009;120(10):1841-4.

19. Wang CT, Young YH. Comparison of the head elevation versus rotation methods in eliciting vestibular evoked myogenic potentials. Ear Hear. 2006;27(4):376-81.

20. Chang CH, Yang TL, Wang CT, et al. Measuring neck structures in relation to vestibular evoked myogenic potentials. Clin Neurophysiol. 2007;118(5):1105-9.

21. Murofushi T, Shimizu K, Takegoshi H, et al. Diagnostic value of prolonged latencies in the vestibular evoked myogenic potential. Arch Otolaryngol Head Neck Surg. 2001;127(9):1069-72.

22. Young YH, Huang TW, Cheng PW. Assessing the stage of Meniere's disease using vestibular evoked myogenic potentials. Arch Otolaryngol Head Neck Surg. 2003;129(8):815-8.

23. Day AS, Lue JH, Yang TH, et al. Effect of intratympanic application of aminoglycosides on click-evoked myogenic potentials in Guinea pigs. Ear Hear. 2007;28(1):18-25.

24. Lue JH, Day AS, Cheng PW, et al. Vestibular evoked myogenic potentials are heavily dependent on type I hair cell activity of the saccular macula in guinea pigs. Audiol Neurootol. 2009;14(1):59-66.

25. Yang TH, Liu SH, Young YH. Evaluation of guinea pig model for ocular and cervical vestibular-evoked myogenic potentials for vestibular function test. Laryngoscope. 2010;120(9):1910-7.

26. Yang TH, Liu SH, Young YH. A novel inner ear monitoring system for evaluating ototoxicity of gentamicin eardrops in guinea pigs. Laryngoscope. 2010;120(6):1220-6.

27. Yang TL, Young YH. Radiation-induced otitis media—study by a new test, vestibular evoked myogenic potential. Int J Radiat Oncol Biol Phys. 2004;60(1):295-301.
28. Halmagyi GM, Weber KP, Curthoys IS. Vestibular function after acute vestibular neuritis. Restor Neurol Neurosci. 2010;28(1):37-46.
29. Lin CM, Young YH. Identifying the affected branches of vestibular nerve in vestibular neuritis. Acta Otolaryngol. 2011;131(9):921-8.
30. Okuno T, Sando I. Localization, frequency, and severity of endolymphatic hydrops and the pathology of the labyrinthine membrane in Mènière's disease. Ann Otol Rhinol Laryngol. 1987;96(4):438-45.
31. Huang CH, Wang SJ, Young YH. Localization and prevalence of hydrops formation in Mènière's disease using a test battery. Audiol Neurootol. 2011;16(1):41-8.
32. Kuo SW, Yang TH, Young YH. Change of vestibular evoked myogenic potentials after Meniere attack. Ann Otol Rhinol Laryngol. 2005;114(9):717-21.
33. Manzari L, Tedesco AR, Burgess AM, et al. Ocular and cervical vestibular-evoked myogenic potentials to bone conducted vibration in Mènière's disease during quiescence vs during acute attacks. Clin Neurophysiol. 2010;121(7):1092-101.
34. Chen CH, Young YH. Vestibular evoked myogenic potentials in brainstem stroke. Laryngoscope. 2003;113(6):990-3.
35. Su CH, Young YH. Differentiating cerebellar and brainstem lesions with ocular vestibular-evoked myogenic potential test. Eur Arch Otorhinolaryngol. 2011;268(6):923-30.
36. Ushio M, Iwasaki S, Murofushi T, et al. The diagnostic value of vestibular-evoked myogenic potential in patients with vestibular schwannoma. Clin Neurophysiol. 2009;120(6):1149-53.
37. Murofushi T, Matsuzaki M, Mizuno M. Vestibular evoked myogenic potentials in patients with acoustic neuromas. Arch Otolaryngol Head Neck Surg. 1998;124(5):509-12.
38. Day AS, Wang CT, Chen CN, et al. Correlating the cochleovestibular deficits with tumor size of acoustic neuroma. Acta Otolaryngol. 2008;128(7):756-60.
39. Rosengren SM, Todd NP, Colebatch JG. Vestibular evoked myogenic potentials evoked by brief interaural head acceleration: properties and possible origin. J Appl Physiol. 2009;107(3):841-52.
40. Brantberg K, Westin M, Löfqvist L, et al. Vestibular evoked myogenic potentials in response to lateral skull taps are dependent on two different mechanisms. Clin Neurophysiol. 2009;120(5):974-9.

Chapter
8

LARYNGEAL ELECTROMYOGRAPHY

Lucian Sulica

ABSTRACT

Electromyography is uniquely suited to address several questions that arise commonly in evaluation of the larynx. These include diagnosing nerve injury or dysfunction, distinguishing mechanical movement limitation from neurogenic, prognosis of paralysis and paresis, intraoperative monitoring and guidance of therapeutic botulinum toxin injection. Used circumspectly, with an understanding of its limitations as well as its potential, it is an important complement to office laryngoscopy and stroboscopy.

INTRODUCTION

Electromyography (EMG) is a means of studying electrical activity in muscle; as such, is uniquely suited to address several questions that arise commonly during evaluation of the larynx (Table 8.1). As the only diagnostic tool which can reveal laryngeal neurologic activity in vivo, EMG has greatly expanded its clinical scope in the decades since the seminal work of Faaborg-Andersen and Buchtal in the late 1950s.[1,2] Despite widespread acceptance,[3] though, some misunderstandings persist about its capabilities and as a result, its potential as well as some of its limitations may be ignored.

TABLE 8.1: Clinical applications of laryngeal EMG

1.	Diagnosis of laryngeal paralysis or paresis
2.	Differentiation of neurogenic versus mechanical immobility
3.	Prognosis of laryngeal paralysis
4.	Evaluation of synkinesis or other phenomena of misdirected reinnervation
5.	Diagnosis of laryngeal involvement from other neurologic disease, e.g., tremor, myasthenia, spasmodic dysphonia
6.	Intraoperative recurrent laryngeal nerve monitoring
7.	Therapeutic injection of intrinsic laryngeal muscles

PRINCIPLE AND TECHNIQUE

Electromyography measures electrical activity by means of electrodes. All EMG techniques require three electrodes: (i) a ground electrode which helps to reduce interference, (ii) a reference electrode, and (iii) a recording electrode. The last two are designated positive and negative electrodes by convention (which should not imply that they carry a charge), and the visual signal generated by EMG represents the difference in electrical potential between them. Electrodes may be placed on the surface of the body, overlying the muscle in question, or into the muscle itself by means of needles or fine wires. In the larynx, where muscles are small, deep, and close together, precision demands needle examination techniques.

For general clinical use, needle electrodes are available in monopolar and concentric configurations. The monopolar needle is solid and insulated except for its tip, and it is used to measure potential differences between the tip and a reference electrode on the skin. The concentric needle is hollow with a fine wire in its lumen. It records differences between the outer cannula, functioning as a reference electrode, and the inner wire. The area of muscle sampled is smaller than that sampled by a monopolar electrode, and thus data obtained using one type of electrode is not directly comparable to that collected using the other. Concentric needle examination is generally held to yield less "noise" and more precise information about individual motor unit action potentials (MUAPs). These considerations are especially important in the evaluation of myopathy. For clinical assessment of neuropathies, both techniques appear to be of approximately equal utility.

Single-fiber electrodes, generally used for research purposes or to evaluate neuromuscular transmission disorders, have a small recording surface on the shaft of the needle just behind the tip and use the needle cannula as the reference. This yields a tightly-circumscribed recording area that encompasses the electrical activity of one or two muscle fibers, a feature which gives the technique its name.

In the larynx, muscles are small, and activity such as a swallowing or a cough can easily displace a needle out of the muscle to be sampled. The problem of needle movement can be overcome with hooked-wire electrodes. In this technique, a 30-gauge wire is bent and placed through the shaft of a needle that is then placed into muscle. The outside needle is then removed, and recording can be done from the retained wire. Hooked-wire electrodes are particularly important for measurements over a prolonged period of time across different activities, or in simultaneous examination of multiple muscles.[4-6]

At our center, the percutaneous concentric needle technique is the standard. In cases of vocal fold immobility, the examination at the least includes both cricothyroid and thyroarytenoid muscles in order to investigate superior and recurrent laryngeal nerve integrity on each side. These muscles are not necessarily assessed simultaneously. Local anesthesia is used subcutaneously at the puncture site, but not intratracheally, as the procedure is only mildly uncomfortable and the anesthetic agent may produce artifact.[7] The patient is placed in a semirecumbent position with the neck extended. A ground electrode is placed over the sternum, and the reference lead is placed over the cheek.

To reach the cricothyroid muscle, the needle is passed through the skin overlying the cricothyroid membrane just off the anterior midline, and directed along the outside of the cricoid cartilage superiorly and laterally until electrical activity is identified. Placement is checked by confirming recruitment during high-pitched sustained vowel phonation.

The thyroarytenoid muscle complex is reached by passing the needle through the skin and the cricothyroid membrane near the midline (Fig. 8.1). It may then be advanced superiorly and laterally until it pierces the muscle complex and crisp potentials are identified during phonation. The skilled examiner will usually be able to place the needle without entering the lumen of the trachea, and thus avoid stimulating the sensory receptors of the laryngeal mucosa which is unpleasant for the patient. Gentle manipulation of the needle allows sampling at multiple sites within the muscle.

Occasionally, it may be useful to test the posterior cricoarytenoid muscle if there are specific questions about vocal fold abduction. This muscle may be reached in two ways (Figs 8.2A and B). Most commonly, the larynx is rotated away from the investigator and the posterior edge of the thyroid lamina is palpated with the thumb of the non-injecting hand. The needle is inserted along the lower half of the posterior edge of the thyroid cartilage, traversing the inferior constrictor, and advanced until it stops against the cricoid. The needle is then pulled back slightly and the patient is asked

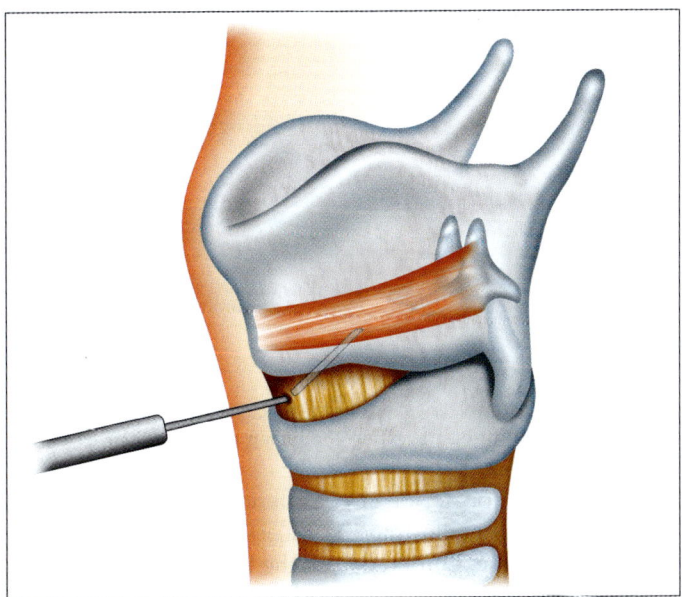

Fig. 8.1: The thyroarytenoid muscle is reached via percutaneous puncture of the cricothyroid membrane just off the midline

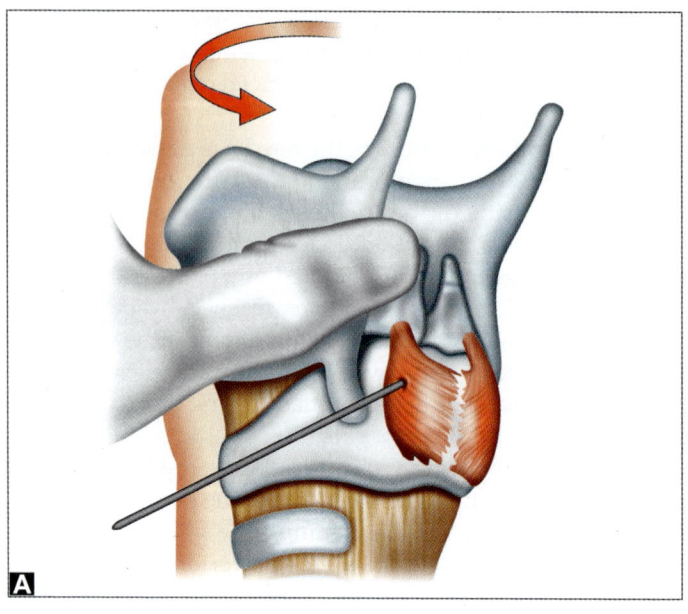

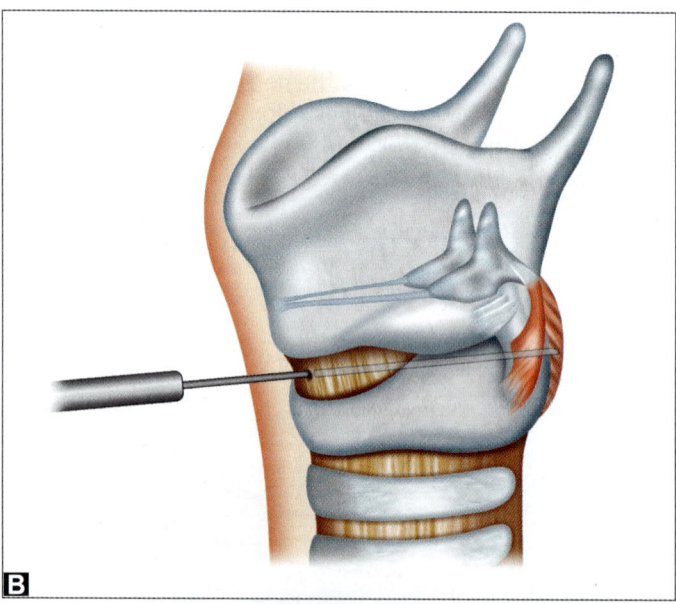

Figs 8.2A and B: The posterior cricoarytenoid muscle may be approached laterally by: (A) rotating the larynx; (B) or by traversing the lumen of the trachea

to sniff to activate the posterior cricoarytenoid in order to check placement. Alternately, the needle may be inserted through the cricothyroid membrane in the midline, guided across the lumen of the subglottic space (again identified by the characteristic airway "buzz"), and through the posterior lamina of the cricoid cartilage to one side or the other of midline.[8] The electrical signal on the far side of the cartilage represents posterior cricoarytenoid muscle. This approach is most useful in the younger patient whose cartilage has not undergone extensive calcification.

It is also possible to test lateral cricoarytenoid and interarytenoid muscles, but in cases of vocal fold immobility, these rarely yield additional information.

Correct needle placement is obviously essential for an accurate examination. Validating maneuvers, detailed above for each muscle, confirm that the needle lies in the appropriate muscle. In cases of vocal fold paresis or paralysis, however, diminished or absent electrical activity can render these unhelpful, and synkinesis can create misleading signals. To minimize the possibility of error in such situations, the examiner must probe extensively in the area of the target muscle with the needle electrode before accepting any ambiguous signal as valid. Extensive sampling is important in any EMG examination, but it is especially so in vocal fold paralysis.

PHYSIOLOGY AND PATHOLOGY

An EMG yields a visual signal of electrical activity in muscle, either via oscilloscope or a digital trace in most recent systems. The electrical signal is coupled to a speaker and produces audible output. Different types of potentials have specific acoustic signals that are readily identifiable to the experienced examiner, and the audible signal is an important part of the EMG examination. There are four characteristics of electrical activity in muscle: (i) morphology (waveform), (ii) amplitude, (iii) duration, and (iv) frequency. Acoustically, amplitude of an electric potential generally corresponds to loudness, and duration and rise time correspond to pitch.[9]

Electrical activity in muscle is the result of changes in the strong negative resting potential of the muscle cell that in turn result from other electrical or chemical factors. Normally, depolarization is the result of neural stimulation via acetylcholine to the motor endplates of a muscle fiber. All muscle fibers innervated by a given motoneuron form a motor unit. The electrical summation of all their potentials forms a motor unit action potential—(MUAP, also called a muscle action potential); the basic electrophysiologic component of striated muscle.

Electrical activity seen during the EMG examination may be divided into three types depending on the circumstance in which it appears: (i) insertional, (ii) spontaneous, and (iii) voluntary. Upon insertion, irritation by the needle itself usually causes a few individual fibers to depolarize which yields a short-lived burst of spike discharges. Any such activity persisting more than 400 milliseconds after needle movement is considered prolonged and a sign of pathologic muscle membrane instability.

Spontaneous activity in normal muscle at complete rest is minimal, usually limited to subthreshold non-propagated depolarizations at the endplate that produce very brief, irregular, and low-amplitude electrical signals. They make a characteristic hissing or white-noise type sound, and have an initial negative deflection (by convention, an upward deflection of the trace is negative). This distinguishes them from fibrillation potentials, which have an initial positive deflection and are pathologic. In laryngeal muscles, measurement of spontaneous activity is difficult because complete silence is rarely achieved. Unlike limb muscles, which can be completely relaxed, laryngeal muscles are continuously active in respiration.[10] In the larynx, electrical silence in itself suggests pathology.

Voluntary activity is examined by having the patient contract the muscle in which the electrode rests. In the larynx, this consists of an action appropriate for the muscle in question: (i) voicing or a Valsalva maneuver for the thyroarytenoid, (ii) sniffing for the posterior cricoarytenoid, or (iii) high-pitched phonation for the cricothyroid. Contraction results in the appearance of the MUAP. Each MUAP has its own characteristics and is thus identifiable throughout the examination. The normal MUAP is usually bi- or triphasic in shape, phases counted by noting the number of times the potential crosses the baseline and adding one. Greater than four phases is considered abnormal and termed "polyphasic." This reflects a loss of organization and synchrony among the endplates that make up a motor unit, and is a hallmark of reinnervation.

Duration and amplitude of a normal MUAP depend on the muscle studied and in general, are proportional to the muscle size. Quantitative characterizations of human laryngeal MUAPs have been made by Faaborg-Andersen, Buchtal and others.[1,2,10,11] Amplitude is also affected by the distance of the needle from the muscle fibers, and an examiner may check this distance by measuring the rise time of a MUAP — the time between the onset of the first negative deflection and its peak. For observations to be valid, the rise time should be less than 200 microseconds.[6,12] In practice, the examiner is more likely to make a qualitative judgment based on the waveform and the crispness of the "pop" noise made by MUAPs during contraction.

Frequency of MUAPs is determined by the force of contraction. Besides increasing the frequency of discharge from an individual motor unit, increasing contraction will result in the activation of adjacent motor units. This phenomenon is known as recruitment. At a high level of contraction, multiple motor units will be firing at high frequency, making it impossible to distinguish the features of any single MUAP either visually or acoustically. This is known as a full interference pattern, because the baseline becomes completely obscured, and is normally achieved at about 30% of maximum isometric contraction.[9] Inability to attain this suggests pathology.

Like normal findings, abnormalities in EMG may also be classified as insertional, spontaneous and voluntary. Prolonged insertional activity is suggestive of muscle membrane instability, as in polymyositis and other myopathies. Spontaneous firing of individual muscle fibers at rest suggests denervation or myopathy. This may appear either as spike fibrillations or positive sharp waves, both of which carry similar significance. Both are marked by an initial positive (downward) deflection and fire with a regular periodicity. High-frequency runs of spike fibrillations or positive sharp waves, usually triggered by needle movement, that wax and wane in amplitude and frequency are called myotonic discharges, and occur in a variety of intrinsic disorders of muscle such as myositis, myotonic dystrophy, glycogen storage diseases, hyperparathyroidism and so forth. Fasciculation potentials are the result of spontaneous discharge of all or part of an entire motor unit, which they resemble, except that they occur singly rather than in trains, and at rest rather than with movement. They are a typical finding in amyotrophic lateral sclerosis, but may appear in any condition of chronic denervation. MUAPs that occur in repetitive runs, but are generally constant in duration and amplitude, are termed myokymia. These occur in the presence of a number of factors that alter the biochemical environment of the nerve, such as demyelination, edema, or toxins.

Voluntary contraction may yield abnormal MUAPs. In general, large amplitude, long-duration MUAPs suggest neurogenic disease whereas small, short-duration MUAPs suggest myopathy. There are several exceptions to this, like early reinnervation potentials and potentials of chronic severe myopathy.

As is evident, the spectrum of abnormal findings in EMG is broad and reflects the disordered physiology of the disease under investigation. Most findings can occur in a variety of conditions; none is pathognomonic. Whether they are significant depends on the frequency with which they occur and their clinical context. For this reason, there are few lists of strict diagnostic criteria for specific diseases in the EMG literature. Although EMG yields measurable data, it is in essence qualitative—a fact that may not be immediately evident to the physician unfamiliar with the test.

CLINICAL APPLICATIONS

Laryngeal EMG is useful in separating the mechanical from neurogenic causes of vocal fold immobility.[13-18] Cricoarytenoid arthritis, arytenoid dislocation and posterior glottic scarring generally yield normal EMGs, although Yin and colleagues have cautioned that patterns of myopathy or neuropathy may occur in longstanding arytenoid dislocation, and have emphasized the importance of adequate muscle sampling.[19] Neurogenic vocal fold immobility, on the other hand, can show a wide variety of abnormal activity, as reviewed above. EMG has been found to be more reliable than computed tomography scanning for this purpose,[16] and offers a safer and less costly alternative to operative laryngoscopy.

In cases of denervation, comparison of findings in the cricothyroid muscle, innervated by the superior laryngeal nerve, and the thyroarytenoid muscle can indicate the site of the lesion.[13,20] Abnormal findings in both suggest an injury proximal to the branching of the superior laryngeal nerve from the main trunk of the vagus, whereas abnormalities isolated to the thyroarytenoid direct investigation into the lower neck and mediastinum.

More widespread use of laryngeal EMG has created a new appreciation for the entity of laryngeal paresis, including superior laryngeal nerve palsy.[21-25] Both conditions may cause subtle glottic insufficiency, and EMG can help between that caused by these neurologic factors and from glottic insufficiency caused by other factors such as atrophy, sulcus vocalis and postsurgical scarring.

Laryngeal EMG is an essential tool in the investigation of disorders of vocal fold mobility associated with a variety of systemic neurologic conditions. These include hereditary sensory and motor neuropathies,[26,27] postpolio syndrome,[28,29] and the Parkinson-plus syndromes.[30,31] Laryngeal EMG can be used to distinguish upper from lower motor neuron lesions.[32] With multiple muscle samples, bulbar palsy (anterior horn cell disease), primary lateral sclerosis, Arnold-Chiari malformation, or syringomyelia can be identified.[33] Repetitive firing of laryngeal MUAPs in synchrony with those of palatal and pharyngeal muscles can help diagnose myoclonus. Regular 4–8 Hz repetitive activation can help identify and distinguish essential tremor from other movement disorders (Fig. 8.3). Once again, the evaluation of extralaryngeal muscles may be helpful. Decrease in amplitude and numbers of MUAPs with repetitive function or repetitive stimulation may suggest myasthenia gravis.

Electromyography can be used for intraoperative monitoring of the recurrent laryngeal nerve during surgeries that place this structure at risk. Hooked-wire electrodes may be placed into the thyroarytenoid muscle complex endoscopically, or surface electrodes can be placed in the postcricoid area or attached to the endotracheal tube at the level of the glottis to provide warning when the recurrent nerve is stimulated.[33-35] Surgeons should be aware that anesthetic agents including paralytics and local anesthetics, inhibit electrical activity in muscle, and can compromise the utility of the EMG in this context.

Electromyography has proved to be the ideal method of guiding therapeutic injection of botulinum toxin. A hollow needle is used as a monopolar electrode to inject toxin where the electrical signal is crisp, loud and high-pitched—indicating that motor end plates and therefore, nerve

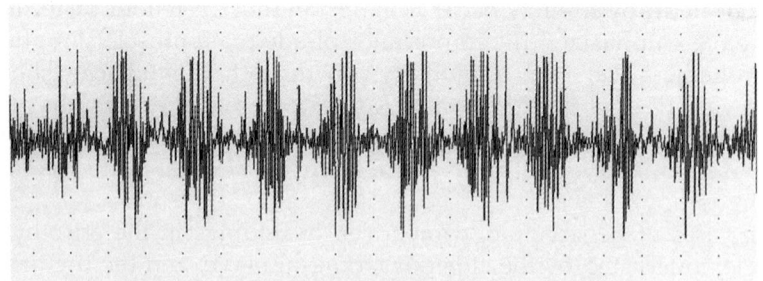

Fig. 8.3: This EMG recording of the thyroarytenoid muscle of a patient with essential voice tremor during sustained /i/ phonation clearly reveals the rhythmic waxing and waning activation of the muscle typical of tremor, at a rate of 5 Hz in this case. Normally, muscle activation should be continuous during this activity (each horizontal division = 100 msec; each vertical division = 100 µVolts)

terminals are nearby. Because these are the sites of action of botulinum toxin, laryngeal EMG serves to minimize the dose needed for therapeutic effect and increases the accuracy of placement, thereby reducing diffusion and unintended effects.

Finally, surface EMG is an evolving tool in biofeedback therapy of both speech and swallowing disorders.[36]

EMG FOR PROGNOSIS IN VOCAL FOLD PARALYSIS

Of all clinical uses for laryngeal EMG, prognostication in cases of vocal fold paralysis is undoubtedly the most frequently discussed and debated. Critics claim that EMG criteria for return of function are "subjective" and that, as a result, findings cannot be used to inform clinical decision-making. The highly variable rates of correct prediction of return of vocal fold motion reported in the literature[37-43] have only added to the confusion about the capabilities of EMG in this role.

Criteria for assignment of prognosis vary but generally, preservation of normal unit waveforms, activation of motor units during appropriate voluntary tasks, and preservation of a brisk degree of recruitment have been indicative of good prognosis. The presence of spontaneous activity and the absence of normal motor unit waveforms and recruitment are signs of poor prognosis. Time is a highly relevant factor; the earlier favorable signs are identified, the more likely it is that spontaneous recovery will take place, although extremely early EMG assessment may exaggerate the degree of injury.[40,44]

It is true that certain aspects of laryngeal EMG are subjective, particularly judgments regarding subtle impairment of recruitment with voluntary activity sometimes used to identify paresis. However, most electromyographic findings such as fibrillations, positive sharp waves, and polyphasic motor unit potentials are clear both in appearance and significance. EMG might more properly be described as qualitative rather than subjective; findings require interpretation by a knowledgeable physician. In this regard, it does not differ from most other common diagnostic procedures in otolaryngology like laryngoscopy and stroboscopy for example, except inasmuch as training and familiarity allows otolaryngologists to use these studies routinely and comfortably in daily practice. Strictly speaking, in fact, EMG exceeds both laryngoscopy and stroboscopy in its ability to definitively—and objectively—diagnose vocal fold paralysis as opposed to immobility.

The practical clinical difficulty has been that laryngeal EMG appears to be unreliable in predicting recovery. That is, the appearance of unambiguous signs of reinnervation does not always lead to return of function. In fact, both animal and human studies have shown that a paralyzed vocal fold is not always a denervated fold.[45-47] In many—perhaps most—cases, vocal fold muscles are reinnervated, but that reinnervation is often dysfunctional. This is not limited to misdirected adductor and abductor innervation—the traditional notion of "synkinesis"—but appears to involve changes in neural organization both peripherally and centrally.[48] The laryngeal neuromotor system is complex and highly specialized; this sophistication probably leaves many ways in which reinnervation may miscarry. Laryngeal EMG is not able to reveal all of these subtleties, so that electromyographic evidence of nerve regrowth is not synonymous with vocal fold motion.

To date, investigators have focused their attention on laryngeal EMG as a positive predictor, and may have overlooked its power as a predictor of failure of reinnervation. In the latter context, there are no physiologic ambiguities, and electromyographic findings may reflect glottic function more reliably. Characteristic electrical features of denervation—fibrillations and other types of spontaneous activity—leave little to be misinterpreted, and strongly suggest that: (i) the initial injury is profound and (ii) there is little reinnervation of any sort. The more time that elapses from injury, the more definitive the finding becomes. Although potentially misleading very early in the course of the paralysis,[40] spontaneous activity with absent or scant voluntary motor unit activation appears to be a reasonably accurate predictor of non-recovery significantly earlier than 6 months.[39,41-43,49] A review of comparable studies of electromyographic assessment of vocal fold paralysis of less than 6 months duration reveals that accurate prediction of recovery does not exceed 80%, and has been reported to be as low as 13% when strict criteria for recovery of full range of motion are used. However, when determination of poor prognosis rests on the presence of spontaneous activity and absence (or scant presence) of motor units, laryngeal EMG is a more accurate predictor of the failure of recovery (75–100%).[50]

This is clinically useful information which can be used to identify patients for early definitive intervention, eliminating a several-month wait, or eliminating the need for a temporary intervention when a definitive one is likely to be ultimately necessary. At our centers, failure of reinnervation as demonstrated by EMG has been a reliable finding as early as 3 months. Appropriately designed studies are needed to refine this observation further, and determine more precisely how early such findings may be deemed to be significant.

FURTHER QUESTIONS

One problem in managing vocal fold paralysis with the aid of EMG lies in the fact that EMG as studied to date does not directly answer the central clinical question: will the patient's voice improve substantially without surgical intervention? Vocal fold motion rather than voice function has uniformly been used as a measure of outcome. Yet, it is clear in some cases that adequate glottic closure for phonation returns even in the absence of vocal fold motion. Retrospective studies suggest that this is due to maintenance or restoration of muscle bulk and tone in the immobile vocal fold by dysfunctional reinnervation.[45,51] Such reinnervation is an observable phenomenon in EMG, and a prospective study to assess the practical significance of this finding would be useful.

In most peripheral neuropathies, electrodiagnosis is a two-part undertaking comprising of both EMG and nerve-conduction studies. In the larynx, nerve-conduction techniques are not in routine clinical use, perhaps because of technical challenges to nerve stimulation imposed by anatomy. The accessible portion of the superior laryngeal nerve is relatively short and lies near other nerves that can create confusing results, and the recurrent nerve is deep and difficult to reach reliably outside of the operating room. Comparison of laryngeal nerve anatomy with that of the facial nerve, routinely assessed by means of nerve conduction testing, reveals the obvious anatomic difficulties presented by the former. Efforts at a noninvasive method of stimulation have included use of surface electrodes, a vibratory stimulator[52] and magnetic stimulation.[53] Isolated reports of needle stimulation techniques have appeared in the literature,[38,54] but the techniques have not been widely adopted despite promising results especially with respect to prognosis. The absence of nerve conduction testing leaves important limitations in electrodiagnosis of laryngeal disorders.

Traditionally, vocal fold paralysis has been regarded as an all-or-none phenomenon largely because the field has lacked the means to distinguish more subtle abnormalities. However, it stands to reason that laryngeal neuropathy should be a graded phenomenon like most peripheral neuropathy. Once again, otolaryngologists may find a useful analogy in the clinical spectrum of facial nerve dysfunction. EMG has made the identification of laryngeal nerve paresis or weakness possible.[23,24] Despite general acceptance of the clinical entity of paresis, which can involve both superior and recurrent nerves, its significance remains a matter of debate. Points of disagreement include incidence, etiology, clinical course, endoscopic appearance—if indeed there are consistent findings—and effect upon voice and other laryngeal functions. EMG as currently used may permit diagnosis but as a qualitative technique, it is poorly suited to investigating these more subtle issues. Their resolution awaits the development and application of quantitative electrodiagnostic techniques.

As experience with laryngeal EMG accumulates, it becomes more evident that our understanding of laryngeal neurophysiology is incomplete. Recent work has raised the possibility of greater variation among individuals than was previously thought, physiologically distinct compartments within laryngeal muscles, and variations in motor unit firing patterns.[55-58] Because a normal EMG signal is a composite of multiple superimposed MUAPs, individual motor units are difficult to distinguish during voluntary activity. Investigative techniques which are able to untangle the composite signal like computer-assisted vector EMG,[59] thus revealing the behavior of individual motor units as well as relations among them, are necessary to expand knowledge in this field, and refine the use of clinical EMG.

CONCLUSION

Laryngeal EMG has become a useful tool for the otolaryngologist in the 4 decades since the pioneering work of Faaborg-Anderson and Buchtal. It is able to distinguish between mechanical limitation and denervation in an immobile vocal fold. In the paralyzed vocal fold, it can guide workup by pointing to the site of lesion. And in the hands of a circumspect clinician, it can provide clinically valuable information regarding prognosis. EMG is also an integral part of the investigation of neurologic disorders affecting the larynx. Intraoperatively, it can be used to monitor the recurrent laryngeal nerves during procedures in which they are at risk. EMG is the standard method of directing therapeutic injection of botulinum toxin, and has been used in biofeedback therapy for speech and swallowing disorders.

The most important benefit of clinical use of laryngeal EMG may be that it has catalyzed and broadened interest in laryngeal neurophysiology in the same way that stroboscopy has focused attention on the structure and function of the vocal fold lamina propria. The continuing refinement of electrodiagnostic approaches to the larynx that has resulted including quantitative, single-fiber and vector laryngeal EMG, and evolving methods of nerve-conduction testing, will continue to yield important insights into mechanisms of neural control that are likely to drive developments in the treatment of vocal fold paralysis in the future.

REFERENCES

1. Faaborg-Andersen K. Electromyographic investigation of intrinsic laryngeal muscles in humans. Acta Physiol. 1957;41(Suppl 140):1-149.
2. BUCHTAL F. Electromyography of intrinsic laryngeal muscles. Q J Exp Physiol Cogn Med Sci. 1959;44(2):137-48.
3. Halum SL, Patel N, Smith TL, et al. Laryngeal electromyography for adult unilateral vocal fold immobility: a survey of the American Broncho-Esophagological Association. Ann Otol Rhinol Laryngol. 2005;114(6):425-8.
4. Hirano M, Ohala J. Use of hooked-wire electrodes for electromyography of the intrinsic laryngeal muscles. J Speech Hearing Res. 1969;12(2):362-73.
5. Lovelace RE, Blitzer A, Ludlow C. Clinical laryngeal electromyography. In: Blitzer A, Brin MF, Sasaki CT, Fahn S, Harris K (Eds). Neurological Disorders of the Larynx. New York: Thieme Medical Publishers; 1992. pp. 66-82.
6. Hillel AD. The study of laryngeal muscle activity in normal human subjects and in patients with laryngeal dystonia using multiple fine-wire electromyography. Laryngoscope. 2001;111(Pt 2 Suppl 97):1-47.
7. Chitkara A, Meyer T, Cultrara A, et al. Dose response of topical anesthetic on laryngeal neuromuscular electrical transmission. Ann Otol Rhinol Laryngol. 2005;114(11):819-21.
8. Mu LC, Yang SL. A new method of needle-electrode placement in the posterior cricoarytenoid muscle for electromyography. Laryngoscope. 1990;100(10 Pt 1):1127-31.
9. Campbell WW. Needle electrode examination. In: Campbell WW (Ed). Essentials of Electrodiagnostic Medicine. Maryland: Williams & Wilkins; 1999: pp. 93-116.

10. Knutsson E, Mårtensson A, Mårtensson B. The normal electromyogram in human vocal muscles. Acta Otolaryngol. 1969;68(6):526-36.
11. FAABORG-ANDERSEN K, BUCHTAL F. Action potentials from internal laryngeal muscles during phonation. Nature. 1956;177(4503):340-1.
12. Aminoff MJ. Clinical electromyography. In: Aminoff MJ (Ed). Electrodiagnosis in Clinical Medicine, 4th edition. Philadelphia: Churchill Livingstone; 1999. pp. 2223-52.
13. Koufman JA, Postma GN, Whang CS, et al. Diagnostic laryngeal electromyography: The Wake Forest experience 1995-1999. Otolaryngol Head Neck Surg. 2001;124(6):603-6.
14. Woo P, Arandia H. Intraoperative laryngeal electromyographic assessment of patients with immobile vocal fold. Ann Otol Rhinol Laryngol. 1992:101(10):799-806.
15. Rontal E, Rontal M, Silverman B, et al. The clinical differentiation between vocal cord paralysis and vocal cord fixation using electromyography. Laryngoscope. 1993;103(2):133-7.
16. Sataloff RT, Bough ID Jr, Spiegel JR. Arytenoid dislocation: diagnosis and treatment. Laryngoscope. 1994;104(11 Pt 1):1353-61.
17. Hoffman HT, Brunberg JA, Winter P, et al. Arytenoid subluxation: diagnosis and treatment. Ann Otol Rhinol Laryngol. 1991;100(1):1-9.
18. Miller RH, Rosenfield DB. The role of electromyography in clinical laryngology. Otolaryngol Head Neck Surg. 1984;92(3):287-91.
19. Yin SS, Qiu WW, Stucker FJ. Value of electromyography in differential diagnosis of laryngeal joint injuries after intubation. Ann Otol Rhinol Laryngol. 1996;105(6):446-51.
20. Quiney RE. Laryngeal electromyography: a useful technique for the investigation of vocal cord palsy. Clin Otolaryngol Allied Sci. 1989;14(4):305-16.
21. Simpson DM, Sternman D, Graves-Wright J, et al. Vocal cord paralysis: clinical and electrophysiologic features. Muscle Nerve. 1993;16(9):952-7.
22. Dursun G, Sataloff RT, Spiegel JR, et al. Superior laryngeal nerve paresis and paralysis. J Voice. 1996;10(2):206-11.
23. Dray TG, Robinson LR, Hillel AD. Idiopathic bilateral vocal fold weakness. Laryngoscope. 1999;109(6):995-1002.
24. Koufman JA, Postma GN, Cummins MM, et al. Vocal fold paresis. Otolaryngol Head Neck Surg. 2000;122(4):537-41.
25. Tanaka S, Hirano M, Chijiwa K. Some aspects of vocal fold bowing. Ann Otol Rhinol Laryngol. 1994;103(5 Pt 1):357-62.
26. Dray TG, Robinson LR, Hillel AD. Laryngeal electromyographic findings in Charcot-Marie-Tooth disease type II. Arch Neurol. 1999;56(7):863-5.
27. Sulica L, Blitzer A, Lovelace RE, et al. Vocal fold paresis of Charcot-Marie-Tooth disease. Ann Otol Rhinol Laryngol. 2001;110(11):1072-6.
28. Driscoll BP, Gracco C, Coehlo C, et al. Laryngeal function in postpolio patients. Laryngoscope. 1995;105(1):35-41.
29. Robinson LR, Hillel AD, Waugh PF. New laryngeal muscle weakness in postpolio syndrome. Laryngoscope. 1998;108(5):732-4.
30. Guindi GM, Bannister R, Gibson WP, et al. Laryngeal electromyography in multiple system atrophy with autonomic failure. J Neurol Neurosurg Psychiatry. 1981;44(1):49-53.

31. Isozaki E, Osanai R, Horiguchi S, et al. Laryngeal electromyography with separated surface electrodes in patients with mulitple system atrophy presenting with vocal cord paralysis. J Neurol. 1994;241(9):551-6.

32. Palmer JB, Holloway AM, Tanaka E. Detecting lower motor neuron dysfunction of the pharynx and larynx with electromyography. Arch Phys Med Rehabil. 1991;72(3):214-8.

33. Lovelace RE, Blitzer A, Ludlow C. Clinical laryngeal electromyography. In: Blitzer A, Brin MF, Sasaki CT, Fahn S, Harris K (Eds). Neurological Disorders of the Larynx. New York: Thieme Medical Publishers; 1992. pp. 66-82.

34. Khan A, Pearlman RC, Bianchi DA, et al. Experience with two types of electromyography monitoring electrodes during thyroid surgery. Am J Otolaryngol. 1997;18(2):99-102.

35. Lipton RJ, McCaffrey TV, Litchy WJ. Intraoperative electrophysiologic monitoring of laryngeal muscle during thyroid surgery. Laryngoscope. 1988;98(12):1292-6.

36. Hillel AD, Robinson LR, Waugh P. Laryngeal electromyography for the diagnosis and management of swallowing disorders. Otolaryngol Head Neck Surg. 1997;116(3):344-8.

37. Hirano M, Nozoe I, Shin T, et al. Electromyography for laryngeal paralysis. In: Hirano M, Kirchner JA, Bless DM (Eds). Neurolaryngology: Recent Advances. California: Singular Publishing; 1991. pp. 232-48.

38. Thumfart W. Endoscopic electromyography and neurography. In: Samii M, Janetta PJ (Eds). The Cranial Nerves. Berlin: Springer-Verlag; 1981. pp. 597-605.

39. Parnes SM, Satya-Murti S. Predictive value of laryngeal electromyography in patients with vocal cord paralysis of neurogenic origin. Laryngoscope. 1985;95(11):1323-6.

40. Gupta SR, Bastian RW. Use of laryngeal electromyography in prediction of recovery after vocal cord paralysis. Muscle Nerve. 1993;16(9):977-8.

41. Min YB, Finnegan EM, Hoffman HT, et al. A preliminary study of the prognostic role of electromyography in laryngeal paralysis. Otolaryngol Head Neck Surg. 1994;111(6):770-5.

42. Sittel C, Stennert E, Thumfart WF, et al. Prognostic value of laryngeal electromyography in vocal fold paralysis. Arch Otolaryngol Head Neck Surg. 2001;127(2):155-60.

43. Munin MC, Rosen CA, Zullo T. Utility of laryngeal electromyography in predicting recovery after vocal fold paralysis. Arch Phys Med Rehabil. 2003;84(8):1150-3.

44. Munin MC, Murry T, Rosen CA. Laryngeal electromyography: diagnostic and prognostic applications. Otolaryngol Clin North Am. 2000;33(4):759-70.

45. Blitzer A, Jahn AF, Keidar A. Semon's law revisited: an electromyographic analysis of laryngeal synkinesis. Ann Otol Rhinol Laryngol. 1996;105(10):764-9.

46. Crumley RL, McCabe BF. Regeneration of the recurrent laryngeal nerve. Otolaryngol Head Neck Surg. 1982;90(4):442-7.

47. Zealear DL, Hamdan AL, Rainey CL. The effects of denervation on posterior cricoarytenoid muscle physiology and histochemistry. Ann Otol Rhinol Laryngol. 1994;103(10):780-8.

48. Zealear Dl, Billante CR. Synkinesis and dysfunctional reinnervation of the larynx. In: Sulica L, Blitzer A (Eds). Vocal Fold Paralysis. Heidelberg: Springer; 2006. pp. 17-32.

49. Mostafa BE, Gadallah NA, Nassar NM, et al. The role of laryngeal electromyography in vocal fold immobility. ORL J Otorhinolaryngol Relat Spec. 2004;66(1):5-10.

50. Rickert S, Childs L, Carey BT, et al. Laryngeal electromyography for prognosis of vocal fold palsy: a meta-analysis. Laryngoscope. In press.

51. Crumley RL. Laryngeal synkinesis revisited. Ann Otol Rhinol Laryngol. 2000;109(4):365-71.

52. Yin SS, Qiu WW, Stucker FJ, et al. Laryngeal evoked brainstem responses in humans: a preliminary study. Laryngoscope. 1997;107(9):1261-6.

53. Ludlow CL, Yeh J, Cohen LG, et al. Limitations of electromyography and magnetic stimulation for assessing laryngeal muscle control. Ann Otol Rhinol Laryngol. 1994;103(1):16-27.

54. Satoh I. Evoked electromyographic test applied for recurrent laryngeal nerve paralysis. Laryngoscope. 1978;88(12):2022-31.

55. Sanders I, Rai S, Han Y, et al. Human vocalis contains distinct superior and inferior subcompartments: possible candidates for the two masses of vocal fold vibration. Ann Otol Rhinol Laryngol. 1998;107(10 Pt 1):826-33.

56. Sanders I, Wu BL, Mu L, et al. The innervation of the human larynx. Arch Otolaryngol Head Neck Surg. 1993;119(9):934-9.

57. Sanders I, Wu BL, Mu L, et al. The innervation of the human posterior cricoarytenoid muscle: evidence for at least two neuromuscular compartments. Laryngoscope. 1994;104(7):880-4.

58. Maranillo E, León X, Ibañez M, et al. Variability of nerve supply patterns of the human posterior cricoarytenoid muscle. Laryngoscope. 2003;113(4):602-6.

59. Roark RM, Li JC, Schaefer SD, et al. Multiple motor unit recordings of laryngeal muscles: the technique of vector laryngeal electromyography. Laryngoscope. 2002;112(12):2196-203.

Chapter

9

CURRENT TECHNIQUES IN SLEEP-DISORDERED BREATHING SURGERY

Rodolfo Lugo Saldaña

ABSTRACT

The Otolaryngology view of the sleep disordered breathing patient. A lot of surgical procedures have been developed to treat the upper airway anatomical components causing sleep disordered breathing diseases. The airway pattern and severity of obstruction vary greatly between patients, which affects the success rate of a given surgical procedure, and often with bad results. In general, as the severity of obstructive sleep apnea increases, so does the invasiveness of the required procedure to achieve a successful surgical outcome. The most principal factor, in all types of these surgeries, is the diagnosis of any sleep disordered breathing disease based on sleep-study results and in a systematized approach with special care in the upper airway anatomy. The surgeon's role change from being the adversary of positive pressure respiratory therapy (CPAP) to be the best ally when through surgery, decreases airway resistance and improving the compliance and adherence to CPAP. And, we gave a lot of therapeutic option in those patients with poor acceptance to the CPAP. In this chapter, we will see an overview of the sleep disordered breathing diseases like the simple snoring, upper airway resistance syndrome, and the obstructive sleep apnea syndrome and their surgical treatment from office-based procedures to multilevel surgery. In conclusion, the tailored treatment is essential in these patients, and the otolaryngologist should be able to handle all aspects of sleep-disordered diseases from a systematic approach to the multiple treatments available, from oral devices, positive pressure respiratory therapy to the most advanced surgical techniques.

Rodolfo Lugo Saldaña MD Otolaryngologist. Director Ronquido Monterrey Clinic. www.ronquidomonterrey.com www.oidosnarizygarganta.com

The otolaryngologist so far has played a supporting role in the treatment of sleep-disordered breathing (SDB) patients. In performing upper airway surgery, the otolaryngologist sometimes gives too much importance to postsurgical results (often failed), measured by "snoring as noise." While important to the patient, this focus does not adequately consider apnea, hypopnea, desaturation and arousals in addition to the many variations that can occur in a nocturnal respiratory therapy [continuous positive airway pressure (CPAP), autoadjusting positive airway pressure (APAP), and bilevel positive airway pressure (BiPAP)].

In recent years, the role of the otolaryngologist in the field of SDB has grown and become more sophisticated. Presently, several different surgical treatment options are available, with the appropriate surgery being selected based on a precise and systematic questioning, exploration, topodiagnosis, grading and staging of the patient. While positive pressure nocturnal respiratory therapy remains the "gold standard," this increasingly nuanced understanding of SDB belies the accusation that "The ENT doctor wants to operate everything, and does not believe in the CPAP."

In the sixties, Dr. Ikematsu first reported pharyngopalatoplasty which began a boom of corrective surgeries for snoring; however, many of these techniques eventually demonstrated poor results. During that time, success was measured only by the effect on the volume of snoring, with postoperative patients with persistent snoring classified as surgical failures.

In 1979, a psychiatrist from France, Dr. Christian Gilleminault, first described obstructive sleep apnea syndrome (OSAS). He emphasized the effects on cardiovascular and cognitive symptoms.[1]

In 1981, Dr. Fujita, in Japan, reported good results after uvulopharyngoplasty. This technique became very popular, but offered unpredictable results and significant postoperative complications.

In the same year, a pulmonologist from Sidney, Dr. Colin Sullivan, performed the first positive air pressure treatment in patients with OSAS. Because of its efficacy and since the only other treatment available for severe OSAS at that time was tracheotomy, CPAP became the "gold standard" treatment.

During the 1980s, many investigators published articles exploring OSAS variations and patterns. These investigations demonstrated the important roles played by various sites of obstruction in OSA patients, and offered insight into the multifactorial causes of the airway obstruction. In addition, multiple metabolic and cardiovascular effects were demonstrated in patients with OSA. Additionally, a wide range of emotional and cognitive effects were shown including a relationship between OSAS and attention deficit hyperactivity disorder in pediatric patients.

In 1990, Dr. Murray Johns developed the Epworth Sleepiness Scale in the Epworth Hospital in Melbourne, Australia and it is one of the most used in the sleep medicine practice.[2]

In 1990, Dr. Ives Kamami published positive results, more than 80%, with his technique of laser assisted uvulopalatoplasty, taking the advantage of not requiring general anesthesia or present complications presented by the original technique of uvulopalatopharyngoplasty (UPPP), but at the end of the decade it began to develop complications such as palate stenosis in patients who had exaggerated tissue resection and more complications. This technique is actually only suggested in simple snoring with no OSA.

In 1990, Dr Guilleminault described the upper airway resistance syndrome (UARS) in the article "obstructive sleep apnea syndrome or abnormal upper airway resistance during sleep?" in the Journal of Clinical Neurophysiology.[3]

In 1993, Fujita, who previously described UPPP, started to focus on his classification of obstructive area. Fujita had previously reported palate surgery, after seeing that a percentage of their patients still had symptoms and had no improvement, began to focus on the different levels of narrowing of the upper airway and described his classification, marking the basis of what later become known as the topodiagnosis, or narrowness multisegmental location in the patients with sleep-disordered breathing diseases.

Katsantonis determined the level of obstruction by monitoring the pressure of the upper airway. He found that 55% had obstruction of the palate and tongue, 25% in palate only, 10% tongue and 10% supraglottis. With these results, researchers began to focus on topodiagnosis as the principal issue in patient work up and treatment.

Recent studies have shown that the combination of positive pressure breathing therapy and surgery in patients suffering from SDB increased their survival. It has also been observed in patients treated with APAP, CPAP or BiPAP that the functional nasal surgery decreased pressure required and increased adherence and tolerance to this treatment. This understanding may represent the most important step in the history of OSAS treatment.[4]

It is important to point out that surgery is not in tension with positive pressure respiratory treatment. Rather, the roles of these therapies are potentially complimentary in the vast majority of cases. Take the example of a patient diagnosed with OSAS for whom CPAP use was recommended. Upon titration, apneas were extinguished at 17 cm/H_2O, leading to poor mask compliance. In this case, a treating physician who does not have surgical options available in their arsenal is unable to offer more than nasal sprays and oral decongestant medication to try to relieve the high resistance and improve compliance with nasal CPAP. The otolaryngologist who is trained to explore the upper airway and understand the functional relationships among the nose, nasopharynx and hypopharynx, and retropalatine space is able to detect functional pathology in this region which results in intolerance to the CPAP mask. In such cases, a functional nasal surgery can diminish the titration pressure and optimize utilization of CPAP.

In the actual approach of the patient with some SDB disease, very important is the topodiagnosis and the sleep study. With these results, you can tailor the treatment and make a better medical or surgical, or both decisions.

For its part, the otolaryngologist is trained to explore the upper airway and can see the functional integrity of the nose, nasopharynx, hypopharynx and retropalatine space, the "topodiagnosis," so to detect functional nasal pathology which is one of the most common causes of intolerance to the use of CPAP mask.[5]

In this case we suggest to the patient a nasal surgical treatment, not as a definitive treatment but as an auxiliary treatment for better utilization and adaptation to the positive pressure breathing therapy. The functional nasal surgery is the natural ally for the ideal treatment for this patient.

The most difficult issue in the sleep apnea patient is detecting the areas of narrowing in the upper respiratory tract. Since the 1970s, investigators have performed nasovideoendoscopy during normal and chemically induced sleep. Its use is controversial because the medication effects on normal sleep physiology.

However, this study offers the most reliable view of the anatomical areas of interest during sleep. It is recommended in difficult patients with many comorbidities and without clear diagnosis.[6]

THE TAILORED TREATMENT

The most important point is choosing the appropriate procedure. The goal of treatment is to expand the limited space in the upper airway. This can be difficult because each patient has unique anatomy and collection of contributing factors. In order to help assess this, it is always necessary to perform a sleep study, or polysomnography. Computed tomography, a detailed history, the Epworth Sleepiness Scale measurements (Friedman), body mass index (BMI), neck circumference and understanding relevant comorbidities are all important. If the patient data and polysomnography present a picture of severe OSAS, this patient may require CPAP, upper airway surgery, as well as hyoid and mandibular advancement, if results a severe case of obstructive sleep apnea, which does not adaptate, does not tolerate or do not want the positive pressure respiratory therapy (CPAP), you can suggest a multilevel surgical treatment.

The SDB treatment is based in three types:

Type 1: Behavioral
Type 2: Devices to be worn
Type 3: Surgery

▌ Type 1: The Behavioral Treatment

The behavioral treatment is indicated in all patients with OSA and SDB problems. It is important to address sleep hygiene, and avoidance of alcohol and fatty meals before bedtime. Sedating medicines and alcoholic beverages may exacerbate OSA. Patients with insomnia should be counseled to avoid physical exercise and coffee or tea near bedtime, and avoid activities such as reading or watching television in bed.

In obese patients, considering weight loss is important since, in most patients, there is a threshold level of weight above which they have symptoms and below which they do not. There are many additional medical benefits to be gained from weight loss. It is an important count in the sleep laboratory or sleep apnea clinic to a nutrition specialist.

The sleep hygiene: Sedating medicines and alcoholic beverages may exacerbate OSA. Patients with insomnia should be counseled to avoid physical exercise and coffee or tea near to sleep time and avoid activities such as reading or watching television in bed. Lastly, since OSA is usually worse when supine, some patients may benefit from simple measures such as sewing a raquetball or tennis ball into the back of a pajama shirt to avoid sleeping in the supine position.

■ Type 2: Devices to be Worn

Oral Appliances

Oral appliances can be effective in relieving OSA symptoms. These work by mechanically displacing the jaw or tongue forward and opening the retrolingual space. No single appliance has been shown to be superior to another. Some have been shown to be effective to relieve the airway obstruction in patients with apnea/hypopnea index (AHI) under 20 without comorbidities. Exist a lot of models like the adjustable tongue advancement is feasible and some patients find them difficult to use; however, in general, compliance is superior to CPAP, and is relatively safe way to reduce the AHI and snoring in selected patients with moderate to severe OSA and CPAP intolerance.

There are many such types of oral appliances, and they have some potential advantages over CPAP in that they are unobtrusive, make no noise, do not need a power source and are potentially less costly. There is a growing evidence base to support the use of oral appliances in the management of OSA.

Oral appliances have become established treatment devices for simple snoring and mild or moderate sleep apnea. Substantial scientific evidence has demonstrated that mandibular repositioning appliances are effective.[7]

Positive Pressure Appliances

Given its ability to overcome obstructive apneas in all degrees of OSAS severity and avoidance of risk related to surgery, positive pressure devices are considered the "gold standard" among OSAS therapies. If a patient is a candidate for continuous positive air pressure therapy, this represents the first-line intervention. Some centers perform a split night adaptation study while other centers perform diagnostic studies first with titration studies being performed at a separate, later time. In our center, we prefer trials over 3 or 4 days using two or three different types of masks. Compliance is considered adequate when CPAP is used greater than or equal to 4 hours per night when averaged over all nights observed.

Split Night Studies

Split night studies are recommended in patients with AHI between 20 and 40 over at least 2 hours of study. The diagnostic study and the CPAP mask titration are performed during the same night in sleep laboratory. In some patients with significant comorbidities, it is more difficult to perform this type of study. Split night studies are not recommended in anxious patients.

Multiple Night Trial

One of the most reliable ways to adapt a patient to the APAP, CPAP or BiPAP is to perform a multiple night trial over 3 or 4 days. This type of study generally involves an autoset with humidifier and one or two masks. This allows the patient and physician to assess tolerance and adherence to respiratory devices and masks. This type of study is performed in the patient's home with recording the patient's exam data on the system's storage card for review in the office after 3 or 4 days of use. Air leaks, persistent apneas and hypopneas, and the minimum and maximum pressures are recorded. The pressure at which significant air leakage occurs resulting in worsening titration and an increase of CPAP pressure is considered the highest CPAP, a patient can tolerate during a given sleep stage. Higher pressure is generally more difficult to tolerate.

■ Type 3: Surgery

Surgery for Sleep-Disordered Breathing

Surgery is often considered to be the first-line treatment for simple snoring and mild/moderate OSA. Surgery is considered successful when the AHI drops at least 50% and is below 20 per hour in patients whose presurgical AHI was greater than 20 per hour.For this discussion, we will consider three categories of sleep surgery: surgery to improve compliance with CPAP, surgery to modify the upper airway without the use of tracheostomy or bariatric surgery, and finally surgery that directly alters the upper airway.

The diagnostic focus is to identify narrowed anatomical sites, a task for which the otolaryngologists have ideal tools. Nasal rigid endoscopes can examine the nasal valve, turbinates, septal cartilage and perpendicular plate irregularities. Flexible fiberscopes view the sites of nasopharyngeal and hypopharyngeal narrowing. Some centers also perform sleep nasovideoendoscopy allowing insight into dynamic aspects in this region. However, this study is somewhat difficult and requires medical sedation which may alter normal sleep patterns. Another limitation is that it is performed for only 10 or 15 minutes which does not allow observation of pathological events occurring during all levels of sleep. Additionally, some authors report no relationship between sites of anatomical narrowing identified during sleep nasoendoscopy, the Muller maneuver, or the Mallampati scale and postsurgical outcome.

Nasal Surgery in Sleep-Disordered Breathing

The role of nasal patency in the pathogenesis of OSA is not fully understood. There are conflicting data in the literature regarding the influence of nasal resistance in OSA patients.Controlled radiofrequency (RF) ablative technology has become an important surgical option in the surgical treatment of SDB. Its effectiveness in volumetric reduction of the inferior turbinate and base of tongue in addition to its effect on the palate makes this a useful tool in our therapeutic arsenal. In some centers, controlled RF tongue base reduction has replaced genioglossus advancement (GA). This trend has been driven by a desire to avoid morbidity and possible complications that may arise from GA, while effecting similar surgery outcomes (Fig. 9.1).

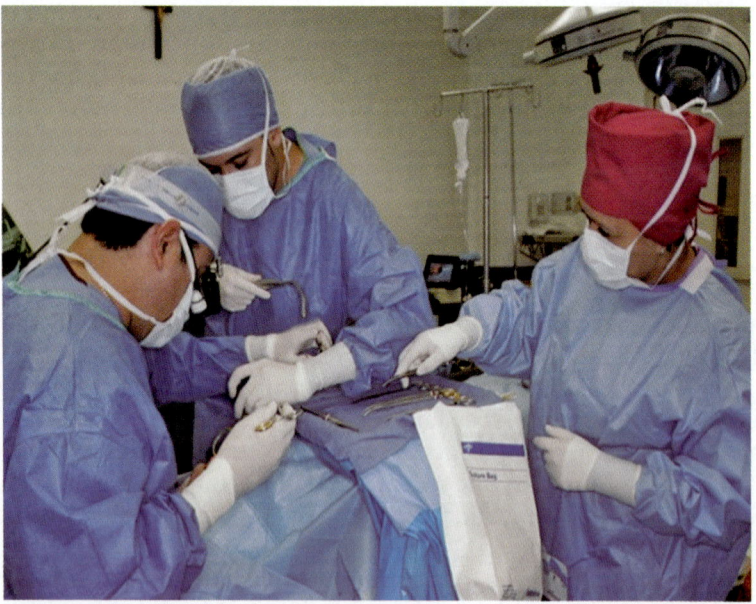

Fig. 9.1: Surgical team during base of tongue and palatal surgery
Source: Courtesy by Rodolfo Lugo Saldaña, MD and Rodolfo Topete, MD

Techniques for Turbinate Reduction

For years the volumetric reduction of the nasal turbinates focused solely on turbinate electrocautery. This technique often results in post-surgical complications like crusting, pain, scarring and bleeding as well as high rates of recurrence. Turbinectomy is indicated in small subset of patients with huge inferior turbinates or compensatory hypertrophy and obstructive symptoms. This technique has several potential post-surgical complications including atrophic rhinitis. Despite this risk, it remains a good technique in some selected patients with numerous articles supporting favorable results when compared to volumetric reduction.

Endoscopic submucosal turbinate reduction with a microdebrider is another technique which has demonstrated good results. It is commonly performed in combination with outfracture of the inferior turbinate. For this procedure, the turbinate is infiltrated presurgically with lidocaine 2% with epinephrine and a small incision is made in the anterior inferior turbinate. Debridement is performed with a 2.5 mm microdebrider blade, paying particular attention to the turbinate head and the medial portion of the turbinate. This is a safe technique with a few complications with emphasis in the mucosa and cilia integrity.

Subjective analysis with questionnaires on daytime fatigue or excessive daytime sleepiness has revealed that nasal surgery is beneficial in the sleep quality of OSAS patients. Corrective nasal surgery or turbinate volume reduction may help patients to tolerate CPAP therapy. Thus, rhinologic procedures may be considered for patients with poor compliance with CPAP therapy. Nasal airway pathology should also be considered when a multilevel surgery is proposed in the patient with OSA.[8]

Palatal Surgery in the Sleep Disordered Breathing

Since Ikematsu and Fujita reported the UPPP in 50s and 80s, palatal surgery has been controversial due to irregular results on snoring noise levels. With the understanding that the number of apneas, hypoapneas, cardiac desaturations, sleep quality and number of arousals are more important than snoring and noise, palatal surgery alone for OSAS has fallen out of favor. However, for patients with simple snoring in the absence of apneas or hypoapneas palatal surgery has an important role to play.

Surgery for Simple Snoring

Simple snoring is the least common among the SDB pathologies. It is very important to complete work up including the superior airway examination and sleep study to assess and confirm that no additional pathology is present. Like other forms of SDB, the etiology is multifactorial. In light of

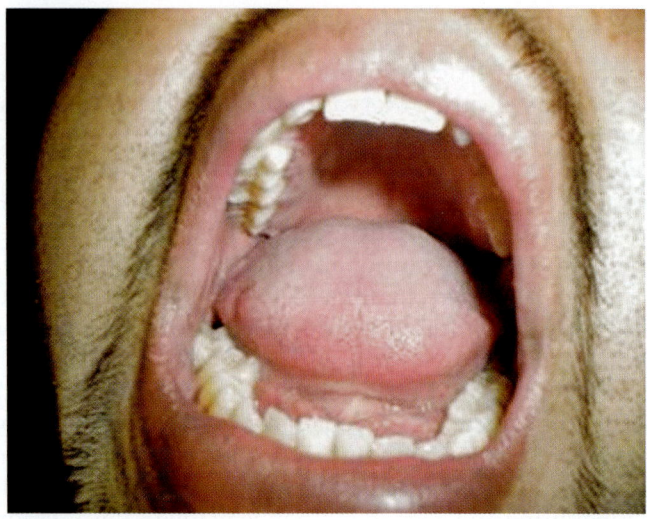

Fig. 9.2: Friedman tongue position III pre-SMILE surgery

this precise, topodiagnosis is important in order to find the affected areas and guide surgical choices.

The Friedman Staging Chart, assessment of the Friedman Tongue Position using nasopharyngoscopy with the tongue in the retracted position, and a sleep endoscopy all help in this assessment (Fig. 9.2).

If the patient is a surgical candidate, the nasal valve and the anterior portion of the inferior turbinate are key areas to address. However, several articles reviewed show little effect in the level of snoring versus preoperation levels. These data are based on nonrandomized and noncontrolled studies. Taken together, this suggests that nasal surgery can be employed in conjunction with other levels of surgery to optimize results in the simple snoring patient.

Patients with a Mallampati I or II, with Grade I or II tonsils, and under 43 cms neck circumference, with 30 or under BMI are ideal candidates for palatal stiffening procedures.

Palatal Stiffening Procedures

To perform palatal stiffening procedures, we need to achieve good local anesthesia. The first step is to anesthetize the palate with lidocaine 10 g/100 ml spray. Following this, benzocaine gel can be applied directly to the soft palate.

It is preferable to inject a small amount of lidocaine 2% at the target points in the soft palate for increased comfort and patient compliance. The goal of palatal stiffening procedures is to achieve increased rigidity and a less collapsibility in the airway. With time, a fibrotic area forms around the treated area resulting in further stiffness to the palate. This can be achieved using a variety of techniques which are further explored below.

Injection Snoreplasty

The injection snoreplasty is a technique in which a sclerosing agent is injected into the soft palate in order to achieve this fibrotic response. Fibrosis results in decreased vibration as air passes. Brietzke and Mair performed a study in 27 patients using the sclerosant Sotradecol. Twenty-five of the 27 patients (92%) reported subjectively diminished snoring noise level at 3 months with persistent effect in 75% at 19 months. Other sclerosants were also investigated by Brietzke and Mair, including ethanol, doxycycline and hypertonic saline. Fifty percent ethanol was found to be the safest of these and achieved similar results to Sotradecol.

In our center, we performed a study of 100 patients with simple snoring treated by injection snoreplasty with 50% ethanol. There was a direct relationship between Mallamapati grade and patient results. Patients with mallamapati Type I or II had higher likelihood of reduction in noise level than patients with Mallampati Type III or IV at 6 months posttreatment.

Like another snoring procedures, the most important point is the topo-diagnosis to ensure the real narrowed airway area.

Cautery-Assisted Palatal Stiffness Operation

This technique is reported for first time by Ellis in 1994 and Mair realized a modification in 2000.

The original technique under local anesthesia is performed with a "diamond style" incision, using electrocautery and removing the mucosa and the uvula. The results often produce a narrowing space postscar to the anterior pillars, with unclear results (Fig. 9.3).

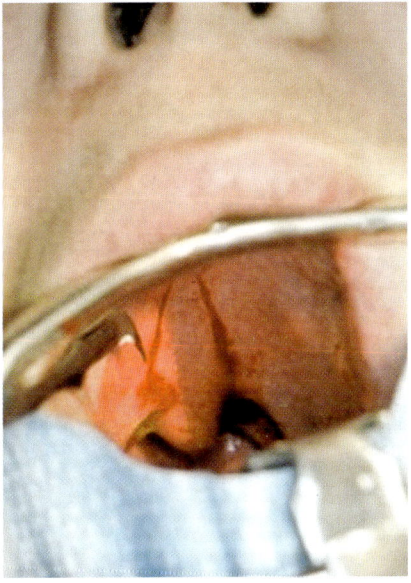

Fig. 9.3: Uvulopalatal Incision with #12 bisturi blade

The modification is under local anesthesia with infiltration of lidocaine 2% with epinephrine and topical benzocaine gel, a uvulectomy is realized and after that a little "rectangle style" mucosa resection is realized about 1 cm in the soft palate midline to produce a upward scarring pattern during the healing process and retracts superiorly and avoid the palatal stenosis (Fig. 9.4).

This procedure is performed under local or general anesthesia in one session, the surgeon realizes the surgery with the cautery in coagulation mode to make the incision in the soft palate and makes a fibrosis secondary to normal cicatrization.

Palatal Radiofrequency Technique

It is basically the same theory like cautery-assisted palatal stiffness operation (CAPSO), but this technique is realized with the controlled RF, and is realized under local anesthesia with topical benzocaine gel in the palate and without uvulectomy.

In this procedure, we need less points in the palate, in a triangle pattern, in the midline part of the soft palate and two or three sessions to obtain good results in the noise levels. We use multiple points of RF in 70–80 grades for 90 seconds per lesion in the soft palate to produce a lesion with the secondary fibrosis to obtain a resistance to the vibration and if the noise is retropalatal, reduce the snoring. This technique often needs more than one session.

It is more reliable to use controlled type RF devices to better results with less discomfort and pain.

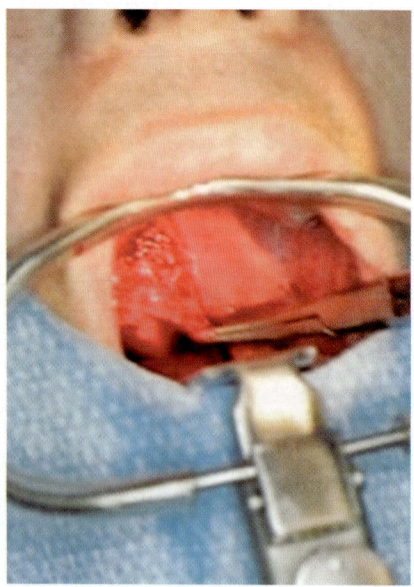

Fig. 9.4: Mucosa resection in uvulopalatal flap

Palatal Implants

Palatal implants involve the placement of three implants in the upper portion of the soft palate under local anesthesia in the office. The implants are designed to stiffen the soft palate to help to diminish the noise level of snoring. It is relatively painless procedure that can be performed in the office under local anesthesia. The target is to stimulate the natural fibrotic response and add structural stiffness to the soft palate and reduce the vibration.These implants are made of a woven polyester material (pillar procedure is a patented brand) 18 mm length and 2 mm of circumference.

The ideal candidate is a simple snoring or mild sleep apnea patient, 20 AHI or minor, with Grade I or II tonsils and Friedman Staging I, with a BMI of 30 or under. If is a patient who underwent a palate surgery, only be to examine whether there is sufficient soft palate to check if is a candidate for pillar palate implants.

One of the major complications is the extrusion. In a study in Manheim in 40 patients, they had 10 patients (13 implants) who partially extruded, uneventfully.

This technique can be used in the minimally invasive multilevel procedures concept to mild sleep apnea patients or simple snoring.

We realize this office-based procedure combined with turbinal RF in almost all cases, if the patient is candidate.

Results in Stiffness Palate Procedures

Injection snoreplasty: Brietzke and Mair reported in their first report that snoring decreased from 92% at 3 months to 75% at 19 months. Our center had a 75% of success, is important to note that patients with Mallampati classification III or IV and Friedman III or IV, or neck circumference>43 cms in general have a worse prognosis.

Cautery-assisted palatal stiffness operation: Mair and Day reported a 77% of success rate in 206 patients of 1-year postoperation, and the original technique had a similar results.

Palatal radiofrequency: Li and the Stanford group report in 2005 in 22 patients a 41% of subjective snoring relapsed in general they need a multiple sessions. In conclusion, the success of the palatal stiffness procedures diminishes with time, as the other surgical techniques of the palate.

Palatal implants (Pillar Palatal System): Maurer and the Manheim group report a study in long term in 40 patients with simple snoring with significant decrease in snoring and daytime sleepiness.

Walker et al. realize a study with 22 patients with good long-term outcome in mild and moderate OSA selected patients.

Palatal Surgery

Uvulopalatopharyngoplasty

Uvulopalatopharingoplasty was first reported by Ikematsu in 1963, and later modified by Fujita in 1981. UPPP is the most commonly performed surgery for OSAS. This technique removes soft tissue from the soft palate in conjunction with tonsillectomy and uvulectomy. Cut mucosal edges are sutured together with absorbable stitches. UPPP aims to enlarge the airway and is performed under general anesthesia in a hospital operating room.

Should UPPP be performed as a stand-alone procedure? The answer to this question appears to be related to patient's BMI, with morbid obesity being a negative predictor of outcome. BMI between 28 and 30 kg/m^2 appears to be the limit for successful UPPP as a stand-alone. Neck circumference greater than 40 cm in females or greater than 43 cm in males is also a negative predictor as are high AHI and high degree of desaturation. For the authors, AHI more than 30 serves as a dividing line above which we prefer multilevel surgery. Additional negative predictors include micrognathia and retrognathia. In these patients, the obstruction often includes the retrolingual space. By contrast, Grade IV tonsils are a positive predictor of success.

Some authors prefer to use coblator, laser or cautery to make mucosal incisions, but we see worse scarring patterns with these techniques. In our hands, "cold" technique is used, making cuts with the scalpel and scissors. Incision technique is an individual surgeon's choice.

After years of study, many complications have been identified with aggressive tissue resection. In some patients, classic UPPP causes narrowing of the palatal structure, with a decrease in the size of the oropharyngeal space. Patients with OSA despite previous tonsillectomy are poor candidates for classic UPPP, owing to absence or scarring of the posterior pillar. Newer, more conservative techniques have been developed, focusing on moderate uvula shortening, in order to avoid some of these complications. UPPP techniques which preserve the muscles and mucosa of the pharynx appear to reduce postsurgical complication rates as well.

Full recovery takes just under 3 weeks, during which time pain is the major factor. As a result, weight loss of 10–15 lbs. is common during this time. Since UPPP is often performed in conjunction with another level of surgery (e.g. base of tongue, rhinologic surgery) hospitalization in the immediate postoperative period is often required. Intravenous analgesia during the first 2 or 3 days can be helpful to shorten recovery time. Additionally, it is important for patients to observe a strict posttonsillectomy diet. A polysomnographic evaluation is necessary 1 year after surgery, or sooner as part of a new CPAP trial.

Uvulopalatal Flap Technique

Uvulopalatal flap (UPF) technique originated from a 1996 Sleep article from the Stanford group entitled "A Reversible Uvulopalatal Flap for snoring and sleep apnea syndrome." The authors later compared the postsurgical results versus uvulopharyngoplasty with similar outcomes. The reported advantage is the reversibility and conservative nature of the technique which reduces the risk of velopharyngeal incompetence.* This technique has gained popularity both because of the favorable outcome, low complication rate and for the lower level of pain. Authors, like the Manheim group, see the advantages over UPPP with similar indications (Figs 9.5 to 9.7).

Technique

The UPF technique is performed under general anesthesia. It begins with tonsillectomy, taking special care to preserve the posterior pillar. The authors prefer the "cold" dissection with scissors and Hurd dissector, foregoing the use of cautery technique or other energy-delivering instrument because the posterior pillar is very important in creating the flap. A small back-cut is made in the superior angle of the tonsillar fossa to avoid the circumferential scarring of the palate. Avoiding this complication is the reason to avoid energy-delivering techniques.

After the initial mucosal dissection, an incision is made on the oral side of the uvula, taking special care to match the size of the palatal dissection to the area of mucosal excision on the uvula. The flap is secured with

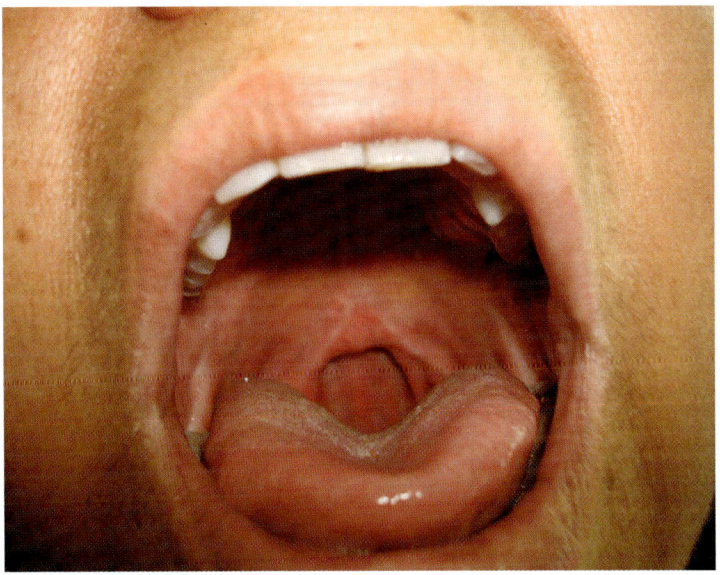

Fig. 9.5: Postuvulopalatal flap

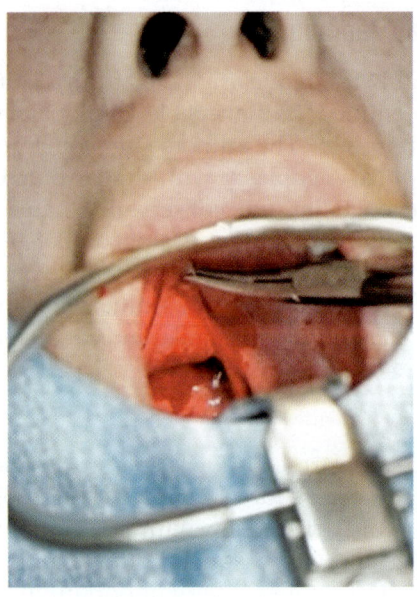

Fig. 9.6: Flap rotation in uvulopalatal flap

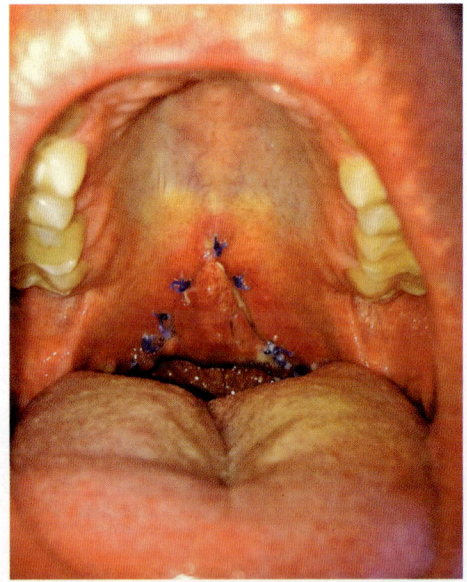

Fig. 9.7: Uvulopalatal flap 5 days postoperation

3-0 Vicryl using a liberal number of sutures to avoid dehiscence of the flap. This surgery is frequently performed in conjunction with surgery at another level (e.g. base of tongue RF, "submucosal minimally invasive lingual excision (SMILE)" of the tongue, or hyoid surgery). Again, the authors prefer patient bed rest and providing analgesia intravenous for the first 3 or 4 days postoperatively. Pain control is very important because the pain is one of the reasons for which this type of procedure can get a bad reputation (Fig. 9.8).[9]

Z-Pharyngoplasty Technique

The Z-pharyngoplasty (ZZP) is ideal to perform in posttonsillectomy patients who need to have their palates addressed, in Friedman Staging Grade II or III, in patients with failed UPPP, inability to tolerate CPAP trials and failure of conservative treatment. Apparent obstruction at the level of the soft palate must be determined by flexible nasopharyngoscopy, and Muller maneuver or snoring effort imitation.

Conceptually, the ZZP is similar to the uvulopalatal flap. The central difference being midline division of the uvula and attachment of the divided sections into the lateral soft palate with muscle incision. This results in widening of the anterolateral retropalatal space. Special care should be taken to minimize the possibility to velopharyngeal insufficiency.

Temporary palatal insufficiency is common, but usually does not last more than 3 months. Typically, the ZZP involves comparable pain level as UPF technique. It is rare to perform this technique as a stand-alone surgery. It is often performed with the base of tongue surgery or hyoid surgery (Fig. 9.9).

Technique

Under general anesthesia, the mucosa is gently dissected with scissors. Only the exact amount is excised to allow the flap to attach. The midline uvula is divided in a horizontal superior line at the anterior tonsillar pillar.

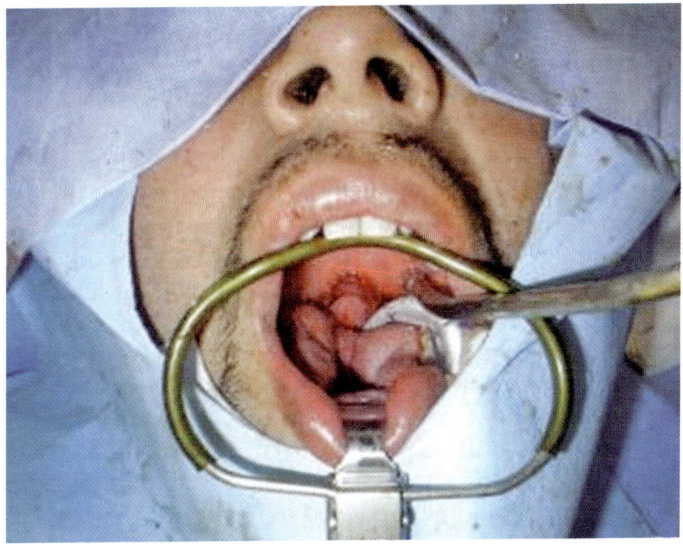

Fig. 9.8: Smile surgery and Uvulopalatal flap postoperative image

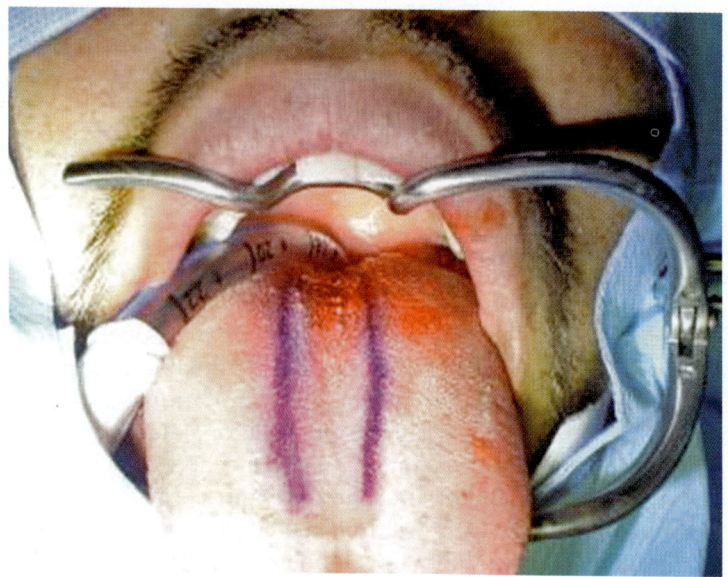

Fig. 9.9: Tongue marks pre-SMILE surgery

The midline bilobulated flap is retracted anterolaterally, which widens the retropharyngeal space. 5-0 Vicryl is used to secure the flap with ample support. Finally, a base of tongue procedure or hyoid surgery is performed.

The pain level is less than with UPPP, while the postsurgical complications are similar. Again, bed rest and IV analgesia are preferred.

▌Transpalatal Advancement Technique

Tucker Woodson and Toohill in 1990 described a technique to reconstruct the upper pharynx by performing a posterior maxillary osteotomy and advancing the soft palate anteriorly with a posterior palatal osteotomy and palatal advancement.

Transpalatal advancement technique is a pharyngeal procedure indicated to structurally enlarge the retromaxillary and retropalatal airway in patients with OSA. This procedure enlarges the proximal pharyngeal space, which is difficult by other procedures other than maxillary advancement.

Results demonstrate both structural and clinical improvements. Compared to more traditional UPPP, postoperative success is dependent on treating all areas of obstruction, including in the results of the topo-diagnosis. Success is dependent on adequate advancement and closure of the soft palate tissue to prevent fistula and dehiscence of the surgery area. Another recent study compared a group of patients with palatal advancement to a group of UPPP patients all of whom were Friedman Stage 3. This group would be predicted to have an 8% success rate with UPPP alone. And, the palatal advancement group demonstrated significant polysomnographic improvement over UPPP.

In conclusion, If the patient has a palatine narrowing space, our choice is about to make a palatine surgery like UPF with tonsillectomy, UPPP or a pharyngoplasty. If the patient doesn't like oral surgeries, and they had a BMI under 30 and not had a Grade IV tonsils, we can suggest the palatal implants or RF stiffness palatal technique or the injection snoreplasty, but this is only suggested in a simple snoring or low AHI with no comorbidities and another complications.

TONGUE SURGERY IN THE SLEEP DISORDERED BREATHING

Many procedures have been reported to address obstruction in the tongue base and include glossectomy, lingualplasty, RF tongue ablation, hyoid suspension, mandibular osteotomy with GA, and maxillary-mandibular advancement.

Radiofrequency of Base of the Tongue

The use of RF devices fit good in the sleep apnea surgery because the concept of "volumetric reduction" is very useful in turbinates, palate, tonsils and base of tongue.

If upper airway exploration asseses the retrolingual narrowed area in OSA patient, you can choose any technique for tongue excision. The more conservative procedure is the RF excision of base of the tongue, with a device from Gyrus ENT, with a hand piece (Fig. 9.10) especially used for tongue surgery. We deliver 85 grades 4 points, 600 joules per side, 1,200 joules total, in the midline with special care so as not to injure the neurovascular bundle.

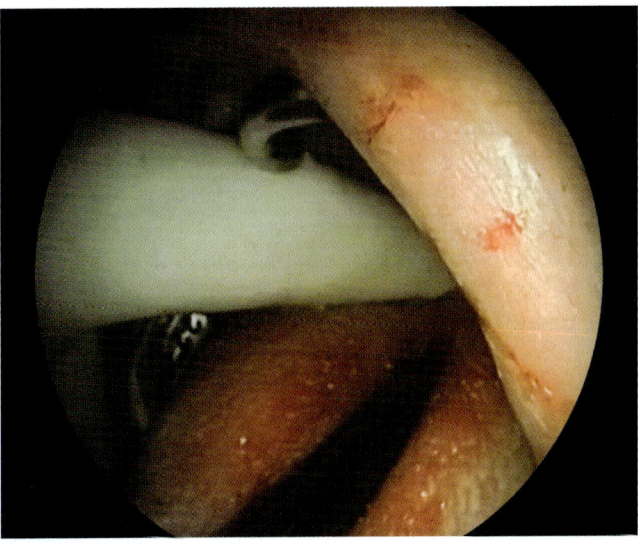

Fig. 9.10: Endoscopic view with the Evac 70 hand piece in the tongue insertion site during a SMILE surgery

Foreign body sensation is one of the postsurgical symptoms, regular pain controlled with paracetamol 500 mgs TID, hematoma and abscess are rare complications.

Tongue Base Suspension

In 1992, Faye Lund reported for the first time the glossopexia as a surgical treatment to OSA, with the use of fascia lata as a sling in the tongue; the ends are attached in the drill holes in the mandible and sutured to each other after maximal anterior suspension of the tongue. This procedure has not become popular because of the difficulty to obtain the exact quantity of fascia for this technique. With the theoric base of this procedure, a company (Influ ENT) patented a new procedure "the repose system."[10]

Repose System (Tongue Suspension)

Considered in patients who are suitable candidates for UPPP with AHI above 20 and moderate base of tongue obstruction on the exploration.

The ideal candidate for this procedure had an AHI greater than 15 and oxygen desaturation of less than 90% with high Epworth scale results or UARS with poor compliance to CPAP.

Technique

Under general anesthesia, incising the floor of mouth posterior to Wharton conducts, the periosteum is elevated over the genial tubercle and the screw inserter is placed through, and attach the suture there with the screw inserter handle that is positioned perpendicular to the angle of the mandible. The suture passer containing a preloaded temporary suture loop is inserted through the floor of the mouth incision to exit the tongue base posterior to the circumvallate papillae and 1 cm lateral to the midline. Polypropylene suture attached to the mandibular screw is loaded into the empty suture passer and is passed through the floor of the mouth incision to exit the contralateral tongue base.

The instruments and the lingual retractor come in the surgical package from the company.

Finally, the repose tongue base suspension is useful in the therapy of retrolingual narrowed space patients. For OSA, the results are comparable with RF of turbinates and RF of the tongue base.

SUBMUCOSAL PARTIAL GLOSSECTOMY TECHNIQUES

Percutaneous Submucosal Tongue Base Excision

Robinson et al. introduced for first time in 2003 this technique for OSA adults patients with the help of a plasma-mediated RF device (coblation), the surgical approach is an invasive suprahyoid neck incision (Figs 9.11 and 9.12).

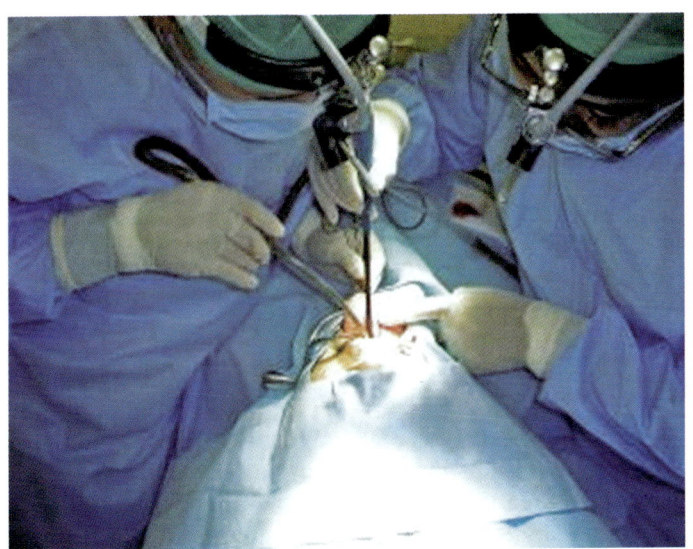

Fig. 9.11: Base of tongue coblation technique
Source: Courtesy by Alberto Labra, MD

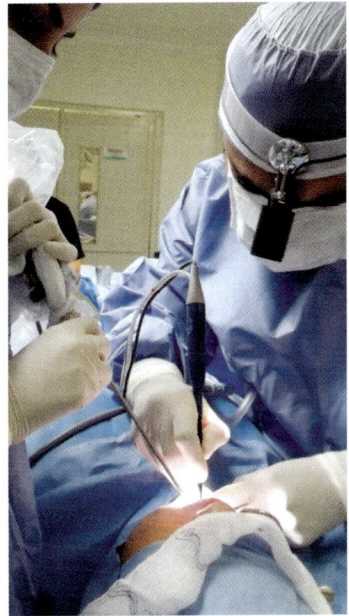

Fig. 9.12: Use of coblator Evac 70 hand piece in base of tongue surgery
Note: the importance of maintain the position in the midline

Although it is a good technique, the complicated approach is the cause of the morbidities, this technique did not became popular because of the approach and its complications.

The results are very similar to those of the tongue wedge excision or another tongue resection techniques. Based on this technique but without the neck incision is the next procedure.

Submucosal Minimally Invasive Lingual Excision

This single intraoral technique, the SMILE procedure is reported by Maturo and Mair in 2006 in treatment for macroglossia in pediatric patients with Down's syndrome or Beckwith-Wiedemann syndrome. Previous ultrasonography localize the neurovascular bundle.

Technique

Under general anesthesia, we realized a small incision in the anterior portion of the tongue (dorsal side); we use a rigid irrigator endoscope to avoid the mouth floor and musculature and with the plasma wand and the coblator devices, initiate the resection with special care to stay medial and advance in posterior direction and moving superior and inferior fashion, but always staying medial to the lingual arteries with a lot of irrigation in the new created cavity, finally, the incision is not closed to let the drain in the first time of the postoperative period. Also is suggested the use of irrigation 0 grades endoscope.

The blood loss is minimal and the edema is treated with IV corticoids. Moreover, oral antibiotics are mandatory, but in this area, infections are rare because of the tongue blood supply. Paracetamol with or without codeine are the painkillers of choice. In pediatric patients, it is very important in the postsurgery recuperation period to take care of the extubation and stay in touch with the anesthesiologist.

Results in Submucosal Partial Glossectomy Techniques

The results in base of tongue partial resection techniques are variable because it is so rare to perform this type of surgery as a unique treatment option. Fujita, in 1991, has shown a 41.7% success rate in a study with a 5–15 month follow up. In another investigation by Woodson and Fujita in 1992 a success rate of 78.6% was reported but they presented a 1.5 months of follow-up period only. Mickelson and Rosenthal in 1997 presented a 46.6% of success with 2.4 months of follow-up, and Chabolle in 1999 presented an 80% success rate with a combination of UPPP.

Mandibular Osteotomy with Genioglossus Advancement

Powell, Riley and Guilleminault group reported in 1986, the use of MO with GA for the treatment of OSA. This must always be used in combination with a hyoid suspension in patients with severe OSA. This technique is not indicated as a unique procedure.

Technique

The ideal approach is intraoral 10-15 mm below the gingivomucosal junction, the symphysis is dissected without lateral exposure, then an osteotomy is performed in the central square, where is the genial tubercle/genioglossus muscle complex are attached in the oral side and with a clamp move to the anterior position and fixed with a screw osteosynthetically. Ultimate you can reduce the bone cortex to avoid a no esthetic profile of the chin, close the incision with vycril with no drains. Complications are intraoral wound dehiscence but healed without problems in a few days, transient lower lip numbness and little pain in lower certral incisors for 1 or 2 months of postoperative dysphagia, for up to 1 week. In general, injuries to the teeth root, mentonian nerve injuries and mandibular fractures are rare complications.

Results in Tongue Surgery for Obstructive Sleep Apnea

Fibbi et al. reported the use of the MO and the tongue suspension at the same time, another surgeon Neruntarat combined in the multilevel concept of the MO with UPF and hyoid suspension, and they had a therapy success of 78.3% after 6 months and of 65.2% after 39 months.

The Manheim group preferred to realize the base of tongue RF than MO and they presented similar postoperative results with less morbidities and complications.

Hyoid Surgery in the Sleep-Disordered Breathing

A lot of studies and articles existed about retropalatal obstruction due to popularity of the UPPP, but only very few reports existed focus in hypopharyngeal constriction. A lack of long-term results may be more complex because of their techniques and their peri- and postoperative morbidity.

The collapse of the base of the tongue which relaxes during the sleep supine position obstructs the upper airway, and some investigators try to treat with the help of a suspension of the hyoid bone to thyroid bone or the chin bone. At the early 1980s, a technique for upper airway using hyoid suspension was demonstrated, first for the animal model. In 1984, Kaya et al. reported the hyoid section as therapeutic surgical technique, and later another investigators made the same technique for humans. Initially, fixation of the hyoid on the chin was reported.

Technique

We can realize with local anesthesia or under general anesthesia in the multilevel surgery concept. The approach is through horizontal incision and careful dissection to the fat tissue in front of the hyoid level. The original technique from Riley et al. sectioned the stylohyoid ligaments from the lesser cornu. The Hormann modification preserved the ligament and the supra hyoid musculature and with little manual drill made two holes in the superior part of the thyroid cartilage. With a Grade III disease, steel wire is passed to medial part of the hyoid bone in the middle part of the muscular junction. With a strong push and pull, you can make the twist to better fixation. We recommend 2 days of drainage with suction.

The complications are a temporary dysphagia of up to 1 month. The postoperative soft diet is very important, a nasal CPAP respiration during the postoperative period is recommended.

There exists only one report in simple snoring: Hormann and Verse from Manheim reported 26 patients with primary snoring or UARS, treated with the hyoid suspension in 2004. Twenty-five of them (96%) reported a "significant reduction" in their snoring after operation. In 1994, Riley et al. reported a 53.3% as only procedure.

We suggest this procedure into the multilevel surgery concept like another technique because the success as unique treatment is poor.[11-16]

Anesthesia in Sleep-Disordered Breathing Patient

It is always very important communication with your anesthesiologist team to report the severity of the OSA or another type of SDB disease, the desaturation level and the mallamapati type.

For the anesthesiologist to maintain the upper airway is essential in patients with OSA. The anesthesia technique choice, the location of the surgery, the severity of symptoms of sleep apnea, availability of monitoring and trained personnel in the postoperative period is important because there are more complications after surgery for more than 3 hours. The use of long-term neuromuscular blockers should be as little as possible because it may exacerbate the collapse of the soft tissues of the upper airway, and that is the reason to suggest the awake intubation with a fiberoptic bronchoscope.

If it is possible, local anesthesia technique or regional blockades should be preferred in these patients.

During the orotracheal intubation, the anesthesiologist must be available in a flexible fiberoptic bronchoscope and laryngeal mask. In the extubation, he should be especially careful to always check the oxygen saturation, and do not fall into apnea.

Finally, the patients with severe OSA and less than 80% of desaturations is recommended the postoperative recovery in intensive care to avoid postoperative respiratory complications and if possible use the CPAP immediately after your procedure.

Complications in Sleep-Disordered Breathing Surgery

Immediate complications are:

Postsurgical edema with possible respiratory depression during the first few hours after surgery is a constant danger, be prepared to reintubation or emergent tracheotomy.

Hemorrhage is similar as the oral and nasal surgery.

Serious cardiorespiratory complications other than death occur in 1.5%.

Infection: preventive antibiotics administered an hour before surgery can help to reduce the risk and postoperation antibiotics like oral cephalexine are good option.

Wound dehiscence is relatively frequent, and is always important to put enough absorbable stitches

The impaired soft palate function is the velopharyngeal insufficiency due to aggressive tissue resection in the soft palate and midline area.

Mucus sensation in the throat is due to uvula resection because this organ had a salivary gland and works like a separator in this area, that is the reason to be more conservative in the midline with the uvula resection.

In the patients, postpalatal stiffness procedures present ulceration or mucosal erosion especially in the point of the needle insertion.

Another complications like voice changes, regurgitation, foreign body sensation and swallowing problems are less common.

The complications like bleeding and anesthesia recovery time can be avoided with special care in the surgical technique and in the postsurgical recovery time with special emphasis in patients with comorbidities like cardiovascular and metabolic diseases and morbid obesity.

The palatal stenosis is due to soft palate aggressive resection with posterior mucosa injury, the correction is very hard and difficult and the reopening is often only by millimeters, the palatal surgery is one of the most popular techniques but the difference than another procedures is the resection tissue removed, if you are aggressive, there exists the stenosis risk.

With the use of energy such as laser, radiofrequency or cautery is sometimes difficult to avoid the palate heals in a circle pattern and that is why we suggest the use of bisturi blade techniques to palatal surgeries.

REFERENCES

1. Guilleminault C. The sleep apnea syndrome. Med Times. 1979;107(6):59-63, 67.
2. Johns MW. A new method for measuring daytime sleepiness: the Epworth sleepiness scale. Sleep. 1991;14(6):540-5.
3. Stoohs R, Guilleminault C. Obstructive sleep apnea syndrome or abnormal upper airway resistance during sleep? J Clin Neurophysiol. 1990;7(1):83-92.
4. Ferris BG Jr, Mead J, Opie LH. Partitioning of respiratory flow resistance in man. J Appl Physiol. 1964;19:653-8.
5. Cole P, Haight JS. Mechanisms of nasal obstruction in sleep. Laryngoscope. 1984;94(12 Pt. 1):1557-9.
6. Kezirian EJ, Hohenhorst W, de Vries N. Drug induced sleep endoscopy: the VOTE classification. Eur Arch Otorhinolaryngol. 2011;268(8):1233-6.
7. Hoffstein V. Review of oral appliances for treatment of sleep disordered breathing. Sleep Breath. 2007;17(1):1-22.

8. Powell NB, Zonato AI, Weaver EM, et al. Radiofrequency treatment of turbinate hypertrophy in subjects using CPAP: a randomized double-blind placebo-controlled clinical pilot trial. Laryngoscope. 2001;111(10):1783-90.

9. Powell N, Riley R, Guilleminault C, et al. A reversible uvulopalatal flap for snoring and sleep apnea syndrome. Sleep. 1996;19(7):593-9.

10. Faye-Lund H, Djupesland G, Lyberg T. Glossopexia—evaluation of a new surgical method for treating obstructive sleep apnea syndrome. Acta Otolaryngol Suppl. 1992;492:46-9.

11. Patton TJ, Thawley SE, Water RC, et al. Expansion hyoidplasty: a potential surgical procedure designed for selected patients with obstructive sleep apnea syndrome. Experimental canine results. Laryngoscope. 1983;93(11 Pt 1):1387-96.

12. Van de Graf WB, Gottfried SB, Mitra J, et al. Respiratory function of hyoid muscles and hyoid arch. J Appl Physiol. 1984;57(1):197-204.

13. Kaya N. Sectioning the hyoid bone as a therapeutic approach for obstructive sleep apnea. Sleep. 1984;7(1):77-8.

14. Riley RW, Powell NB, Guilleminault C. Inferior sagittal osteotomy of the mandible with hyoid myotomy-suspension: a new procedure for obstructive sleep apnea. Otolaryngol Head Neck Surg. 1986:94(5):589-93.

15. Riley RW, Powell NB, Guilleminault C. Maxillofacial surgery and nasal CPAP. A comparison of treatment for obstructive sleep apnea syndrome. Chest. 1990;98(6):1421-5.

16. Riley RW, Powell NB, Guilleminault C. Obstructive sleep apnea and the hyoid: a revised surgical procedure. Otolaryngol Head Neck Surg. 1994;111(6):717-21.

PEDIATRIC VOICE DISORDERS: EVALUATION, PATHOLOGY AND INNOVATIONS

Scott Rickert

INTRODUCTION

The subspeciality of pediatric voice has advanced immensely in recent years. The widespread, simplistic view of the pediatric hoarse voice as something to outgrow is no longer true and it has acted as a disservice to the patients and their families. Voice disorders in children are increasingly being noted as a barrier to success in the school environment in terms of academic achievement and socialization.[1] Significant advances in pediatric voice over the past decade in evaluation, diagnosis, and management of pediatric voice disorders have improved both short-term and long-term outcomes for the dysphonic child.

Voice disorders in the pediatric population are as varied as they are in the adult population. There is a wide spectrum of "normal" voice in the pediatric population which varies by age, sex, and pubertal development. It is important to note that different adults (parents, teachers, speech language pathologists, pediatricians) interacting with the child may perceive the child's voice differently and may not be in agreement as to whether the child is dysphonic and the degree of dysphonia. This range of opinion provides a complicating factor in discerning the presence of a voice disorder and how to manage it appropriately. The prevalence of pediatric dysphonia in the literature is generally 6–9%, with one study noting dysphonia as high as 38%.[2-4] In studies of school-aged children, an incidence of hoarseness of 18–23% had been noted[5-9] with males more frequent than females. Interestingly, there is no difference in incidence in school-aged children identified as "child singers".[10] Parent questionnaires have been shown to score lower incidence than speech language pathologists or clinic evaluation[11] most likely leading to an under diagnosing of voice disorders in children in general. Past advice for the dysphonic child was to "let them outgrow it" which is poor advice. While some children may resolve their dysphonia with time, a longitudinal study of 203 dysphonic children showed that 35% continued to be dysphonic at 1 year and 9% continued to be so 4 years after diagnosis.[12]

General voice disorders may be congenital in nature or acquired. Congenital pathology include glottic web, vocal fold paralysis, glottic/subglottic stenosis, or a neurogenic cause. Acquired voice disorders can be due to trauma, previous intubation, post-surgical, infectious/inflammatory, functional, or via vocal overuse. Of note, Zalzal et al. reported that 15 of 16 patients undergoing laryngotracheal reconstruction were noted to be dysphonic[13] adversely affecting their post-reconstructive quality of life.

EVALUATION OF DYSPHONIA

History and Quality of Life Measurements

Evaluation of the dysphonic child is best done with a multidisciplinary team comprised of an otolaryngologist, a speech language pathologist (SPL), the child's pediatrician, the child's parents, and possibly further specialized care (gastroenterologist, pulmonologist, neurologist, allergist) in voice clinic setting with appropriate office-based equipment. Children are initially oriented to the entire voice clinic team and then are evaluated with a thorough history and physical with the airway nurse or team. A pediatric voice history (see below)[14] including the onset and progression of symptoms, voice variability, developmental history, typical voice activities and psychosocial environment is completed. Particular attention is made to their functional, structural, and neurological basis. Other factors such as allergies, medications, asthma, and reflux are important factors in the presentation of a dysphonic child. The parents also fill out a quality of life study to determine how disabled their child is from their dysphonia. One of these quality of life studies is the Pediatric Voice Handicap Index (pVHI) (Fig. 10.1), a recent

Basic questions of typical pediatric voice history
1. Please describe your child's voice
2. Please describe how your child's voice effects his/her overall ability to communicate within the home
3. Please describe how your child's voice effects his/her ability to communicate in social situations (play, recess, with friends)
4. Please describe how your child's voice effects his/her ability to communicate in educational settings
5. Are you satisfied with the support your child receives from his/her school regarding voice and communication?
6. If your child has a tracheotomy tube, are you satisfied with the level of support and care you receive from the schools?
7. Please describe the physical effort (e.g. gets tired, strains) your child experiences when using his/her voice
8. Do you feel like your child's voice has an impact on his/her general well-being and development? If yes, how?
9. Please describe any concerns your child has about his/her voice (e.g. sometimes embarrassed, sometimes avoids communication, never has a concern)

Pediatric Voice Handicap Index

Subject Number:_____   Date:_____

I would rate my/my child's talkativeness as the following (circle response)

1	2	3	4	5	6	7
Quiet listener			Average talker			Extremely talkative

To be filled out by Staff:
F= _____
P= _____
E= _____
Total= _____
Talkativeness: _____

Instructions: These are statements that many people have used to describe their voices and the effects of their voices on their lives. Circle the response that indicates how frequently you have the same experience.

0=Never   1=Almost never   2=Sometimes   3=Almost always   4=Always

		Rating				
F1	My child's voice makes it difficult for people to hear him/her	0	1	2	3	4
F2	People have difficult understanding my child in a noisy room	0	1	2	3	4
F3	At home, we have difficult hearing my child when he/she calls through the house	0	1	2	3	4
F4	My child tends to avoid communicating because of his/her voice	0	1	2	3	4
F5	My child speaks with friends, neighbors, or relatives less often because of his/her voice.	0	1	2	3	4
F6	People ask my child to repeat him/herself when speaking face-to-face	0	1	2	3	4
F7	My child voice difficulties restrict personal, educational and social activities.	0	1	2	3	4
P1	My child runs out of air when talking	0	1	2	3	4
P2	The sound of my child's voice changes throughout the day	0	1	2	3	4
P3	People ask, 'What's wrong with your child's voice?"	0	1	2	3	4
P4	My child's voice sounds dry, raspy, and/or hoarse	0	1	2	3	4
P5	The quality of my child's voice is unpredictable	0	1	2	3	4
P6	My child uses a great deal of effort to speak (e.g. straining)	0	1	2	3	4
P7	My child's voice is worse in the evening	0	1	2	3	4
P8	My child's voice "gives out" when speaking	0	1	2	3	4
P9	My child has to yell in order for others to hear him/her	0	1	2	3	4
E1	My child appears tense when talking to others because of his or her voice	0	1	2	3	4
E2	People seem irritated with my child's voice	0	1	2	3	4
E3	I find other people don't understand my child's voice problem	0	1	2	3	4
E4	My child is frustrated with his/her voice problem	0	1	2	3	4
E5	My child is less outgoing because of his/her voice problem	0	1	2	3	4
E6	My child is annoyed when people ask him/her to repeat	0	1	2	3	4
E7	My child is embarrassed when people ask him/her to repeat	0	1	2	3	4

Overall Severity Rating of Voice

(Please place "X" mark anywhere along this line to indicate the severity of child's voice; the verbal descriptions serve as a guide)

Normal   Severe

Fig. 10.1: Pediatric voice handicap index (pVHI)

adaption of the adult voice handicap index (VHI). It is a 23 question validated tool created in 2005 for the dysphonic child to evaluate the functional, emotional, and physical impact of a voice disorder on their daily activities.[14] It is a useful tool to follow their dysphonia through medical, surgical, and behavioral modifications. Other quality of life surveys in use include the Pediatric Voice Outcomes Survey (PVOS)[15] and the Pediatric Voice-Related Quality of Life questionnaire (PV-RQOL).[16]

Speech Language Pathology Assessment

An experienced speech language pathologist then performs subjective and objective evaluations of the voice, including an acoustic and perceptual evaluation. Objective assessments of a child's voice include measurements of fundamental frequency (pitch), range, sound pressure (loudness), intensity perturbation (shimmer) and frequency perturbation (jitter). These objective findings and the subjective assessment combine to give an overall impression of the degree of dysphonia of the patient. Voice recordings are non-invasive and generally well-tolerated by the patients. An electroglottography (EGG) uses surface electrodes to measure the glottic cycle and assess basic objective measures such as pitch and jitter. It also measures vocal hyperfunction in the case of incomplete glottic closure. Further aerodynamic measurements can provide a more detailed understanding of the glottic air flows and subglottic pressures. Currently, both PAS and Kay Pentax have aerodynamics equipment in use for adults, but still in the evaluation phase for children. The aerodynamic measurements combined with the objective and subjective voice data give a useful picture of the nature of the voice pathology.

Otolaryngology Assessment

Once the speech language pathologist completes the evaluation, the otolaryngologist then performs a thorough history and physical, including a videostroboscopy (Figs 10.2A and B) to best evaluate vocal fold pathology. Children more commonly have limitations in tolerating rigid stroboscopy than adults. Both rigid videostroboscopy and flexible videostroboscopy/laryngoscopy provide valuable information. Rigid videostroboscopy allows for a very clear picture with a narrow depth of field, but does lead to a higher gagging rate. Flexible videostroboscopy causes less gagging of the patient and allows for better visualization of connected speech. In the past, images from the flexible laryngoscopes were poorer in quality than the rigid ones. However, the recent advent of chip-in-tip technology (Kay Pentax), flexible videostroboscopy has similar image quality in the flexible laryngoscopes compared to that of rigid scopes. Both flexible and rigid stroboscopy are important tools in the evaluation of a dysphonic child (Figs 10.3A to C).

When performing a videostroboscopy, it is important to explain the procedure to the child and caregivers prior to starting. A monitor for viewing is helpful in patient cooperation and can provide initial feed-

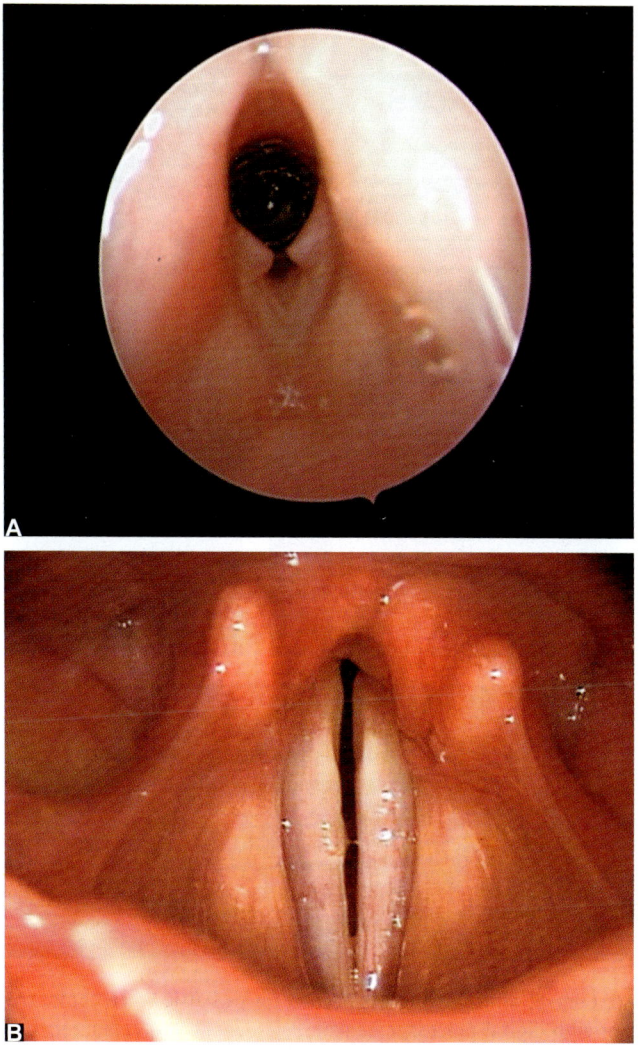

Figs 10.2A and B: Office evaluation images of dysphonia. (A) Bilateral post-intubation granulomas seen within conventional flexible laryngoscopy; (B) Bilateral vocal fold paresis seen with rigid stroboscopy

back therapy. The nasal passage is initially decongested with a mixture of 0.05% oxymetazoline and 1–2% lidocaine with careful attention to the overall dosage. Once the medication is noted to take effect, videostroboscopy is performed and recorded for further analysis. A contact microphone is used to time the stroboscopy appropriately. Specific laryngeal function noted on videostroboscopy include vocal fold motion, glottis closure, mucosal wave abnormalities, vocal fold irregularities, phase symmetry of the vocal fold motion, arytenoids movement, supraglottic compression or compensation, presence of erythema and/or edema and the presence of pooling of secretions adversely affecting the voice. All

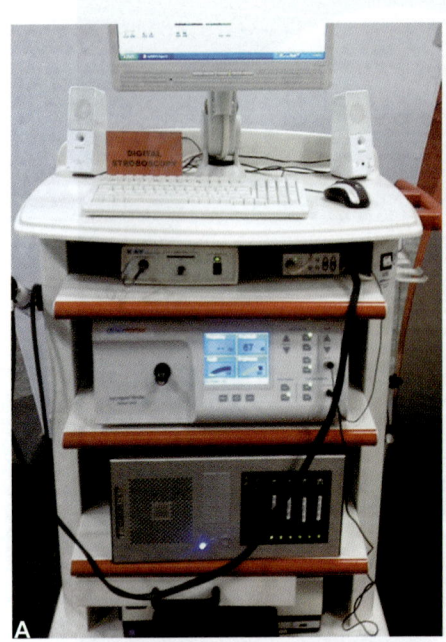
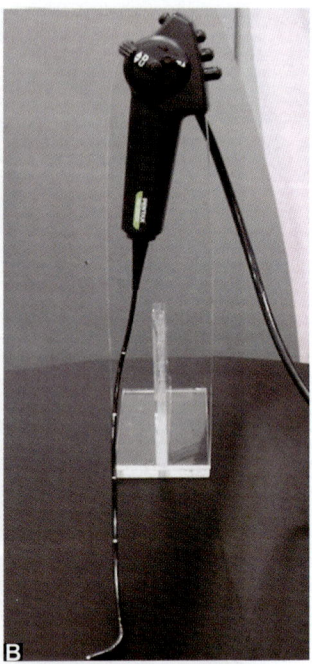
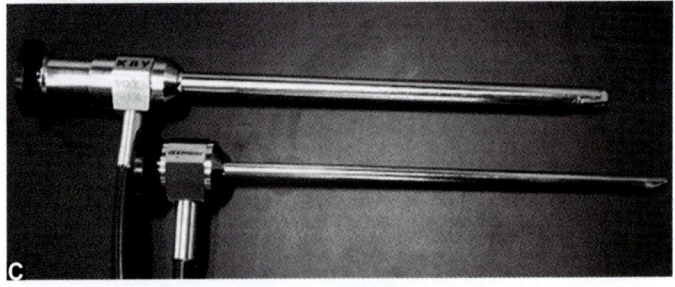

Figs 3A to C: General office equipment needed for pediatric voice clinic. (A) Videostroboscopy tower with digital processor, camera, microphone and computer; (B) Distal chip flexible laryngoscope; (C) Rigid 10-mm and 4-mm stroboscope

exams are recorded for easy analysis, playback and comparison to future and past exams.

Specific tasks have been designed by the speech language pathologist to accommodate children's shorter attention span while providing quick and accurate information of assessing their dysphonia. Oral-motor assessment of facial motion including range of motion, strength, speed and coordination helps assess neurologic involvement of the presenting voice disorder. Sampling of speech allows the speech pathologist to assess the voice quality with the GRBAS scale (Grade, Roughness, Breathiness, Asthenia, Strain).[17] Other perceptual assessments of speech such as the child's alertness, muscle tone, temperament, emotional maturity and social interaction are most easily assessed in interactions with the caregiver or sibling during free play.[18] If the child is unwilling to play freely than a structured activity, such as reading a book or telling a story, can be helpful in the evaluation process. Those noted to have poor attention or trouble socially interacting may need more directed behavioral therapy in conjunction with treatment of their voice disorder.

Observing respiratory breathing patterns during speech can impact speech patterns and produce a breathy voice. Children naturally take more frequent breaths than adults but may not coordinate breathing with speech. History may note a child that uses excessive effort to finish their sentences and/or has increasing hoarseness as the day progresses. Maximum phonation time is very helpful in measuring a child's efficiency of speech and breath support. Pitch and volume measurements can help map out the flexibility of the child's voice. Many with vocal disorders have certain inflexibility in their vocal range that negatively impacts their voice quality. This inflexibility can manifest as pitch inflexibility, volume inflexibility, or an inflection abnormality.

PATHOLOGY OF DYSPHONIA

The above history and exam techniques can help narrow the potential differential diagnosis. The most common pathological causes of dysphonia are further discussed individually.

Benign Lesions of the Vocal Folds

Benign lesions of the vocal folds such as nodules, polyps, or cysts are true physical impediments to good voicing. Vocal fold nodules are the most common cause of dysphonia in children and are more common in boys than girls in a bimodal distribution (3–5 years old and 8–10 years old). They always occur as paired, bilateral lesions. Only fourty-four percent of children with findings of bilateral nodules achieve normal voice by adolescence[19] with few proceeding to surgical intervention. These nodules are composed of fibronectin deposits layered in the superficial lamina propria of the vocal folds and are associated with thickened collagen in the basement membrane. They typically present at the midfold of the vocal fold, where the majority of "whip" is seen. An initial insult begins the process, which is exacerbated by repeated strain on the voice to overcome the dysphonia. This "weighted midfold" then causes further whip-like trauma with repeated use. Due to the large population who fail to resolve their dysphonia up to adolescence, it is important to treat these patients early with voice and behavioral therapy. Vocal fold nodule patients typically present with intermittent dysphonia which worsens with repeated voice use and improves with vocal rest. In assessing these patients, Shah and Nuss noted 75% exhibited significant muscle tension as a compensatory mechanism and 25% exhibited significant reflux.[20] They also noted the size of the nodules corresponded with the extent of muscle tension, which correlates with the idea of a "weighted midfold" causing whip-like trauma with repeated use. The gold standard for diagnosis is direct or indirect visualization of the lesion. Videostroboscopy is useful to distinguish between nodules and cysts, as the mucosal wave remains intact for midmembranous vocal fold nodules. Typical treatment includes voice and behavioral therapy tailored to their age with medical management if reflux is suggestive additive cause. Surgical intervention is extremely rare and may result in scarring and poor outcomes. Vocal fold cysts, congenital or acquired present similarly to vocal fold nodules. Congenital cysts can be mucus retention cysts or epidermal cysts. They are typically unilateral, but may cause a reactive lesion on the contralateral vocal fold. These are distinguished from vocal fold nodules by videostroboscopy as they impair the mucosal wave depending on its size and location. These lesions do not improve with voice and behavior therapy. Surgical excision with microlaryngoscopy is typically required with careful removal of the entire cyst wall to prevent recurrence. Occasionally, mucus-retention cysts are located in the subglottis causing a mild dysphonia. These are removed in a straightforward fashion using cold dissection, electrocautery, or laser. Vocal fold polyps, a gelatinous degeneration of the superficial lamina propria, are similar to vocal fold cysts and are not amenable to voice and behavior therapy. Surgical excision with careful microlaryngoscopy is typically required. Cold dissection is the standard surgical procedure with good results typically afterwards. Malignant lesions of the larynx are uncommon in children but if any suspicion arises, an endoscopic biopsy should be performed. Squamous cell carcinoma and rhabdomyosarcoma are the most frequent lesions in this group and should be treated appropriately if found on biopsy.

Juvenile Recurrent Respiratory Papillomatosis

Juvenile recurrent respiratory papillomatosis (RRP) is the most common neoplasm of the pediatric airway and is a more aggressive variant than the adult-onset type. Children with RRP typically present with dysphonia initially and may progress to stridor and respiratory distress if untreated. Seventy five percent of children with juvenile RRP initially present before age five.[21] Human papilloma virus (HPV) has been linked with the development of RRP[21] with HPV-6 and HPV-11 being the most common RRP-related subtypes.[22] HPV-11 has been noted to be the more aggressive subtype in RRP formation.[22] Control over HPV infectivity is important in treating further spread of disease and the recent advent of the quadrivalent HPV vaccine for women addresses HPV serotypes 6, 11, 16 and 18. The long-term results of this therapy in conjunction with RRP infectivity rates in children remains to be seen. Children with RRP may present with supraglottic, glottic, subglottic and/ or tracheal lesions and a complete visualization of the pharynx and larynx is necessary. Outpatient awake flexible fiberoptic laryngoscopy can give good visualization of the supraglottis and glottis in the patients with a stable airway. Those with airway compromise should be fully evaluated in the more controlled operating room setting. Papillomas can vary from small sessile lesions to large bulky and obstructive lesions. Surgical treatment is the mainstay of treatment for RRP. The challenge is to provide good voice and swallowing while maintaining an excellent airway with a disease known to have a latent, recurrent component. Careful microscopic laryngeal dissection is the gold standard for RRP. Currently, microscopic dissection with cold instrumentation is most commonly used, with the powered microdebrider being the most preferred.[23] Laser resection/ablation with a pulsed-dye laser (PDL) is currently less used due to studies showing poorer functional outcomes, higher cost,[24] and potential infectious particles in the smoke plume due to the laser ablation.[25] While the mainstay of treatment is surgical debulking and removal of clinically significant lesions, adjuvant therapy helps to provide a second layer of therapy targeted to prevent distal spread and increase the time needed between surgical procedures. Adjuvant therapies are typically recommended for children needing four or more surgical interventions a year, which accounts for up to 20% of those with juvenile RRP.[23] Intralesional injection of an antiviral cidofovir has been efficacious against HPV in uncontrolled studies[26] although, there have been reports of vocal scarring after cidofovir use.[27] Other treatments used include systemic interferon alpha, retinoic acid, acyclovir, indole-3-carbinol and heat-shock protein E7. Vaccination of adolescent and early adulthood women with the quadrivalent HPV vaccine is the most promising adjuvant therapy but long-term results of RRP infectivity rates in children remain to be seen.

Laryngeal Webs

Laryngeal webs may be congenital or acquired and typically affect the anterior margin of the vocal fold. In tethering a portion of the vocal folds together, the vibration of the true margin of the vocal fold changes and prevents a normal propagating mucosal wave. Repeated microlaryngoscopy with intervention is the most common cause of acquired laryngeal webs, which tend to be thinner than congenital webs. Congenital airway webs, 75% which are glottic in location, are formed due to a failure in recanalization of the glottis during development. A narrowed cricoid is associated with congenital glottic webs. Velocardiofacial syndrome, a genetic deletion of 22q, is also associated with congenital webs. Therefore, all congenital webs should have a genetic workup in their treatment plan.[28] Laryngeal webs are notoriously difficult to treat, as the goal is to restore a normal vibrating vocal fold with proper propagation of the mucosal wave. Typically, cold sharp dissection is used in an endoscopic fashion, with or without placement of a keel to try and prevent reformation of the glottis web. If the cricoid is severely narrowed, an anterior cricoid split (endoscopic or open) or laryngotracheoplasty may be indicated in addition.

Laryngopharyngeal Reflux

Incidence of gastroesophageal reflux disease (GERD) and laryngo-pharyngeal reflux (LPR) in children is difficult to obtain. Many infants have episodes of "spitting up" yet few present to the otolaryngologist with dysphonia. Young infants who do present with dysphonia should have reflux as a potential factor in their dysphonia. Premature infants have an especially high incidence of GERD, 63% in a study by Marino.[29] Fortunately, 55% resolve their symptoms by 10 months of age and 71% resolve by 18 months of age.[30] Higher incidence of infantile reflux is multifactorial: anatomic (more obtuse angle of His), neurologic (transient LES pressure relaxation) and physiologic (large feeds, supine feeding position). Signs of pharyngeal and laryngeal reflux include erythema/edema in the supraglottis and interarytenoid area, true vocal fold edema and cobblestoning of the trachea. Although objective measurements are not entirely specific or sensitive in the diagnosis of clinically significant GERD/LPR, they can be extremely helpful. Workup of GERD/LPR can include an upper gastroesophageal series, pH probe testing, impedance monitoring and upper endoscopy. An upper GI series includes a barium contrast swallowing while under fluoroscopy to examine the upper aerodigestive tract in real time. The combined team of a speech/swallowing therapist, a radiologist, a gastroenterologist and an otolaryngologist is used to best evaluate these studies. A 24-hour double pH probe is the current gold standard in the evaluation of reflux. This involves placing a probe in the nose with two separate measuring endpoints within the proximal and distal esophagus respectively. The probes measure the number of reflux events (pH < 4), the number of events greater than 5 minutes and the total and percentage of time below a pH of 4.[31] Endoscopic visualization of the aerodigestive tract is useful in assessing whether GERD/LPR played a significant role in the patient's dysphonia, especially in those who have failed medical management. One must examine the interarytenoid area carefully for the potential presence of a laryngeal cleft which would allow for aspiration of acidic contents into the trachea and be a significant chronic aspiration risk. Conservative management of LPR includes: elevation of the head of the bed; avoidance of caffeine, mint and citrus; avoidance of large meals before activity; avoidance of meals at least 2 hours before bedtime. Medical management typically includes: prokinetic medications (cisapride), H_2 receptor antagonists, or proton-pump inhibitors. Those with severe reflux who fail medical management can consider surgical management; typically, a Nissen fundoplication.

Neurogenic Voice Disorders

Neurogenic voice disorders include vocal fold paralysis/paresis and spasmodic dysphonia. Vocal fold paralysis/paresis can be congenital or acquired in nature and are due to: birth trauma, cardiovascular, iatrogenic, neurogenic, infectious, or idiopathic causes. Birth trauma related vocal fold paresis is typically associated with a forceps delivery, which places a traction injury on the recurrent laryngeal nerve. Up to 21% of bilateral vocal fold pareses have been attributed to birth trauma.[32] The neurological supply of the vocal fold musculature is from the vagus nerve, which supplies both the superior laryngeal nerve (SLN) and recurrent laryngeal nerve (RLN). The particularly long pathways of the recurrent laryngeal nerves — the right RLN travelling around the right subclavian and left RLN travelling around the aorta — make the nerves particularly vulnerable to surgical stretch, trauma related stretch injury and vascular abnormalities. Cardiac and vascular abnormalities such as vascular rings, ventricular septal defects and patent ductus arteriosus have been associated with concomitant vocal fold palsies[33] while it is most common to see an iatrogenic vocal fold paresis after the repair is completed. Thirty five percent of children undergoing cardiac surgery have been noted to have a unilateral vocal fold paresis postoperatively.[34] Central neurogenic causes include structural abnormality such as Arnold-Chiari malformation, cerebral palsy, tumors, or leukodystrophies. In the case of Arnold-Chiari, patients frequently present with bilateral vocal fold paresis due to the typical inferior cerebellar tonsil displacement and vagal rootlet traction, although, unilateral paresis has also been reported.[35] Other causes of vocal fold paresis include infectious causes (tuberculosis, West Nile virus, Lyme, poliomyelitis, pneumococcus, other viral infections)[36] intubation,[37] foreign bodies and chemotherapy.[38] Congenital bilateral voice fold paresis has been shown to have a genetic component in an X-linked and autosomal dominant fashion with incomplete penetrance.[39] Idiopathic causes of unilateral vocal fold paresis in children range from 7–41% depending on the study.[40,41] Evaluation of vocal fold paresis involves a detailed birth, family, and surgical history. Exam should note the nature of the stridor and its correlation with respiration (inspiratory stridor vs. expiratory stridor), the presence of suprasternal or substernal retractions and the presence of any craniofacial abnormalities, masses, or surgical scars. A thorough neurological evaluation, particularly the cranial nerve exam, is essential in picking up any more subtle findings. Flexible fiberoptic laryngoscopy allows excellent visualization of the vocal folds and helps to assess vocal fold motion and whether there is any decreased sensation in the supraglottic airway. It can also assess other concomitant issues such as laryngomalacia or the presence of a mass. If a flexible fiberoptic laryngoscopy is not tolerated, a rigid exam in the operating room yields excellent visualization and allows the surgeon to rule out vocal fold fixation by palpating the cricoarytenoid joint. A swallowing evaluation with video fluoroscopic visualization should be performed if there is any history of feeding issues as well. Imaging should be considered if there is no clear iatrogenic etiology of the vocal fold paresis. Laryngeal electromyography (EMG) is another useful tool in distinguishing vocal fold fixation from neurogenic paresis. This is easily done in the awake, cooperative adult, but relies on percutaneous placement of EMG needles for monitoring. In children, it is rare for such cooperation and general anesthesia or sedation is more commonly used if an EMG is deemed necessary. Treatment of vocal fold paresis depends on the etiology of the paresis. Many mild cases only need observation while the majority of more severe cases need surgical intervention. An honest, open discussion of the potential interventions as well as the need for voice therapy and postoperative care is important to the success of the intervention. Injection laryngoplasty, in which a "filler" material is injected into the paraglottic space, helps medialize the immobile vocal fold. This allows for better closure and better voicing, but does narrow the airway. Materials for injection include: autogenous fat, several formulations of hydroxylapatite and absorbable gelatin foam. Teflon was a material used in the past, but is rarely being used currently due to the risk of granulation formation.[42] Medialization thyroplasty (type I) is a more permanent solution to medializing the vocal fold by directly placing a permanent implant in the paraglottic space through an open procedure done under mild sedation. Implants materials include cartilage, silastic and Gore-Tex. In children, it is important to note that the vocal folds lie more inferior within the thyroid cartilage relative to an adult. This procedure can be combined with an arytenoid adduction if deemed necessary by the anatomy. Medialization thyroplasty has been done successfully in children[43] with good results, due its ability to precisely place the implant. Laryngeal reinnervation surgery through a primary neurorrhaphy can help provide tone and subsequent bulk to the deinnervated laryngeal musculature. Multiple nerves have been brought to anastomose with the recurrent laryngeal nerve including the ansa cervicalis or phrenic, as a bare nerve neurorrhaphy or with a muscle pedicle. Ansa cervicalis is the typical nerve of choice and it is identified just deep to the omohyoid muscle in the neck and anastomosed with the RLN proximal to the larynx. This anastomosis provides neurogenic signals to the laryngeal musculature providing tone and bulk, but not specific motion. This combination with an injection laryngoplasty provides immediate relief followed by decreased rate of atrophy over time. Studies have shown improvement in voice outcomes and better approximation of the vocal folds over time.[44] For patients with bilateral vocal fold paresis, many have a tracheotomy due to their airway compromise. There are several surgical interventions that can be implemented to provide a larger airway, sacrificing some voicing in the hopes of possible decannulation. Endoscopic resection such as laser posterior cordectomy or arytenoidectomy (typically using CO_2 laser) allows for a more appropriate airway while preserving the anterior margin of the true vocal fold for vibration and formation of reasonable voice. External lateralization and expansion laryngotracheoplasty also can be used to allow a more adequate airway. Both provide a larger airway by lateralizing the vocal fold (one directly and one indirect by placement of a midline graft), sacrificing quality of voice in the process.

Functional Voice Disorders

Functional voice disorders, those without structural or neurologic etiology, are more uncommon in children than in adults. Up to 40% of adult patients have functional voice disorders[45] while only 7% of children had a functional etiology.[46] Functional disorders affecting the voice include muscle tension dysphonia, psychogenic dysphonia and puberphonia. Muscle tension dysphonia is believed to be an imbalance in the laryngeal and perilaryngeal muscular activity, due to excessive vocal demand, altered adaptation, increased afferent tone, or psychological reasons. These patients have a history of periods of dysphonia or aphonia followed by periods of normal voice. Their voice typically has a strained quality, reduced volume and a disordered pitch. On physical exam, many are tender in the thyrohyoid space, but endoscopic exams have not elicited a standardized pattern of dysregulated closure.[47,48] Those with muscle tension dysphonia have been shown to have higher levels of anxiety, depression and emotionality than those with other voice disorders.[49] Psychogenic dysphonia is believed to be a subtype of muscle tension dysphonia brought on by psychological causes and leads to a similar imbalance of laryngeal musculature. Successful treatment of muscle tension dysphonia relies on behavioral therapy, psychological therapy if necessary and rebalancing of the laryngeal musculature. Massage of the laryngeal and perilaryngeal musculature[47] and topical lidocaine spray to the larynx[50] to decrease excessive sensitivity have proven to be effective further interventions. Puberphonia presents in adolescent males and is mainly characterized through its pitch instability. It can present in early adolescent and persist into early adulthood. The dysphonic voice is typically weak, thin, breathy and/or hoarse,[48] with the habituated use of falsetto with pitch breaks. Many consider puberphonia a distinct type of muscle tension dysphonia, as there is frequent tenderness of the thyrohyoid space. Behavioral therapy is the typical treatment for puberphonia, with attempts to relax the musculature and lower the laryngeal positioning, which has been shown to be successful in recent studies.[51] Botulinum toxin can be used in particularly resistant cases to relax the musculature.[52]

Paradoxical Vocal Fold Motion

Paradoxical vocal fold motion(PVFM) is a challenging problem in pediatric dysphonia. PVFM, also known as vocal cord dysfunction (VCD), is an episodic, inappropriate adduction of the vocal folds during respiration causing glottic obstruction. Frequently these patients are misdiagnosed with asthma. There are many defined etiologies for PVFM: (i) GERD/LPR, (ii) neurologic (brainstem compression, lower motor neuron, dystonias), and (iii) psychogenic (malingering or conversion). Typically reflux is more likely to be associated with laryngospasm than PVFM, but there are documented cases of PVFM with GERD/LPR as the only cause. Respiratory dystonias similar to spasmodic dysphonia (which causes a strained dysphonia in adductor spasmodic dysphonia and a breathy dysphonia in abductor spasmodic dysphonia), affects the respiration more than the voice. It may be accompanied by other dystonic movements such as spasmodic dysphonia, blepharospasm, oromandibular dystonia, torticollis, or tremors. These patients demonstrate consistent patterns of adduction during inspiration as well as during respiratory and speech tasks, which worsen with stress and exertion. They differ from patients with LPR induced laryngospasm, who have acute episodes of adduction rather than chronic adduction. They also differ from psychogenic patients who are not consistent in their adduction when not being actively observed. Other neurologic causes such as cortical injury, lower motor neuron disease, brainstem compression must be worked up appropriately as well. Psychogenic causes of dysphonia/PVFM are especially difficult to assess and are usually brought out by severe stress or anxiety. If the patient has any past history of psychiatric disease, this etiology must be considered. Organic causes must be ruled out first. Although psychogenic PVFM is most common in young woman and people in healthcare, it is not exclusively in those groups and must be considered for all patients. Other psychiatric disorders such as anxiety, depression and personality disorders may be present as well. Up to 70% of PVFM patients have a concomitant psychiatric diagnosis.[53] A classic finding is the worsening of symptoms when being actively observed. This can be due to a conversion disorder or due to malingering for secondary gain. The presence of PVFM is confirmed through adduction of the vocal folds during inspiratory phase of respiration. Typically, the anterior two third of the vocal folds medialize during inspiration while the posterior aspect forms a "posterior glottic chink". Since it presents intermittently, it can be difficult to visualize. Some use physical activity (such as a stationary bike) to stress the body and help bring out the disorder. Laryngeal EMG can be helpful in determining the laryngeal muscular contractility and synchronicity. Flow volume loop spirometry shows a typical inspiratory flattening of an extra-thoracic obstruction when symptomatic. Their flow volume loops are normal when asymptomatic.[54] Treatment depends on the cause, but visual biofeedback[55] remains a mainstay of treatment. Other noninvasive therapies with success include respiratory retraining, psychological education and behavior modification techniques. When a psychological component is involved, it is important to not initially imply it is the only cause. Initial treatment should begin with a speech language pathologist while treating the psychological and emotional component in tandem once the initial treatment has begun. Botulinum toxin has been used successfully to treat respiratory dystonias[56] with four of seven patients describing outstanding relief of symptoms post-injection. More aggressive surgical procedures such as arytenoidectomy or cordectomy are reserved for the very rare recalcitrant case.

Trauma and Laryngeal Reconstruction

Trauma, surgical trauma and/or reconstruction can affect the voice significantly, as most of these patients have significantly stenotic airways. As the subglottic airway is altered, the turbulent airflow adversely affects the ability for vocal fold vibration and proper respiration. Frequently, these patients prior to reconstruction need a tracheotomy for a safe and adequate airway. There are many different types of voicing disorder that arise from dysphonic patients after trauma, including glottic insufficiency, supraglottic compensation and phonation and pitch difficulties. The initial goals for those with stenotic airway are reconstruction with a reasonable airway for successful decannulation, safe swallowing and adequate voicing ability. And while patients with stenotic airways expectedly have poor voice quality, after-reconstruction voicing is not normal either. Zalzal notes 15 of 16 patients after laryngotracheoplasty had abnormal voicing.[13] However, as the quality of the surgical reconstruction improved, the quality of life measure of voicing ability has become more important in the postoperative management. Prior to reconstruction, it is important to systematically note the child's communication ability, condition of the laryngeal framework and the potential for voicing. If the child has a tracheotomy tube during the more formative years of language development, they may show signs of delay regardless of the quality of the reconstruction. A multidisciplinary team compromised of an otolaryngologist, a SPL, the child's pediatrician, the child's parents and possibly further specialized care (gastroenterologist, pulmonologist, neurologist, allergist) is essential for management success before and after reconstructive surgery. Initial evaluation must assess the child's ability to communicate (cry, babble, etc.), potential for voicing, and whether they have the ability to tolerate phonation with a one-way valve (Passy-Muir valve). An awake flexible fiberoptic laryngoscopy gives essential information of the anatomic structure of the laryngeal framework, and its mobility during attempted phonation. Once the surgical reconstructive intervention has been performed, it is important to provide effective guidance and treatment postoperatively. Specific school accommodations should be made for the child to be effectively heard and understood if their voice is dysphonic post-reconstruction. Quality of life rating scales help to assess the impact of the patient's dysphonia functionally and socially. These include the pVHI,[14] the PVOS,[15] and the PV-RQOL.[16] Postoperatively, patients undergo acoustic evaluation with voice recording and endoscopic laryngoscopy to try and catch postoperative dysphonic compensation mechanisms prior to them becoming a poor habit. This allows for voice therapy to be more effective and productive when needed. Future directions are geared towards prevention of surgical scarring and innovation of new technologies to provide both better airway and voice post-reconstruction.

In summary, potential treatments modalities are listed below.

Potential Treatment Modalities:
• *Voice Therapy:* Vocal hygiene and abuse reduction, hydration, increase/decrease glottal closure, decrease muscular tension, respiration, easy onset, improve coordination of respiration and phonation, resonance/voice placement, decrease ventricular phonation, raise/lower pitch, increase/decrease loudness, lower laryngeal placement, reinforce reflux treatment.
• *Medical Therapy:* Hydration, environmental allergies, allergic rhinitis, (avoidance of anti-histamines, use of intranasal steroid sprays), asthma (inhaled steroid preparations), gastroesophageal reflux disease [basic GERD precautions, antacids, prokinetic drugs (cisapride), H_2-receptor antagonists, proton-pump inhibitors (omeprazole)].
• *Surgical Therapy:* Conservative excision of benign lesions, "cold" techniques, microlaryngeal instruments, avoidance of laser on true vocal folds, submucosal infusion technique, management of laryngeal papillomas, medialization laryngoplasty, management of laryngeal fracture.

CONCLUSION

Pediatric voice disorders remain a varied and challenging evolving field. Voice disorders in children are increasingly being noted as a barrier to success in the school environment in terms of academic achievement and socialization.[1] As the evaluation of pediatric dysphonia is becoming more sophisticated, the potential treatment therapies. Comprehensive voice evaluation in children with subjective markers (voice history questionnaires, QOL studies) and objective markers (acoustic and perceptual evaluation, videostroboscopy, laryngoscopy) is essential in properly assessing pediatric dysphonia. And, while treatment for voice disorders has improved both short-term and long-term outcomes for the dysphonic child, there is still significant room for improvement. Further outcomes studies are needed to demonstrate the efficacy of the current and future comprehensive regiments (surgical, non-surgical, combined) toward pediatric dysphonia in this new and evolving field.

REFERENCES

1. Hirschberg J, Dejonckere PH, Hirano M, et al. Voice disorders in children. Int J Pediatr Otorhinolaryngol. 1995;32 Suppl:S109-25.
2. Carding PN, Roulstone S, Northstone K, et al. The prevalence of childhood dysphonia: a cross-sectional study. J Voice. 2006;20(4):623-30.
3. Lee L, Stemple JC, Glaze L, et al. Quick screen for voice and supplementary documents for identifying pediatric voice disorders. Lang Speech Hear Serv Sch. 2004;35(4):308-19.
4. Leeper L. Diagnostic examination of children with voice disorders: a low-cost solution. Lang Speech Hear Serv Sch. 1992;23:353-60.
5. Baynes RA. An incidence study of chronic hoarseness among children. J Speech Hear Disord. 1966;31(2):172-6.

6. Silverman EM. Incidence of chronic hoarseness among school-age children. J Speech Hear Disord. 1975;40(2):211-5.
7. Casper M, Abramson AL, Forman-Franco B. Hoarseness in children: summer camp study. Int J Pediatr Otorhinolaryngol. 1981;3(1):85-9.
8. Maddem BR, Campbell TF, Stool S. Pediatric voice disorders. Otolaryngol Clin North Am. 1991;24(5):1125-40.
9. Sederholm E, McAllister A, Dalkvist J, et al. Aetiologic factors associated with hoarseness in ten-year-old children. Folia Phoniatr Logop. 1995;47(5):262-78.
10. Bonet M, Casan P. Evaluation of dysphonia in a children's choir. Folia Phoniatr Logop. 1994;46(1):27-34.
11. McKinnon DH, McLeod S, Reilly S. The prevalence of stuttering, voice, and speech-sound disorders in primary school students in Australia. Lang Speech Hear Serv Sch. 2007;38(1):5-15.
12. Powell M, Filter MD, Williams B. A longitudinal study of the prevalence of voice disorders in children from a rural school division. J Commun Disord. 1989;22(5):375-82.
13. Zalzal GH, Loomis SR, Derkay CS, et al. Vocal quality of decannulated children following laryngeal reconstruction. Laryngoscope. 1991;101(4 Pt 1): 425-9.
14. Zur KB, Cotton S, Kelchner L, Baker S, Weinrich B, Lee L. Pediatric Voice Handicap Index (pVHI): a new tool for evaluating pediatric dysphonia. Int J Pediatr Otorhinolaryngol. 2007;71(1):77-82. Epub 2006 Oct 13.
15. Hartnick CJ. Validation of a pediatric voice quality-of-life instrument: the pediatric voice outcome survey. Arch Otolaryngol Head Neck Surg. 2002;128(8):919-22.
16. Boseley ME, Cunningham MJ, Volk MS, et al. Validation of the Pediatric Voice-Related Quality-of-Life Survey. Arch Otolaryngol Head Neck Surg. 2006;132(7):717-20.
17. Hirano M. Clincial Examination of the Voice. New York: Springer-Verlag Wein; 1981.
18. Batshaw ML. Children with Disabilities, 5th edition. Maryland: Paul H. Brookes Publishing Company; 1997.
19. De Bodt MS, Ketelslagers K, Peeters T, et al. Evolution of vocal fold nodules from childhood to adolescence. J Voice. 2007;21(2):151-6.
20. Shah RK, Woodnorth GH, Glynn A, et al. Pediatric vocal nodules: correlation with perceptual voice analysis. Int J Pediatr Otorhinolaryngol. 2005;69(7):903-9.
21. Derkay CS, Darrow DH. Recurrent respiratory papillomatosis. Ann Otol Rhinol Laryngol. 2006:115(1):1-11.
22. Wiatrak BJ, Wiatrak DW, Broker TR, et al. Recurrent respiratory papillomatosis: a longitudinal study comparing severity associated with human papilloma viral types 6 and 11 and other risk factors in a large pediatric population. Laryngoscope. 2004;114(11 Pt 2 Suppl 104):1-23.
23. Schraff S, Derkay CS, Burke B, et al. American Society of Pediatric Otolaryngology members' experience with recurrent respiratory papillomatosis and the use of adjuvant therapy. Arch Otolaryngol Head Neck Surg. 2004;130(9):1039-42.

24. El-Bitar MA, Zalzal GH. Powered instrumentation in the treatment of recurrent respiratory papillatomatosis: an alternative to the carbon dioxide laser. Arch Otolaryngol Head Neck Surg. 2002;128(4):425-8.

25. Kashima HK, Kessis T, Mounts P, et al. Polymerase chain reaction identification of human papillomavirus DNA in CO2 laser plume from recurrent respiratory papillomatosis. Otolaryngol Head Neck Surg. 1991;104(2):191-5.

26. Pransky SM, Magit AE, Kearns DB, et al. Intralesional cidofovir for recurrent respiratory papillomatosis in children. Arch Otolaryngol Head Neck Surg. 1999;125(10):1143-8.

27. Lee AS, Rosen CA. Efficacy of cidofovir injection for the treatment of recurrent respiratory papillomatosis. J Voice. 2004;18(4):551-6.

28. Miyamoto RC, Cotton RT, Rope AF, et al. Association of anterior glottis webs with velocardiofacial syndrome (chromosome 22q11.2 deletion). Otolaryngol Head Neck Surg. 2004;130(4):415-7.

29. Marino AJ, Assing E, Carbone MT, et al. The incidence of gastroesophageal reflux in preterm infants. J Perinatol. 1995;15(5):369-71.

30. Khalaf MN, Porat R, Brodsky NL, et al. Clinical correlations in infants in the neonatal intensive care unit with varying severity of gastroesophageal reflux. J Pediatr Gastroenterol Nutr. 2001;32(1):45-9.

31. Sutphen JL. Pediatric gastroesophageal reflux disease. Gastroenterol Clin North Am. 1990;19(3):617-29.

32. Emery PJ, Fearon B. Vocal cord palsy in pediatric practice: a review of 71 cases. Int J Pediatr Otorhinolaryngol. 1984;8(2):147-54.

33. Dedo DD. Pediatric vocal cord paralysis. Laryngoscope. 1979;89(9 Pt 1):1378-84.

34. Truong MT, Messner AH, Kerschner JE, et al. Pediatric vocal fold paralysis after cardiac surgery: rate of recovery and sequelae. Otolaryngol Head Neck Surg. 2007;137(5):780-4.

35. de Gaudemar I, Roudaire M, François M, et al. Outcome of laryngeal paralysis in neonates: a long term retrospective study of 113 cases. Int J Pediatr Otorhinolaryngol. 1996;34(1-2):101-10.

36. Amin AR, Koufman JA. Vagal neuropathy after upper respiratory infection: a viral etiology? Am J Otolaryngol. 2001;22(4):251-6.

37. Cohen SR. Pseudolaryngeal paralysis: a postintubation complication. Ann Otol Rhinol Laryngol. 1981;90(5 Pt 1):483-8.

38. Burns BV, Shotton JC. Vocal fold palsy following vinca alkaloid treatment. J Laryngol Otol. 1998;112(5):485-7.

39. Cunningham MJ, Eavey RD, Shannon DC. Familial vocal cord dysfunction. Pediatrics. 1985;76(5):750-3.

40. Cohen SR, Geller KA, Birns JW, et al. Laryngeal paralysis in children: a long-term retrospective study. Ann Otol Rhinol Laryngol. 1982;91(4 Pt 1):417-24.

41. Zbar RI, Smith RJ. Vocal fold paralysis in infants twelve months of age or younger. Otolaryngol Head Neck Surg. 1996;114(1):18-21.

42. O'Leary MA, Grillone GA. Injection laryngoplasty. Otorlaryngol Clin North Am. 2006;39(1):43-54.

43. Link DT, Rutter MJ, Liu JH, et al. Pediatric type I thyroplasty: an evolving procedure. Ann Otol Rhinol Laryngol. 1999;108(12):1105-10.

44. Tucker HM. Long-term preservation of voice improvement following surgical medialization and reinnervation for unilateral vocal fold paralysis. J Voice. 1999;13(2):251-6.

45. Roy N. Functional dysphonia. Curr Opin Otolaryngol Head Neck Surg. 2003;11(3):144-8.

46. Campbell TF, Dollaghan CA, Yaruss JS. Disorders of language, phonology, fluency, and voice in children: indicators for referral. In: Bluestone CD, Stool SE (Eds). Pediatric Otolaryngology, 4th edition. Philadelphia: Saunders; 2003. pp. 1773-87.

47. Roy N, Ford CN, Bless DM. Muscle tension dysphonia and spasmodic dysphonia: the role of manual laryngeal tension reduction in diagnosis and management. Ann Otol Rhinol Laryngol. 1996;105(11):851-6.

48. Morrison MD, Rammage LA. The Management of Voice Disorders. California: Singular Publishing Group; 1994.

49. Roy N, Bless DM, Heisey D. Personality and voice disorders: a multitrait-multidisorder analysis. J Voice. 2000;14(4):521-48.

50. Dworkin JP, Meleca RJ, Simpson ML, et al. Use of topical lidocaine in the treatment of muscle tension dysphonia. J Voice. 2000;14(4):567-74.

51. Dagli M, Sati I, Acar A, et al. Mutational falsetto: intervention outcomes in 45 patients. J Laryngol Otol. 2008;122(3):277-81.

52. Woodson GE, Murry T. Botulinum toxin in the treatment of recalcitrant mutational dysphonia. J Voice. 1994;8(4):347-51.

53. Altman KW, Mirza N, Ruiz C, et al. Paradoxical vocal fold motion: presentation and treatment options. J Voice. 2000;14(1):99-103.

54. Guss J, Mirza N. Methacholine challenge testing in the diagnosis of paradoxical vocal fold motion. Laryngoscope. 2006;116(9):1558-61.

55. Bastian RW, Nagorsky MJ. Laryngeal image biofeedback. Laryngoscope. 1987;97(11):1346-9.

56. Brin MF, Blitzer A, Stewart C, et al. Treatment of spasmodic dysphonia (laryngeal dystonia) with local injections of botulinum toxin: review and technical aspects. In: Blitzer A, Brin M, Sasaki C (Eds). Neurological Disorders of the Larynx. New York: Thieme; 1993. pp.225.

Chapter

11

WHAT'S NEW IN OTITIS MEDIA

Abbas A Anwar, Anil K Lalwani

ABSTRACT

Otitis media (OM) is a common infection in children throughout the world. Ongoing clinical and basic science research has led to an evolution in our understanding of the pathophysiology, diagnosis, and treatment of OM. The goal of this chapter is to explore recent development in the field of OM. Specifically, the role of biofilms in the pathogenesis of OM, the evolving bacteriology of OM, the effects of vaccination, the controversies regarding the use of antibiotics in the treatment of OM, and the potential short and long-term complications will be reviewed.

OVERVIEW

Otitis media is the leading cause for physician visits by children in the United States,[1] and continues to be the most common reason for childhood antimicrobial therapy.[2] Despite advances in public health and medical care, middle ear infections are still prevalent around the world.[3] Even more, annual costs in the US for OM management are estimated to be between $3 billion and $5 billion,[4] with indirect costs likely being considerably higher.[5] Consequently, accurate diagnosis, appropriate treatment, and up-to-date knowledge of OM can help to significantly optimize health care utilization and expenditures.

Acute otitis media (AOM) and otitis media with effusion (OME) are the main classifications of the OM continuum.[6] The pathophysiology of both conditions is multifactorial, but involves Eustachian tubal dysfunction with impaired clearance and pressure regulation of the middle ear.[1] Impairment of these functions can result in a middle ear effusion, which establishes an environment that is conducive to bacterial growth. If the effusion persists, and drainage and aeration are not restored, AOM can ensue. AOM is defined as an acute inflammation of the middle ear associated with a rapid onset of signs and symptoms, such as otalgia and fever. Otoscopic examination of AOM is most frequently characterized by redness and bulging of the tympanum, suggesting the presence of a middle ear effusion. While viruses alone account for 20% of the AOM cases, coinfection with bacteria is more prevalent and is seen in about 65% of the cases.[7] Among the viruses, respiratory syncytial virus, adenovirus and rhinovirus are most commonly associated with AOM[8-10] while the most prevalent bacteria include *Streptococcus pneumoniae*, non-typeable *Haemophilus influenzae* and *Moraxella catarrhalis*.[11]

Otitis media with effusion is defined as an effusion of the middle ear that is not associated with any symptoms of acute inflammation, such as pain or fever. Instead, symptoms may include mild conductive hearing loss and aural fullness, although asymptomatic OME is not uncommon. Examination often reveals an opacification of the tympanic membrane and pneumatic otoscopy will frequently show a retracted or convex tympanum with impaired mobility.[6] The inciting factor leading to OME is frequently residual inflammation and infection after an initial bout of AOM, although de novo OME from tubal dysfunction can also occur.[12] Like AOM, *H. influenzae, S. pneumoniae* and *M. catarrhalis* are the most frequent microorganisms isolated from OME.[13] However, unlike AOM, influenza virus and enterovirus have been shown to be the most common viral pathogens.[10] Furthermore, the idea of bacterial biofilms, which will be discussed further in this chapter, is a field of growing interest and may also play a significant role in the pathogenesis of OME.[14]

In the end, despite years of clinical experience with OM, the pathophysiology, diagnosis, and treatment of this common disorder remains challenging and controversial. Abundant research continues to be undertaken leading to a constantly evolving understanding of OM. This chapter will discuss the controversies and recent developments in the field of OM. Specifically, we will explore the role of biofilms in the pathogenesis of OM, the evolving bacteriology of OM and the effects of vaccination, the controversies regarding the use of antibiotics in the treatment of OM, and the potential short and long-term complications.

BIOFILMS

Otitis media with effusion was long thought to be noninfectious in nature as bacteria could rarely be cultured from the middle ear.[15,16] In fact, it was once suggested that OME was actually a sterile inflammatory process that was the result of a persistence of endotoxin or cytokines in the middle ear after bacterial eradication by antimicrobials.[17] However, more recently, techniques using polymerase chain reaction (PCR) have shown that a large proportion of OME fluid actually harbor viable pathogenic bacteria up to 4 weeks after antibiotic therapy.[18-20] This persistent infection in the setting of negative cultures is often seen in other chronic infections caused by an entity known as bacterial biofilms, and thus, led to the hypothesis that similar bacterial biofilms may have a significant role in the pathogenesis of OME.[18]

Bacterial biofilms are an organized community of metabolically quiescent bacteria usually adherent to a surface and embedded in a matrix rich in extracellular polymeric substances (Fig. 11.1).[21] They are often found in natural environments and are increasingly being discovered in the human body, both on implanted devices and on certain tissue surfaces. Their unique structure and metabolic properties not only make them difficult to culture, but also extremely resistant to common antibiotics, as they have been implicated in several chronic bacterial infections.[22,23]

Initial studies exploring the role of bacterial biofilms in OME examined chinchillas with experimentally induced H. influenzae OM.[14,24] These studies found direct visual evidence by scanning electron microscopy that bacterial biofilms form on the animal's middle-ear mucosa (MEM). A more recent study involving humans examined MEM biopsies from 26 children undergoing tympanostomy tube placement for OME and 8 MEM specimens from control patients undergoing cochlear implantation.[25] This study found direct visual evidence of bacterial biofilms in 92% of biopsy samples from those children with OME, while all 8 control specimens showed no evidence of biofilm growth. Since then, several other studies have shown similar results, and have led to growing support and acceptance of the integral role of bacterial biofilms in the pathogenesis and chronicity of OME.[26-28]

More investigations are currently being performed to gain a better understanding of biofilm development in an effort to optimize treatment

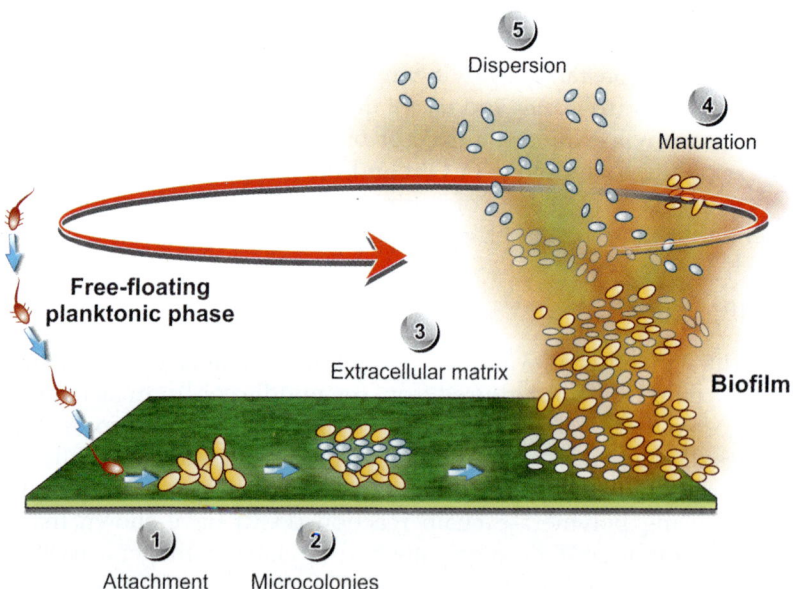

Fig. 11.1: Biofilm formation. Bacterial biofilm formation requires the attachment of the bacteria to host surface, formation of microcolonies, deposition of extracellular matrix by the microcolonies, maturation of the biofilm within the extracellular matrix, and its subsequent dispersion that could lead to further infection or biofilm formation

strategies. Current research has aimed at exploring a possible association between adenoidal biofilms and chronic middle ear infections. A recent study utilizing *16SrRNA* gene-based pyrosequencing analysis to characterize microbial communities in the middle ear, adenoid and tonsils of pediatric patients with OME found that the adenoid microbiota was the most complex, and demonstrated the greatest overlap with the tonsil and the middle ear.[29] These results suggest that the adenoid may actually serve as a bacterial reservoir for both middle ear and tonsillar disease. Although this hypothesis has not been definitively proven, it has been shown that the adenoid tissues of children with OME contain denser surface biofilms compared with those without OME.[30] Even more, a recent review article found a significant benefit of adenoidectomy in terms of resolving middle ear effusions in OME.[31] Thus, further investigation may reveal whether adenoidectomy may be beneficial in preventing or eradicating biofilm formation in the middle ear and whether it is warranted as an adjunct to tympanostomy tube placement (Fig. 11.2).

Research evaluating the efficacies of various antibiotics has also been performed, although a recent review article specifically examining the treatment options available for biofilms in otolaryngologic infections

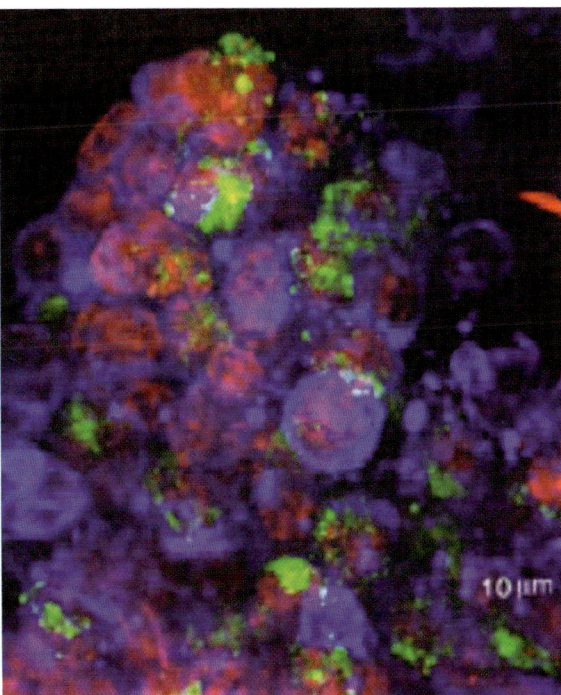

Fig. 11.2: Adenoidal Bacterial Biofilm. In situ bacterial distribution and localization within human pediatric adenoidal tissue visualized by 16 S FISH using the eubacterial 338 probe (green) showing both intracellular bacterial aggregates and extracellular bacterial biofilms. The eukaryotic F-actin cytoskeleton is stained with phalloidin (purple), and the nuclei are stained with Syto 59 (red)

Source: Figure courtesy of Garth D. Ehrlich, Laura Nistico and J. Christopher Post

showed that the utility of antibiotics alone in the treatment of biofilm-related infections is minimal.[32] The same study found that mupirocin irrigation, gentian violet and thiamphenicol glycinate acetylcysteine effectively eradicated biofilms, while physical disruption, surfactants and probiotics were also beneficial. In addition, there has been some promising research aimed at targeting bacterial communication within biofilms as a potential means to disrupt polymicrobial biofilm development in OM.[33] As it stands now though, further research must be done to gain a better understanding of the pathophysiology of biofilms in OME and the potential therapeutic targets that may exist.

BACTERIOLOGY OF OM AND THE EFFECTS OF VACCINATION

OM is a polymicrobial disease, with three different bacteria that have persisted as the predominant pathogens—*Streptococcus pneumoniae*, non-typeable *Haemophilus influenzae*, and *Moraxella catarrhalis*.[11] The introduction of the 7-valent pneumococcal conjugate vaccine (PCV7) in the US in 2000 resulted in rapid shifts in the microbiology of OM (Table 11.1). Before the introduction of the vaccine, multiple studies identified *S. pneumoniae* as the most common AOM pathogen (25–40% of all AOM cases), with non-typeable *H. influenzae* second (23–30%) and *M. catarrhalis* third

Table 11.1: Past and present vaccines and their effects		
Vaccine	*Coverage*	*Consequences/Notes*
PCV7	Serotypes 4, 6B, 9V, 14, 18C, 19F, and 23F	• Licensed by FDA in 2000 • Reduced the rate of invasive pneumococcal disease and pneumococcal AOM • Reduced detection of pneumococcal strains included in the vaccine • Resulted in the emergence of pneumococcal strains not included in the vaccine and *H. influenzae* • 6–7% reduction in overall AOM episodes • More substantial reduction in OM-related healthcare costs
PCV13	Serotypes 1, 3, 4, 5, 6A, 6B, 7F, 9V, 14, 18C, 19A, 19F, and 23F	• Licensed by FDA in Feb 2010 • Supplants PCV-7 and expands coverage to 6 additional serotypes • Further studies necessary to monitor efficacy
PHiD-CV	Serotypes 1, 4, 5, 6B, 7F, 9V, 14, 18C, 19F, 23F + Protein D from *H. influenzae*	• Protects against both pneumococcal OM and *H. influenzae* OM • Shown to reduce the overall occurrence of AOM by 34% • Currently, not licensed in the US, but has been approved in over 40 countries

(10–15%).[34,35] However, early studies after the initiation of the vaccine demonstrated that strains of *S. pneumoniae* expressing capsular subtypes included in the PCV7 were detected less often as causes of AOM and invasive pneumococcal disease (IPD).[36,37] In fact, it has been proven that the vaccine effectively reduced the overall incidence of both IPD and pneumococcal AOM.[38-40]

Non-typeable *H. influenzae* then emerged as the most common AOM pathogen between 2001 and 2003.[41] However, since the PCV7 did not include all pneumococcal capsular subtypes, non-PCV7 serotypes began to emerge, most notably serotype 19A.[42,43] These studies found that the prevalence of pneumococcal serotype 19A actually increased by up to 34% between 2000 and 2005. And a more recent study, examining new patterns in otopathogens 6–8 years after the introduction of PCV7 showed that the frequency of non-PCV7 pneumococcal serotypes is now essentially equal to that of non-typeable *H. influenzae*.[44]

Thus, although *S. pneumoniae* strains expressing vaccine-type serotypes virtually disappeared in vaccinated children,[44] the emergence of non-PCV7 pneumococcal serotypes and non-typeable *H. influenzae* cast some doubt upon the true efficacy of the vaccine in reducing the overall incidence of AOM episodes. In fact, a recent review article consisting of over 46,000 patients found only a marginal 6–7% reduction in overall AOM episodes since the introduction of the PCV7.[45] Even such small reductions, however, were shown to substantially reduce OM-related healthcare utilization and antibiotic prescriptions.[46,47] Nevertheless, additional studies found that many non-PCV7 pneumococcal serotypes were becoming penicillin resistant.[43,48-50] Thus, the initial benefits of the vaccine appeared to be eroding, not only for OM but also for IPD,[51] and a more comprehensive vaccine was likely necessary.

Consequently, in February 2010, a novel 13-valent pneumococcal conjugate vaccine (PCV13) was licensed for use among US children aged 6 weeks to 71 months. In addition, a 23-valent pneumococcal polysaccharide vaccine was also approved for targeted use in children aged 2–18 years who have underlying medical conditions that increase their risk for contracting pneumococcal disease or experiencing complications of pneumococcal disease, if infected.[52] The PCV13 supplants PCV7 and expands its coverage by including six additional capsular polysaccharide antigens not included in the original vaccine.[52] Pre-licensure studies demonstrated this new vaccine to be at least as immunogenic as PCV7 for common serotypes, and to induce comparable levels of antibodies for serotypes unique to PCV13.[53,54] While the efficacy of the new vaccine against IPD and OM has not yet been evaluated, one study has estimated that the introduction of the PCV13 may result in a nearly 90% reduction in IPD from baseline (1998–1999) in children.[55] Further studies will be required to monitor the new vaccine's efficacy in reducing the prevalence of pneumococcal disease and OM, in general.

Recently, a new 10-valent pneumococcal non-typeable *Haemophilus influenzae* protein D conjugate vaccine (PHiD-CV) was introduced and has been licensed in more than 40 countries, including nations in Europe.[56] This vaccine is unique in that it contains both polysaccharides derived from 10 different strains of pneumococcal bacteria as well as protein D from non-typeable *H. influenzae*. By using protein D as an active carrier protein for pneumococcal polysaccharides, PHiD-CV has been shown to not only protect against pneumococcal OM, but also against OM due to non-typeable *H. influenzae*, and thus reduce the overall occurrence of AOM by 34%.[57] In addition, the vaccine has proven to be immunogenic in infants and has a safety profile similar to that of the PCV7.[56] And although it has not been approved in the US, a large European study examining the outcome and cost of this vaccine in four countries found that the PHiD-CV prevented more deaths and resulted in lower costs when compared with the PCV-7.[58]

As these new vaccines begin to be implemented, further studies must be undertaken to monitor their efficacies, and determine the evolution and susceptibilities of the associated otopathogens. Research to compare the efficacies and cost-effectiveness of the new PCV13 and the PHiD-CV may also be beneficial. Furthermore, the possibility of developing a tri-bacterial vaccine that confers protection against *S. pneumoniae*, *H. influenzae* and *M. catarrhalis* is not beyond reality, as several recent studies have been examining the structure of *M. catarrhalis* for potential vaccine antigens.[59,60] In the end, as OM is a costly disease associated with a high degree of morbidity and antibiotic consumption, prevention may be the most prudent strategy. As additional knowledge is gathered concerning the bacteriology and immune mechanisms in the middle ear, a more comprehensive vaccine that effectively targets the true polymicrobial nature of OM may help to significantly reduce the disease burden globally.

CONTROVERSIES OF ANTIBIOTIC THERAPY IN OM

The use of antibiotics for the treatment of AOM has been the primary mode of therapy since the 1950s, when initial studies showed that antimicrobial therapy improved patient outcome.[61] Since then, AOM has quickly become the most commonly cited indication for antibiotic therapy in children.[62] However, with growing concern for rising costs and antimicrobial resistance, studies have now called for these agents to be used judiciously in the treatment of AOM.[63-65] Nevertheless, there is still no consensus regarding the optimal treatment strategy.[66]

The clinical decision to treat or not to treat children with AOM has been the main controversy revolving around AOM therapy, as the choice is not always clear.[67] A watchful waiting strategy, in which medications are withheld from children unless they do not improve spontaneously, has long been utilized in several European nations.[68] For example, guidelines in the UK suggest immediate antibiotic therapy only for children younger than 2 years of age, with bilateral AOM or for children presenting with ottorhea. All other patients, according to these guidelines, should not be prescribed antibiotics initially.[69] The widespread adoption of this strategy was based on the results of several clinical trials that showed a relatively high rate of spontaneous improvement in children with AOM.[68,70,71]

As more studies began to advocate the use of this watchful waiting strategy,[72-74] the approach began to gain interest in the US. As a result, in 2004, the American Academy of Pediatrics (AAP) and the American Academy of Family Physicians (AAFP) jointly released a clinical practice guideline for the management of AOM in children aged 6 months to 12 years (Table 11.2).[75] A watchful waiting strategy was included in the guideline for children 2 years of age or older without severe symptoms or with an uncertain diagnosis. However, more notably, the guideline also included a watchful waiting approach in younger children from the ages of 6–23 months in whom a diagnosis of AOM was uncertain and in whom the illness was "non-severe" which was defined as the presence of mild otalgia and a temperature of less than 39°C during the preceding 24 hours. If the patient failed to improve within 48–72 hours, antibacterial therapy could then be initiated. The guideline also made specific antibiotic recommendations on the basis of illness severity and treatment response, with amoxicillin as the first-line therapy due to its safety, low cost and narrow microbiologic spectrum.[76] Finally, the guideline strongly recommended analgesic therapy for those patients experiencing pain.

Although the AAP/AAFP guidelines are still in effect today, their true implementation by clinicians in the US may be questionable. For example, one survey found that while most primary care physicians agreed with the watchful waiting approach, they infrequently chose it.[77] Furthermore, a larger and more recent study found that the percentage of pediatric AOM visits during which an antibiotic was not prescribed did not increase significantly since the release of the guidelines, shifting only from 11% to 16%.[78] This apparent reluctance in employing the guideline's recom-

Table 11.2: Current management of AOM (US guidelines)		
Age	Antibiotics	Watchful waiting
< 6 months	• Amoxicillin 80–90 mg/kg/day for 10 days • If severe illness[a]: amoxicillin (90 mg/kg/d)-clavulanate (6.4 mg/kg/d)	• No watchful waiting option
6 months–2 years	• Antibiotics as above, if certain diagnosis[c] or severe illness	• Watchful waiting, if uncertain diagnosis and non-severe illness[b]
≥ 2 years	• Antibiotics as above, if severe illness	• Watchful waiting, if uncertain diagnosis or non-severe illness

a Severe illness: moderate to severe otalgia or fever ≥39°C in the past 24 hours
b Non-severe illness: mild otalgia and fever < 39°C
c Certain diagnosis: meets all of the following three criteria: (1) rapid onset; (2) signs of middle ear effusion, and (3) signs and symptoms of middle ear inflammation

mendations may be due to physicians' perceptions of parental unwilling-ness to accept an observational strategy and subsequent difficulties with follow-up care.[77]

To complicate matters even further, recent studies have begun to question the use of this watchful waiting approach, especially in children younger than 2 years of age. Although several studies have appeared to appropriately justify the strategy,[79] some experts have suggested that many of these clinical trials suffered from important limitations, such as the inclusion of only a small number of young children, the use of subop-timal antimicrobial agents or dosages, and perhaps most importantly, the lack of stringent diagnostic criteria.[80-82] These methodological flaws may have biased many of the studies to include either children who did not truly have AOM as a result of over- or mis-diagnosis, or children who were more likely to recover spontaneously, such as older children or those with more mild disease.[75,83]

Thus, in order to avoid these potential flaws, a recently published randomized, double-blind, placebo-controlled trial by Tähtinen et al. utilized a specific set of stringent diagnostic criteria for AOM, in order to ensure proper diagnosis and patient selection.[84] The criteria included specific pneumatic otoscopic findings suggestive of middle-ear fluid, explicit signs of acute middle ear inflammation and other acute symptoms, such as fever, otalgia or respiratory difficulties. The study then compared the use of amoxicillin-clavulanate or placebo for 7 days in children 6–35 months of age who specifically met these diagnostic standards. In the end, the trial appeared to reaffirm the use of immediate antibiotic therapy in younger children, as it found that amoxicillin-clavulanate was superior to placebo for the treatment of AOM with respect to the duration of acute signs of illness. In fact, the antibacterial agent reduced the risk of treatment failure by 62%, as there was a significantly better treatment result with respect to both overall condition and otoscopic signs as compared with placebo. Moreover, based on this study, the number needed to treat for 1 child to benefit from antimicrobial therapy was 3.8, which is much lower than the 7–17 that has been cited in previous meta-analyses.[68,70,71,79] The authors attributed this greater beneficial effect compared with previous trials primarily to methodologic differences, most notably, a stringent diagnostic standard that assured only those with true AOM were included in the study.

Results from another recent clinical trial by Hoberman et al. with simi-larly strict diagnostic criteria appeared to further question the use of the watchful waiting strategy in younger children.[85] This study found that among children 6–23 months of age with AOM, treatment with amoxi-cillin-clavulanate for 10 days, as compared with placebo, resulted in consistently more favorable short-term outcome, an absence of otoscopic evidence for a persistent middle ear infection and a reduced rate of residual middle-ear effusion. Furthermore, the study utilized a symptom severity scale[86,87] for each patient and found that the short-term benefits of antibiotic therapy were present irrespective of the apparent severity of

AOM. In other words, antimicrobial therapy was superior to placebo even in children with less severe disease. However, the authors emphasized that the greater beneficial effect of antibiotics that was seen in this trial as compared to past studies was not because of better outcome among children treated with antibiotics, but instead, because of higher rates of clinical failure among the children who received placebo. Thus, much like the study by Tähtinen et al. the authors attributed this finding of higher antibiotic efficacy to the stringent diagnostic criteria that was used to ensure only children with a definitive diagnosis of AOM were included.

These two studies,[84,85] which both illustrated the beneficial effects of antibiotic therapy over placebo in younger children, may result in a re-evaluation of the watchful waiting approach, especially for children younger than 2 years of age. Nevertheless, the authors do emphasize that the apparent benefits of immediate antibiotic therapy must be weighed against the potential harms. For example, one of the studies found that the patients receiving amoxicillin-clavulanate had a 16.7% higher incidence of adverse events, most notably diarrhea.[84] In addition, the development of bacterial resistance is always a concern with extensive antibacterial therapy.[88,89]

However, perhaps the most essential point that can be gained from these recent studies is the importance of an accurate diagnosis of AOM in order to ensure appropriate disease management. Unfortunately, several studies have suggested that physicians are uncertain of their diagnosis of AOM as much as 40% of the time.[90] Even worse, another study found that three out of four physicians will prescribe antibiotics even when they believe that odds that a patient actually has AOM are 50% or less.[91] These uncertainties may be due, in part, to the continuing debate over which tools and methods are best for obtaining an accurate diagnosis.[92] Therefore, perhaps the first step in resolving the controversy between watchful waiting and immediate antibacterial therapy is to determine which diagnostic strategies are most precise, and subsequently, ensuring that physicians become familiar and experienced with these methods through both standardized guidelines and education. From there, clinicians will be able to more confidently and accurately establish a diagnosis of AOM, and predict which patients may have a poorer prognosis, both of which are essential to improving disease management, limiting antibiotic overuse, and therefore, reducing antibiotic resistance.[92,93] In this way, with a higher diagnostic acumen, physicians may be able to more reliably make the decision to treat AOM or not to treat AOM, although the clinical variability that often characterizes the disease may never make the choice absolutely clear-cut.

COMPLICATIONS OF OM

The complications of OM can generally be classified into two groups; intratemporal (also referred to as extracranial) and intracranial (Table 11.3). Intratemporal complications of OM, which occur due to the progression

Table 11.3: Complications of otitis media	
Intratemporal complications	*Intracranial complications*
Mastoiditis	Meningitis
Cholesteatoma	Extradural abscess
Labyrinthitis	Subdural empyema
Tympanic membrane perforation	Focal otitic encephalitis
Facial paralysis	Intracerebral or subdural abscess
Petrositis	Lateral sinus thrombosis
Perilymphatic fistula	Otitic hydrocephalus

of a middle ear infection into the temporal bone, include acute mastoiditis, cholesteatoma, labyrinthitis and tympanic membrane perforation. Intracranial complications, which occur when the infectious process from the middle ear extends beyond the temporal bone, include meningitis, brain abscess, subdural empyema and lateral sinus thrombosis. This section will focus specifically on the recent developments, controversies and complications associated with acute mastoiditis (AM), which is the most commonly associated complication of AOM.[94]

Most middle ear infections are rarely confined to the middle ear alone, as there is usually some degree of inflammation or infection that occurs in the mastoid process of the temporal bone. This inflammation usually clears with the resolution of the OM episode. However, when the infection becomes more severe and persists, the inflammation and exudate can spread and cause damage throughout the bony architecture of the mastoid cavity, ultimately leading to AM. The most common bacterial isolates from AM include *S. pneumoniae, Pseudomonas aeruginosa, Staphylococcus aureus, Streptococcus pyogenes*, and *Haemophilus influenzae*.[95] Furthermore, it should also be noted that although AM is frequently a complication of OM, it has been shown that AM can present without a preceding OM episode 40–66% of the time.[94,96]

Before the introduction of antibiotics, AOM progressed to AM in up to 20% of patients, the majority of whom required surgical intervention.[97] In fact, during this time, AM was the most common infectious condition requiring hospitalization in infants and children.[98] Then, with the introduction of antimicrobials in the 1940s, the reported incidence declined from 0.4% in 1959[99] to 0.004% in the 1980s.[100] Currently, the annual incidence of AM in children under 14 has been reported to be between 1.2 and 4.2 per 100,000.[101] Nonetheless, many studies have shown an apparent resurgence in the incidence of the disease in recent years,[101-105] although the reports have not been completely universal.[106,107] The possibility of a rising incidence, however, is concerning, given the potentially devastating complications of AM.

This apparent resurgence of AM has been attributed by some authors to an increasing frequency of antibiotic resistance among bacterial pathogens.[108,109] However, although antibiotic resistance has increased over the same time period that AM has apparently re-emerged, studies have found that this cannot fully explain the increased frequency of the disease, as cultures of the mastoid cavity are frequently negative or do not show resistant pathogens.[110,111] Other studies have attributed the increased incidence to the relatively new watchful waiting strategy, in which antibiotics are not prescribed for certain patients with uncomplicated AOM.[112,113] These studies argue that although restricting antibiotic use may decrease bacterial resistance, such a strategy may be associated with a somewhat higher incidence of AM due to the progression of untreated AOM.[112] However, studies have been unable to definitively prove whether a missed diagnosis of AOM or delayed antibiotic therapy can directly contribute to the development of AM.[94,112]

Thus, as a specific explanation has not yet been found for the apparent increase in AM cases, clinicians are currently unable to make explicit changes in AOM management in order to reduce the incidence of AM. However, physicians can continue to be vigilant in closely monitoring and following children with middle ear infections, and appropriately diagnosing AM if it occurs and before it becomes an extensive infection. The diagnosis of AM is mainly clinical, as it should be suspected based on the medical history and clinical examination of the patient.[101] Unfortunately, a recent review article exploring the available diagnostic criteria for the disease found that there is still no consensus regarding the criteria and strategies for diagnosing AM in the pediatric population.[114] Nevertheless, symptoms of AM usually include pain, swelling and tenderness in the mastoid region, as well as otalgia, auricular proptosis, and erythema of the ear and tympanic membrane. Fever and headache are also common, and otorrhea can occur in more severe cases.[115]

In terms of diagnostic imaging, radiographs have not been proven to be useful[116] and the use of CT scans is somewhat controversial. While some authors advocate the use of CT imaging in all cases of suspected AM,[117] others feel that it should be reserved for cases with an uncertain diagnosis, possible complications, failure of conservative medical management or as preparation for a mastoidectomy.[118] Whatever the case may be, once a diagnosis is reached, therapeutic intervention should be initiated as soon as possible.

In the past, AM was invariably a surgical condition as it was usually treated with a cortical mastoidectomy.[101] Now the disease can often be managed medically, although, there is still an open discussion regarding the optimal treatment strategy. Broad-spectrum intravenous (IV) antibiotics are almost always initiated in cases of suspected AM and usually include ampicillin-sulbactam, ceftriaxone or clindamycin, and an antipseudomonal agent if a *P. aeruginosa* infection is suspected.[119] On the other hand, there are conflicting views on the necessity of performing a myringotomy or ventilation tube insertion in AM. Many studies have advocated for a myringotomy during any episode of AM and not exclusively when antibiotic therapy fails.[119-121] These studies argue that early myringotomy will not only provide immediate pain relief due to the drainage of pus and release of middle ear pressure, but it will also allow for the collection of middle ear fluid, and thus, facilitate microbiological diagnosis. In contrast, other studies have noted that conservative medical management with IV antibiotics alone may be sufficient to treat AM.[94,122,123] One study even found that patients who underwent myringotomy for the disease, developed more complications than those who were managed conservatively.[124] Nevertheless, if the infection progresses to coalescent mastoiditis, which is a destructive infection of the mastoid bone and air cell system, IV antibiotics with or without myringotomy may not be sufficient and surgical management with a mastoidectomy may become necessary. This surgical procedure is now generally reserved for more severe or complicated cases of AM, as common indications for the surgery include a slow progression of AM despite medical treatment, the presence of a cholesteatoma, abscessed mastoiditis and intracranial complications.[125-127]

The intracranial complications remain the most feared sequelae of AM. These complications can include sigmoid or lateral sinus thrombosis, epidural abscess, otitic hydrocephalus, subdural empyema and cerebral abscess. Although the rate of mortality from these complications has significantly decreased due to antibiotics and improved medical care, they continue to occur and have a reported incidence between 4.1% and 7.2% of AM cases.[94,127,128] This persistence has been attributed to the masking of symptoms by the use of broad-spectrum antibiotics for AM, rather than the emergence of resistant pathogens.[128] And, much like AM and AOM, the optimal treatment strategy for many of these complications remains unclear. For example, in the event of a sigmoid or lateral sinus thrombosis, some authors advocate for the use of a mastoidectomy followed by a protracted course of antibiotic therapy,[96] while others support the use of surgical decompression of the sinus with anticoagulation to expedite recanalization and prevent septic embolization.[129] However, regardless of which therapy is utilized, early diagnosis of these AM-associated complications and postoperative vigilance are essential to prevent further progression of the disease and possible mortality.

In the end, complications of OM, although relatively rare, can have potentially devastating consequences. As AM remains the most common of these complications, further research must be done to determine both the most efficient diagnostic methods and the best treatment regimens for the disorder. Of course, prevention of AM would be the most pragmatic approach. However, studies have shown that vaccines such as the PCV-7, which have had success in reducing the rate of invasive pneumococcal disease, have not had a significant effect on the incidence of AM.[130] In fact, as noted above, the incidence of AM appears to have made a resurgence in the past decade. Thus, as AM is often a direct complication of OM, perhaps the best method to reduce the rate of the disease would be to either prevent or effectively treat OM before it establishes a persistent infection in the mastoid cavity. In this way, the successful treatment or prevention of OM may reduce the rate of AM in the future.

REFERENCES

1. Rovers MM, Schilder AGM, Zielhuis GA, et al. Otitis media. Lancet. 2004;363(9407):465-73.
2. Physicians AAoF, Otolaryngology-Head AAo, Surgery N, et al. Otitis media with effusion. Pediatrics. 2004;113(5):1412-29.
3. Daly KA, Hoffman HJ, Kvaerner KJ, et al. Epidemiology, natural history, and risk factors: Panel report from the Ninth International Research Conference on Otitis Media. Int J Pediatr Otorhinolaryngol. 2010;74(3):231-40.
4. Bondy J, Berman S, Glazner J, et al. Direct expenditures related to otitis media diagnoses: extrapolations from a pediatric medicaid cohort. Pediatrics. 2000;105(6):e72.
5. Alsarraf R, Jung CJ, Perkins J, et al. Measuring the indirect and direct costs of acute otitis media. Arch Otolaryngol Head Neck Surg. 1999;125(1):12-8.
6. Charles D Bluestone, Jerome O Klein. Otitis Media in Infants and Children, 4th edition. Hamilton, Ontario: BC Decker Inc.; 2007.
7. Segal N, Leibovitz E, Dagan R, et al. Acute otitis media-diagnosis and treatment in the era of antibiotic resistant organisms: updated clinical practice guidelines. Int J Pediatr Otorhinolaryngol. 2005;69(10):1311-9.
8. Alper CM, Winther B, Mandel EM, et al. Rate of concurrent otitis media in upper respiratory tract infections with specific viruses. Arch Otolaryngol Head Neck Surg. 2009;135(1):17-21.
9. Yano H, Okitsu N, Hori T, et al. Detection of respiratory viruses in nasopharyngeal secretions and middle ear fluid from children with acute otitis media. Acta Otolaryngol. 2009;129(1):19-24.
10. Chonmaitree T, Revai K, Grady JJ, et al. Viral upper respiratory tract infection and otitis media complication in young children. Clin Infect Dis. 2008;46(6):815-23.
11. Vergison A. Microbiology of otitis media: a moving target. Vaccine. 2008;26(Supplement 7):G5-10.
12. Alho OP, Oja H, Koivu M, et al. Chronic otitis media with effusion in infancy. How frequent is it? How does it develop? Arch Otolaryngol Head Neck Surg. 1995;121(4):432-6.
13. Pereira MB, Pereira MR, Costa SS, et al. Prevalance of bacteria in children with otitis media with effusion. J Pediatr. 2004;80(1):41-8.
14. Post JC. Direct evidence of bacterial biofilms in otitis media. Laryngoscope. 2001;111(12):2083-94.
15. Giebink GS, Juhn SK, Weber ML, et al. The bacteriology and cytology of chronic otitis media with effusion. Pediatr Infect Dis. 1982;1(2):98-103.
16. Diamond C, Sisson PR, Kearns AM, et al. Bacteriology of chronic otitis media with effusion. J Laryngol Otol. 1989;103(4):369-71.
17. Johnson MD, Fitzgerald JE, Leonard G, el al. Cytokines in experimental otitis media with effusion. Laryngoscope. 1994;104(2):191-6.
18. Rayner MG, Zhang Y, Gorry MC, et al. Evidence of bacterial metabolic activity in culture-negative otitis media with effusion. JAMA. 1998;279(4):296-9.
19. Ueyama T, Kurono Y, Shirabc K, et al. High incidence of Haemophilus influenzae in nasopharyngeal secretions and middle ear effusions as detected by PCR. J Clin Microbiol. 1995;33(7):1835-8.

20. Post JC, Aul JJ, White GJ, et al. PCR–based detection of bacterial DNA after antimicrobial treatment is indicative of persistent, viable bacteria in the chinchilla model of otitis media. Am J Otolaryngol. 1996;17(2):106-11.

21. Post JC, Hiller NL, Nistico L, et al. The role of biofilms in otolaryngologic infections: update 2007. Curr Opin Otolaryngol Head Neck Surg. 2007;15(5):347-51.

22. Costerton JW, Stewart PS, Greenberg EP. Bacterial biofilms: a common cause of persistent infections. Science. 1999;284(5418):1318-22.

23. Costerton W, Veeh R, Shirtliff M, et al. The application of biofilm science to the study and control of chronic bacterial infections. J Clin Invest. 2003;112(10):1466-77.

24. Ehrlich GD, Veeh R, Wang X, et al. Mucosal biofilm formation on middle-ear mucosa in the chinchilla model of otitis media. JAMA. 2002;287(13):1710-5.

25. Hall-Stoodley L, Hu FZ, Gieseke A, et al. Direct detection of bacterial biofilms on the middle-ear mucosa of children with chronic otitis media. JAMA. 2006;296(2):202-11.

26. Lee MR, Pawlowski KS, Luong A, et al. Biofilm presence in humans with chronic suppurative otitis media. Otolaryngol Head Neck Surg. 2009;141(5):567-71.

27. Saunders J, Murray M, Alleman A. Biofilms in chronic suppurative otitis media and cholesteatoma: scanning electron microscopy findings. Am J Otolaryngol. 2011;32(1):32-7.

28. Moriyama S, Hotomi M, Shimada J, et al. Formation of biofilm by Haemophilus influenzae isolated from pediatric intractable otitis media. Auris Nasus Larynx. 2009;36(5):525-31.

29. Liu CM, Cosetti MK, Aziz M, et al. The otologic microbiome: a study of the bacterial microbiota in a pediatric patient with chronic serous otitis media using 16SrRNA gene-based pyrosequencing. Arch Otolaryngol Head Neck Surg. 2011;137(7):664-8.

30. Saylam G, Tatar EC, Tatar I, et al. Association of adenoid surface biofilm formation and chronic otitis media with effusion. Arch Otolaryngol Head Neck Surg. 2010;136(6):550-5.

31. van den Aardweg MT, Schilder AG, Herkert E, et al. Adenoidectomy for otitis media in children. Cochrane Database of Syst Rev. 2010.

32. Smith A, Buchinsky FJ, Post JC. Eradicating chronic ear, nose, and throat infections: a systematically conducted literature review of advances in biofilm treatment. Otolaryngol Head Neck Surg. 2011;144(3):338-47.

33. Armbruster CE, Swords WE. Interspecies bacterial communication as a target for therapy in otitis media. Expert Rev Anti Infect Ther. 2010;8(10):1067-70.

34. Del Beccaro MA, Mendelman PM, Inglis AF, et al. Bacteriology of acute otitis media: a new perspective. J Pediatr. 1992;120(1):81-4.

35. Heikkinen T, Thint M, Chonmaitree T. Prevalence of various respiratory viruses in the middle ear during acute otitis media. N Engl J Med. 1999;340(4):260-4.

36. Eskola J, Kilpi T, Palmu A, et al. Efficacy of a pneumococcal conjugate vaccine against acute otitis media. N Engl J Med. 2001;344(6):403-9.

37. Poehling KA, Talbot TR, Griffin MR, et al. Invasive pneumococcal disease among infants before and after introduction of pneumococcal conjugate vaccine. JAMA. 2006;295(14):1668-74.
38. Whitney CG, Pilishvili T, Farley MM, et al. Effectiveness of seven-valent pneumococcal conjugate vaccine against invasive pneumococcal disease: a matched case-control study. Lancet. 2006;368(9546):1495-502.
39. Eskola J, Kilpi T, Palmu A, et al. Efficacy of a pneumococcal conjugate vaccine against acute otitis media. N Engl J Med. 2001;344(6):403-9.
40. Whitney CG, Farley MM, Hadler J, et al. Decline in invasive pneumococcal disease after the introduction of protein-polysaccharide conjugate vaccine. N Engl J Med. 2003;348(18):1737-46.
41. Block SL, Hedrick J, Harrison C, et al. Community-wide vaccination with the heptavalent pneumococcal conjugate significantly alters the microbiology of acute otitis media. Pediatr Infect Dis J. 2004;23(9):829-33.
42. Huang SS, Hinrichsen VL, Stevenson AE, et al. Continued impact of pneumococcal conjugate vaccine on carriage in young children. Pediatrics. 2009;124(1):e1-11.
43. Richter SS, Heilmann KP, Dohrn CL, et al. Changing epidemiology of antimicrobial-resistant Streptococcus pneumoniae in the United States, 2004–2005. Clin Infect Dis. 2009;48(3):e23-33.
44. Casey JR, Adlowitz DG, Pichichero ME. New patterns in the otopathogens causing acute otitis media six to eight years after introduction of pneumococcal conjugate vaccine. Pediatr Infect Dis J. 2010;29(4):304-9.
45. Jansen AG, Hak E, Veenhoven RH, et al. Pneumococcal conjugate vaccines for preventing otitis media. Cochrane Database Syst Rev. 2009.
46. Grijalva CG, Poehling KA, Nuorti JP, et al. National impact of universal childhood immunization with pneumococcal conjugate vaccine on outpatient medical care visits in the United States. Pediatrics.2006;118(3):865-73.
47. Zhou F, Shefer A, Kong Y, et al. Trends in acute otitis media-related health care utilization by privately insured young children in the United States, 1997-2004. Pediatrics. 2008;121(2):253-60.
48. Tarrago D, Aguilar L, Garcia R, et al. Evolution of clonal and susceptibility profiles of serotype 19A Streptococcus pneumoniae among invasive isolates from children in Spain, 1990 to 2008. Antimicrob Agents Chemother.2011;55(5):2297-302.
49. Hanage WP, Huang SS, Lipsitch M, et al. Diversity and antibiotic resistance among nonvaccine serotypes of Streptococcus pneumoniae carriage isolates in the post-heptavalent conjugate vaccine era. J Infect Dis. 2007;195(3):347-52.
50. Pichichero ME, Casey JR. Emergence of a multiresistant serotype 19A pneumococcal strain not included in the 7-valent conjugate vaccine as an otopathogen in children. JAMA. 2007;298(15):1772-8.
51. Reinert R, Jacobs MR, Kaplan SL. Pneumococcal disease caused by serotype 19A: review of the literature and implications for future vaccine development. Vaccine. 2010;28(26):4249 59.
52. Nuorti JP, Whitney CG. Prevention of pneumococcal disease among infants and children - use of 13-valent pneumococcal conjugate vaccine and

23-valent pneumococcal polysaccharide vaccine - recommendations of the Advisory Committee on Immunization Practices (ACIP). MMWR Recomm Rep. 2010;59(RR-11):1-18.

53. Esposito S, Tansey S, Thompson A, et al. Safety and immunogenicity of a 13-valent pneumococcal conjugate vaccine compared to those of a 7-valent pneumococcal conjugate vaccine given as a three-dose series with routine vaccines in healthy infants and toddlers. Clin Vaccine Immunol. 2010;17(6):1017-26.

54. Kieninger DM, Kueper K, Steul K, et al. Safety, tolerability, and immunologic noninferiority of a 13-valent pneumococcal conjugate vaccine compared to a 7-valent pneumococcal conjugate vaccine given with routine pediatric vaccinations in Germany. Vaccine. 2010;28(25):4192-203.

55. Grijalva CG, Pelton SI. A second-generation pneumococcal conjugate vaccine for prevention of pneumococcal diseases in children. Curr Opin Pediatr. 2011;23(1):98–104.

56. Prymula R, Schuerman L. 10-valent pneumococcal nontypeable Haemophilus influenzae PD conjugate vaccine: Synflorix. Expert Rev Vaccines. 2009;8(11):1479–500.

57. Prymula R, Peeters P, Chrobok V, et al. Pneumococcal capsular polysaccharides conjugated to protein D for prevention of acute otitis media caused by both Streptococcus pneumoniae and non-typable Haemophilus influenzae: a randomised double-blind efficacy study. Lancet. 2006;367(9512):740-8.

58. Talbird SE, Taylor TN, Knoll S, et al. Outcomes and costs associated with PHiD-CV, a new protein D conjugate pneumococcal vaccine, in four countries. Vaccine. 2010;28(Supplement 6):G23-9.

59. Cox AD, St Michael F, Cairns CM, et al. Investigating the potential of conserved inner core oligosaccharide regions of Moraxella catarrhalis lipopolysaccharide as vaccine antigens: accessibility and functional activity of monoclonal antibodies and glycoconjugate derived sera. Glycoconj J. 2011;28(3-4):165-82.

60. Yang M, Johnson A, Murphy TF. Characterization and evaluation of the Moraxella catarrhalis oligopeptide permease A as a mucosal vaccine antigen. Infect Immun. 2011;79(2):846-57.

61. Rudberg RD. Acute otitis media; comparative therapeutic results of sulphonamide and penicillin administered in various forms. Acta Otolaryngol Suppl. 1954;113:1-79.

62. Finkelstein JA, Metlay JP, Davis RL, et al. Antimicrobial use in defined populations of infants and young children. Arch Pediatr Adolesc Med. 2000;154(4):395-400.

63. Rautakorpi UM, Klaukka T, Honkanen P, et al. Antibiotic use by indication: a basis for active antibiotic policy in the community. Scand J Infect Dis. 2001;33(12):920-6.

64. Casey JR. Treating acute otitis media post-PCV-7: judicious antibiotic therapy. Postgrad Med. 2005;118(6 Suppl Emerging):32-3, 24-31.

65. Dowell SF, Marcy SM, Phillips WR, et al. Otitis media - principles of judicious use of antimicrobial agents. Pediatrics. 1998;101(1):165-71.

66. Vergison A, Dagan R, Arguedas A, et al. Otitis media and its consequences: beyond the earache. Lancet Infect Dis. 2010;10(3):195-203.

67. Elden LM, Spiro DM. Acute otitis media—to treat or not to treat? Pediatr Emerg Care. 2006;22(4):283-6.

68. Rosenfeld RM, Vertrees JE, Carr J, et al. Clinical efficacy of antimicrobial drugs for acute otitis media: meta-analysis of 5400 children from thirty-three randomized trials. J Pediatr. 1994;124(3):355-67.

69. Respiratory tract infections – antibiotic prescribing. Prescribing of Antibiotics for Self-limiting Respiratory Tract Infections in Adults and Children in Primary Care. Centre for Clinical Practice at NICE (UK); 2008.

70. Del Mar C, Glasziou P, Hayem M. Are antibiotics indicated as initial treatment for children with acute otitis media? A meta-analysis. BMJ. 1997;314(7093):1526-9.

71. Marcy M, Takata G, Chan LS, et al. Management of acute otitis media. Evid Rep Technol Assess (Summ). 2000;(15):1-4.

72. Rosenfeld RM, Kay D. Natural history of untreated otitis media. Laryngoscope. 2003;113(10):1645-57.

73. Del Mar C, Glasziou P, Hayem M. Are antibiotics indicated as initial treatment for children with acute otitis media? A meta-analysis. BMJ. 1997;314(7093):1526-9.

74. Takata GS, Chan LS, Shekelle P, et al. Evidence assessment of management of acute otitis media: I. The role of antibiotics in treatment of uncomplicated acute otitis media. Pediatrics. 2001;108(2):239-47.

75. American Academy of Pediatrics Subcommittee on Management of Acute Otitis Media. Diagnosis and management of acute otitis media. Pediatrics. 2004;113(5):1451-65.

76. Piglansky L, Leibovitz E, Raiz S, et al. Bacteriologic and clinical efficacy of high dose amoxicillin for therapy of acute otitis media in children. Pediatr Infect Dis J. 2003;22(5):405-13.

77. Vernacchio L, Vezina RM, Mitchell AA. Management of acute otitis media by primary care physicians: trends since the release of the 2004 American Academy of Pediatrics/American Academy of Family Physicians clinical practice guideline. Pediatrics. 2007;120(2):281-7.

78. Coco A, Vernacchio L, Horst M, et al. Management of acute otitis media after publication of the 2004 AAP and AAFP clinical practice guideline. Pediatrics. 2010;125(2):214-20.

79. Sanders SL, Glasziou PP, Del Mar CB, et al. Antibiotics for acute otitis media in children. Cochrane Database of Syst Rev. 2004.

80. Pichichero ME, Casey JR. Diagnostic inaccuracy and subject exclusions render placebo and observational studies of acute otitis media inconclusive. Pediatr Infect Dis J. 2008;27(11):958-62.

81. Vergison A, Dagan R, Arguedas A, et al. Otitis media and its consequences: beyond the earache. Lancet Infect Dis. 2010;10(3):195-203.

82. Wald ER. Acute otitis media: more trouble with the evidence. Pediatr Infect Dis J. 2003;22(2):103-4.

83. Marchant CD. Acute otitis media, antibiotics, children and clinical trial design. Pediatr Infect Dis J. 2002;21(10):891-3.

84. Tähtinen PA, Laine MK, Huovinen P, et al. A placebo-controlled trial of anti-microbial treatment for acute otitis media. N Engl J Med. 2011;364(2):116-26.

85. Hoberman A, Paradise JL, Rockette HE, et al. Treatment of acute otitis media in children under 2 years of age. N Engl J Med. 2011;364(2):105-15.

86. Shaikh N, Hoberman A, Paradise JL, et al. Development and preliminary evaluation of a parent-reported outcome instrument for clinical trials in acute otitis media. Pediatr Infect Dis J. 2009;28(1):5-8.

87. Shaikh N, Hoberman A, Paradise JL, et al. Responsiveness and construct validity of a symptom scale for acute otitis media. Pediatr Infect Dis J. 2009;28(1):9-12.

88. Greenberg D, Hoffman S, Leibovitz E, et al. Acute otitis media in children: association with day care centers—antibacterial resistance, treatment, and prevention. Paediatr Drugs. 2008;10(2):75-83.

89. Beekmann SE, Heilmann KP, Richter SS, et al. Antimicrobial resistance in Strep-tococcus pneumoniae, Haemophilus influenzae, Moraxella catarrhalis and group A beta-haemolytic streptococci in 2002–2003. Results of the multinational GRASP Surveillance Program. Int J Antimicrob Agents. 2005;25(2):148-56.

90. Rosenfeld RM. Diagnostic certainty for acute otitis media. Int J Pediatr Otorhinolaryngol. 2002;64(2):89-95.

91. Gonzalez-Vallejo C, Sorum PC, Stewart TR, et al. Physicians' diagnostic judgments and treatment decisions for acute otitis media in children. Med Decis Making. 1998;18(2):149-62.

92. Grevers G. Challenges in reducing the burden of otitis media disease: an ENT perspective on improving management and prospects for prevention. Int J Pediatr Otorhinolaryngol. 2010;74(6):572-7.

93. Klein JO. Is acute otitis media a treatable disease? N Engl J Med. 2011;364(2):168-9.

94. Benito MB, Gorricho BP. Acute mastoiditis: increase in the incidence and complications. Int J Pediatr Otorhinolaryngol. 2007;71(7):1007-11.

95. Pang LHY, Barakate MS, Havas TE. Mastoiditis in a paediatric population: a review of 11 years experience in management. Int J Pediatr Otorhinolar-yngol. 2009;73(11):1520-4.

96. Mallur PS, Harirchian S, Lalwani AK. Preoperative and postoperative intracranial complications of acute mastoiditis. Ann Otol Rhinol Laryngol. 2009;118(2):118-23.

97. House HP. Otitis media; a comparative study of the results obtained in therapy before and after the introduction of the sulfonamide compounds. Arch Otolaryngol. 1946;43:371-8.

98. Bluestone C, Stool S, Dohar J. Pediatric Otolaryngology, 4th edition. Phila-delphia, PA: Saunders; 2003.

99. Palva T, Pulkkinen K. Mastoiditis. J Laryngol Otol. 1959;73:573-88.

100. Faye-Lund H. Acute and latent mastoiditis. J Laryngol Otol. 1989; 103(12):1158-60.

101. Navazo-Eguia AI, Conejo-Moreno D, De-La-Mata-Franco G, et al. Acute mastoiditis in the pneumococcal vaccine era. Acta Otorrinolaringol Esp. 2011;62(1):45-50.

102. Finnbogadóttir AF, Petersen H, Laxdal T, et al. An increasing incidence of mastoiditis in children in Iceland. Scand J Infect Dis. 2009;41(2):95-8.

103. Katz A, Leibovitz E, Greenberg D, et al. Acute mastoiditis in Southern Israel: a twelve year retrospective study (1990 through 2001). Pediatr Infect Dis J. 2003;22(10):878-82.

104. Ho D, Rotenberg BW, Berkowitz RG. The relationship between acute mastoiditis and antibiotic use for acute otitis media in children. Arch Otolaryngol Head Neck Surg. 2008;134(1):45-8.

105. Benito MB, Gorricho BP. Acute mastoiditis: increase in the incidence and complications. Int J Pediatr Otorhinolaryngol. 2007;71(7):1007-11.

106. Stenfeldt K, Hermansson A. Acute mastoiditis in southern Sweden: a study of occurrence and clinical course of acute mastoiditis before and after introduction of new treatment recommendations for AOM. Eur Arch Otorhinolaryngol. 2010;267(12):1855-61.

107. Kvaerner KJ, Bentdal Y, Karevold G. Acute mastoiditis in Norway: no evidence for an increase. Int J Pediatr Otorhinolaryngol. 2007;71(10):1579-83.

108. Croche Santander B, Porras Gonzalez A, Madrid Castillo MD, et al. [Unusually high frequency of complications in acute otitis media]. An Pediatr (Barc). 2009;70(2):168-72.

109. Antonelli PJ, Dhanani N, Giannoni CM, et al. Impact of resistant pneumococcus on rates of acute mastoiditis. Otolaryngol Head Neck Surg. 1999;121(3):190-4.

110. Mallur PS, Harirchian S, Lalwani AK. Preoperative and postoperative intracranial complications of acute mastoiditis. Ann Otol Rhinol Laryngol. 2009;118(2):118-23.

111. Thorne MC, Chewaproug L, Elden LM. Suppurative complications of acute otitis media: changes in frequency over time. Arch Otolaryngol Head Neck Surg. 2009;135(7):638-41.

112. Van Zuijlen DA, Schilder AG, Van Balen FA, et al. National differences in incidence of acute mastoiditis: relationship to prescribing patterns of antibiotics for acute otitis media? Pediatr Infect Dis J. 2001;20(2):140-4.

113. Bahadori RS, Schwartz RH, Ziai M. Acute mastoiditis in children: an increase in frequency in northern Virginia. Pediatr Infect Dis J. 2000;19(3):212-5.

114. Van Den Aardweg MT, Rovers MM, De Ru JA, et al. A systematic review of diagnostic criteria for acute mastoiditis in children. Otol Neurotol. 2008;29(6):751-7.

115. Hoppe JE, Koster S, Bootz F, et al. Acute mastoiditis—relevant once again. Infection. 1994;22(3):178-82.

116. Harley EH, Sdralis T, Berkowitz RG. Acute mastoiditis in children: a 12-year retrospective study. Otolaryngol Head Neck Surg. 1997;116(1):26-30.

117. Stahelin-Massik J, Podvinec M, Jakscha J, et al. Mastoiditis in children: a prospective, observational study comparing clinical presentation, microbiology, computed tomography, surgical findings and histology. Eur J Pediatr. 2008;167(5):541-8.

118. Tamir S, Schwartz Y, Peleg U, et al. Acute mastoiditis in children: is computed tomography always necessary? Ann Otol Rhinol Laryngol. 2009;118(8):565-9.

119. Spratley J, Silveira H, Alvarez I, et al. Acute mastoiditis in children: review of the current status. Int J Pediatr Otorhinolaryngol. 2000;56(1):33-40.

120. Zapalac JS, Billings KR, Schwade ND, et al. Suppurative complications of acute otitis media in the era of antibiotic resistance. Arch Otolaryngol Head Neck Surg. 2002;128(6):660-3.

121. Tamir S, Shwartz Y, Peleg U, et al. Shifting trends: mastoiditis from a surgical to a medical disease. Am J Otolaryngol.2010;31(6):467-71.

122. Nussinovitch M, Yoeli R, Elishkevitz K, et al. Acute mastoiditis in children: epidemiologic, clinical, microbiologic, and therapeutic aspects over past years. Clin Pediatr (Phila) 2004;43(3):261-7.

123. Luntz M, Brodsky A, Nusem S, et al. Acute mastoiditis — the antibiotic era: a multicenter study. Int J Pediatr Otorhinolaryngol. 2001;57(1):1-9.

124. Geva A, Oestreicher-Kedem Y, Fishman G, et al. Conservative management of acute mastoiditis in children. Int J Pediatr Otorhinolaryngol. 2008;72(5):629-34.

125. Taylor MF, Berkowitz RG. Indications for mastoidectomy in acute mastoiditis in children. Ann Otol Rhinol Laryngol. 2004;113(1):69-72.

126. Trijolet JP, Bakhos D, Lanotte P, et al. Acute mastoiditis in children: can mastoidectomy be avoided? Ann Otolaryngol Chir Cervicofac. 2009;126(4):169-74.

127. Zanetti D, Nassif N. Indications for surgery in acute mastoiditis and their complications in children. Int J Pediatr Otorhinolaryngol. 2006;70(7):1175-82.

128. Go C, Bernstein JM, De Jong AL, et al. Intracranial complications of acute mastoiditis. Int J Pediatr Otorhinolaryngol. 2000;52(2):143-8.

129. Kuczkowski J, Dubaniewicz-Wybieralska M, Przewozny T, et al. Otitic hydrocephalus associated with lateral sinus thrombosis and acute mastoiditis in children. Int J Pediatr Otorhinolaryngol. 2006;70(10):1817-23.

130. Choi SS, Lander L. Pediatric acute mastoiditis in the post-pneumococcal conjugate vaccine era. Laryngoscope. 2011;121(5):1072-80.

SIALOENDOSCOPY IN THE MANAGEMENT OF SALIVARY GLAND DISEASE

Anthony G Del Signore and Vivek Gurudutt

ABSTRACT

Technological advances continually shape the face of medicine. The use of endoscopy for salivary disease has undergone much transition and development, and has emerged as a viable alternative for diagnosis and treatment. Employing increased miniaturization and improved optics, the field of sialoendoscopy has opened up a new approach to the myriad of salivary disease states.

Anatomic and physiologic considerations of the respective salivary glands play a role in the interventions selected. Salivary duct obstruction is a product of many disease pathologies ranging from parenchymal and ductal inflammation, particle deposition within ductules, and strictures due to ductal wall hypertrophy. Diverse instrumentation has been developed over the years to address the pathology encountered.

Sialoendoscopy includes the preparation and entry into the affected salivary duct, diagnosis and visualization of the offending pathology, and deployment of selected intervention. Complications include infection, transient swelling, ranula formation, and ductal perforation and stenosis. Absolute contraindications include acute infection/inflammation and complete distal duct obliteration, while relative contraindications include large sialoliths and small ductal diameter.

Compared to previous modalities, sialoendoscopy allows for therapeutic benefit with substantially less morbidity and retention of salivary function. Given the robust armamentarium available to address the various ductal pathologies and the vigorous data associated with minimally invasive techniques, open total gland excision should be reserved when all other measures have been exhausted.

INTRODUCTION

With the dawn of miniaturization and technological advances, patients continually demand for the most state of the art treatments. Gone are the days of open surgical excision being the only option offered to patients after unsuccessful treatment with conservative therapy.[1,2] Sialoendoscopy has taken a lead role as a minimally invasive technique allowing for intraluminal inspection of the major salivary glands via the utilization of narrow-diameter, fiber optic endoscopes.[3-5] Endoscopic visualization of ductal and glandular tissue permits the elucidation of various pathologic states and delivery of treatment while preserving a physiologically intact salivary gland. With the increased miniaturization and improved optics in today's scopes, the field of sialoendoscopy has opened up a new horizon for diagnostic and therapeutic modalities of salivary gland disease.

HISTORY

The dawn of sialoendoscopy began in the early 1990s with Katz, who first reported exploiting flexible endoscopes to visualize sialoliths. Once visualization was established the new device provided a viable intervention to relieve salivary obstruction site. In the initial description, a wire basket system was successfully employed to retrieve the obstructing stone. For the first time, the anatomy of the interductal system was cataloged showcasing the nuances of the respective salivary glands that would drive further improvement in technique and equipment.[6] With direct visualization available, clinicians no longer had to rely upon radiologic and ultrasound localization of salivary gland obstruction.

The field quickly flourished with the advancement of technology to include variable rigidity and increasingly smaller endoscopes. This progression can be recounted by the work of Nahlieli et al.[7-11] Initially, endoscopic size was based on already available scopes that were commonly utilized for arthroscopic procedures. Originally, the therapeutic 2.7 mm rigid scope was utilized, but eventually replaced by the smaller diagnostic and therapeutic scopes. As endoscopic equipment improved, anatomic studies were performed examining various normal and pathologic glands. Ductal diameters were surveyed within the major salivary ducts. Mean ductal diameters were reported to range between 0.5 mm and 1.4 mm for parotid gland ducts and 0.5–1.5 mm for the submandibular ductal system. Early recommendations for the upper limit of scope diameter design were issued to be a maximum of 1.2 mm in order to prevent complications of ductal scarring.[12,13] Currently, due to improvements in endoscopic techniques, scope diameters have surpassed the 1.2 mm limit previously quoted. The larger bore scope has allowed for the delivery of various interventional modalities at the site of obstruction. Novel sialolith extrusion techniques were developed, including basket removal, forcep manipulation, laser and ultrasound fragmentation. The combination of these novel techniques with endoscopy allowed greater visualization compared to the previously utilized radiological "blind" approaches. Shortly after, algorithms were developed to help clinicians systematically approach various scenarios. Early protocols provided a decision tree based on sialolith size. The determination to proceed with extraction using basket retrieval initially was reserved for stones 3–4 mm in size. Larger stones were initially treated with shock or laser lithotripsy and subsequently extracted.[14]

ANATOMICAL AND PHYSIOLOGICAL CONSIDERATIONS

Sialoendoscopy has primarily been studied for intervention in pathology affecting parotid and submandibular glands. These are paired glands that provide the oral cavity with a mixture of mucous and serous secretions, aiding digestion, lubrication and hygiene. The major salivary glands develop during weeks 6–8 of gestation as outpouchings of ectoderm into the surrounding mesenchymal cells. The development of the parotid gland plays an important role in the subsequent treatment considerations. As the parotid enlarges and grows in a posterior direction, it eventually meets and envelops the facial nerve. This ultimately can put the facial nerve at risk during manipulation and treatment, specifically with transoral cut down procedures.

The parotid gland, averages about 6 cm by 4 cm, making it the largest salivary gland with an average weight of 14 grams. The gland is divided into two main compartments, deep and superficial lobe, which the facial nerve allows for a clear boundary. The enveloping space can be classified as the parotid compartment or the parapharyngeal space. Of the two, the parapharyngeal space is used much more commonly and has its borders defined as an inverted triangle. The base and apex are established by the skull base and greater cornu of the hyoid bone respectively. The medial border is formed by pharyngeal wall and laterally by the mandibular ramus and medial pterygoid muscles.

The majority of the gland (> 80%) overlies the masseter muscle, which is important given the ductal outflow of glandular products. Stensen's duct arises approximately 1.5 cm inferiorly from the inferior margin of the zygomatic arch. It measures about 4–6 cm with an average 5 mm diameter. As it courses towards the oral cavity, its path is parallel to the zygomatic arch and superficial to the masseter muscle. It eventually makes a 90° medial turn piercing the buccinators muscle and entering the oral cavity at the levels of the second maxillary molar. Important anatomic considerations include the buccal branch of the facial nerve which runs parallel with the parotid duct. Also the terminal branches of the facial nerve run superficial so caution should be heeded for any open procedure.

The paired submandibular glands weigh approximately half of the parotid gland. The gland is situated in the submandibular triangle, formed by the anterior and posterior digastric muscles and inferior margin of the mandible. The body of the gland clinches the mylohyoid muscle, lending to a natural division between the superficial and deep lobes. The marginal mandibular branch of the facial nerve plays an important landmark to consider with respect to the gland. It courses over the submandibular gland forming a natural landmark between it and the overlying platysma.

The submandibular secretions are drained via Wharton's duct which exits on the medial side of the gland. The duct courses between the mylohyoid and hyoglossus muscles and eventually through the genioglossus muscle to enter the intraoral cavity just lateral to the lingual frenulum. The average duct length is about 5 cm and has important anatomical considerations regarding the close vicinity of the lingual and hypoglossal nerves making it imperative for accurate identification. The lingual nerve is especially important in the sensory innervation of the tongue, the course takes it from the lateral to medial portions of the duct. The hypoglossal nerve, important for the motor innervation of the tongue, courses parallel and inferior to the submandibular duct. These relationships play important roles in cases of endoscopic assisted techniques and converted open procedures.

Another consideration with regards to possible complications given the anatomy of the submandibular gland is the possibility of ranula formation. A ranula is defined as a mucocele or retention cyst of the sublingual gland. The subsequent ranula may be simple or plunging, where by the latter is much more severe and found to plunge inferior through the mylohyoid muscle and deep into the neck.

The two aforementioned glands contain acinar cells, which primarily produce serous secretions. These secretions are delivered to the oral cavity via a complex interconnected ductal system, primarily controlled by the autonomic nervous system. Dysfunction in glandular innervation can lead to impaired flow and salivary stasis, contributing to the possibility of precipitation and stone formation. This was confirmed by work performed by Harrison et al. whereby glands were parasympathectomized and there was an increased sialolith formation.[15]

MAJOR SALIVARY GLAND DUCTAL OBSTRUCTION

Much of the early work regarding salivary gland pathogenesis and causes of obstruction was initially based upon microscopic observations of Kuttner in the late 1890s.[16] Over the last 120 years our understanding has flourished to involve microscopic, histological and anatomical investigations of salivary gland obstruction.[17,18] The following is a brief discussion of the various causes of salivary gland obstruction, thus providing a treatment rationale for the various interventions offered by sialoendoscopy.

Sialadenitis

Sialadenitis is multifactorial disease state, but ultimately develops from obstruction of salivary flow. There are many causes that can possibly lead to the stagnation of salivary flow as will be discussed below (Table 12.1). Ultimately patients present with a myriad of symptoms, which commonly includes recurrent painful swelling primarily during consumption of meals, fever, abscess formation, purulence and malaise. The most distressing and worrisome for clinicians is the onset of floor of mouth swelling or Ludwig's Angina. The swelling and infection present in the gland may permeate into surrounding tissue causing generalized inflam-

Table 12.1: The various causes of sialadenitis

• Obstruction
   – Sialolithiasis
   – Mucous plugs
   – Strictures/Kinks
   – Microliths

• Autoimmune
   – Systemic lupus erythematousus
   – Sjogrens disease
   – IgG-4 related sclerosing disease
   – Sialodochitis fibrinosa

• Radioiodine-induced sialadenitis
• Neoplasm
• Juvenile recurrent parotitis

mation of musculature, engorging tissue leading to the possibility of airway compromise.

Sialolithiasis

Obstruction of secretory flow within the ductal systems caused by sialolithiasis is one of the main causes of sialadenitis, accounting for up to 50% of major salivary disease.[19] Postmortem studies have revealed a prevalence of approximately 1.2%,[20] while population studies have stated an incidence of disease 0.45%.[21] The average age of patients affected were typically younger in the submandibular disease versus parotid disease.[22] Sialolithiasis typically occurs in adults, but can also be diagnosed in children.[23]

Many theories exist regarding the formation and propagation of microliths into symptomatic sialoliths. The list includes pure obstruction, decreased salivary flow, dehydration, changes in salivary pH, precipitation of crystalloid material from salivary products and retrograde migration of food and bacteria.[24,25] Other hypotheses have also been described. The first is based upon intracellular microcaliculi that when excreted in the ductal environment may become the nidus for additional calcification to be deposited.[26] The second hypothesis alludes to particles, substances and bacteria present in the oral cavity, which migrate into the salivary ducts and become the inciting factor for further deposition to occur.[25] For this migration to occur, secretory inactivity is usually present allowing for the ascent of bacteria and precipitation of materials.

The collection of this deposited material is a varying mixture of organic and inorganic compounds. The organic compounds include glycoproteins, lipids and cellular debris. The inorganic compounds include calcium carbonate and calcium phosphate. Depending on the ratio of calcium and phosphorous, varying amounts of each can allow formation of apatite versus whitlockite.[27] With this high mineral content, the majority of sialoliths are radiopaque, with a range of approximately 56–98% able to be visualized on radiograph (Fig. 12.1).[8] If the stone does in fact contain a higher content of inorganic material, it would lend to radiolucent stone. For these nonopaque stones, further radiographic studies such as sialography may show the presence of a filling defect present.

Significant differences exist with the incidence of the affected glands with 80–90% affecting the submandibular gland, while 5–10% affect the parotid.[28] The hypothesis regarding this discrepancy is thought to lie in the anatomical and physiological differences, with submandibular glands having a much sharper and angulated ductal system secreting primarily mucinous products. The sharp bend in the submandibular duct arises as it passes over the posterior free margin of the mylohyoid muscle as it enters the gland. While the parotid duct has more serpiginous course, with an initial 90° bend at the transition of deep to superficial gland and subsequently as it courses around the masseter muscle.[29] Typically, the location of calculi is fairly consistent with a majority involving the hilum and major ducts of the glands, while only rarely affecting the smaller intraparenchymal ducts (Figs 12.2 and 12.3).[30]

▎Obstruction not Caused by Lithiasis

Obstruction may also be noted with various anomalies and deformities of duct anatomy. They are typically characterized by the the percent encroachment into the ductal lumen. Typically strictures that occupy less

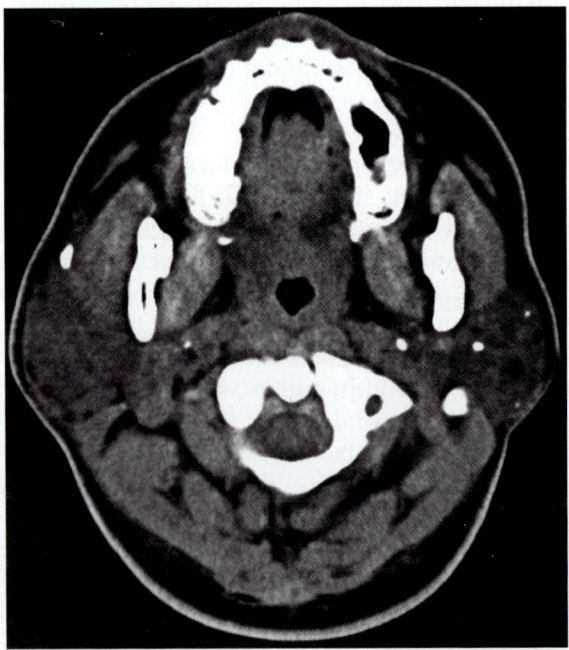

Fig. 12.1: Parotid sialoliths as noted on a noncontrast CT scan. Note the possibility of multiple stones in either one or both parotid glands

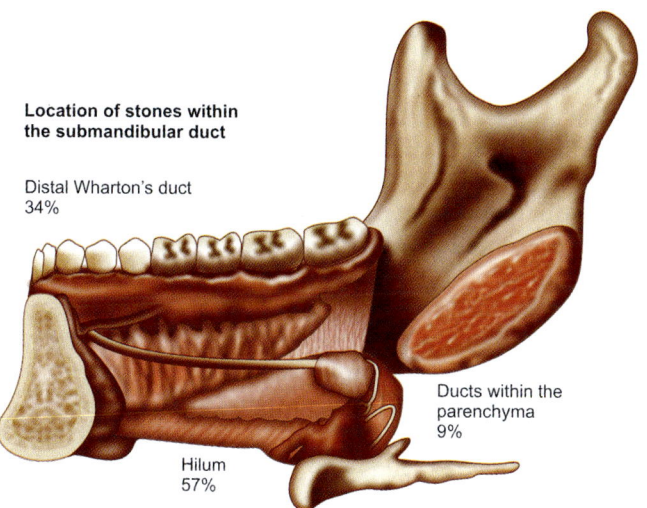

Location of stones within the submandibular duct

Distal Wharton's duct
34%

Ducts within the parenchyma
9%

Hilum
57%

Fig. 12.2: Location and associated frequency of submandibular stones

Source: Koch M, Zenk J, Iro H. Algorithms for treatment of salivary gland obstructions. Otolaryngol Clin North Am. 2009;42:1173-92.

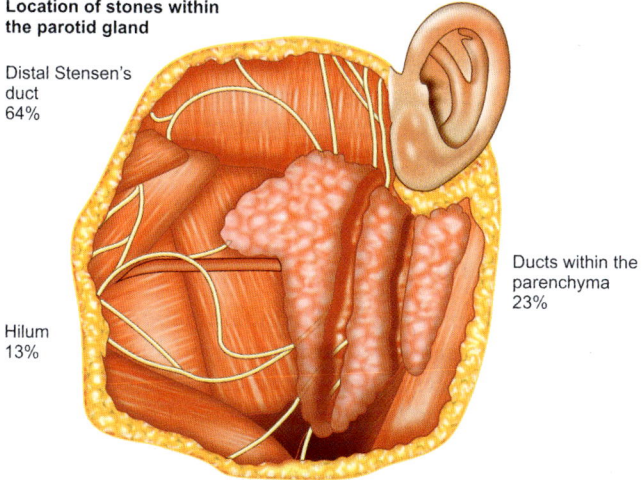

Location of stones within the parotid gland

Distal Stensen's duct
64%

Ducts within the parenchyma
23%

Hilum
13%

Fig. 12.3: Location and associated frequency of parotid stones

Source: Koch M, Zenk J, Iro H. Algorithms for treatment of salivary gland obstructions. Otolaryngol Clin North Am. 2009;42:1173-92.

that 50% of the ductal diameter can be classified as partial obstruction, while greater than 50% are subtotal obstructions.[31] Strictures can also be described with regards to frequency, which can be located in a short single site, occurring over multiple discreet points, or found in a continuous stretch of the duct.[29]

Each of these findings may also be associated with different imaging characteristics, which may aid in diagnosis. For instance in the case of single site obstruction, sialography may show only one stricture site. This finding is best illustrated with the anatomical factors associated with kink production. These have been described with the acute bending of Wharton's duct as it courses over the lingual nerve and mylohyoid muscle. In cases with multiple discrete points of obstruction, a sialography may show multiple areas of alternating patent and stenotic ducts. This pathology may be due to ductal polyps or invaginations.[3,11]

The clinical presentation of strictures is quite different than the obstructive sialolith counterpart. Salivary swelling is a main component, but instead of being exacerbated by food intake, it typically presents worse upon wakening with gradual development of symptoms over several days. The swelling that is evident is secondary to the stagnation of fluid and saliva within the ducts. There is often a sudden release of the fluid with rapid regression of swelling. Endoscopic findings often show gel like material and thick mucous plugs within the ducts.[29]

Fiber like substances and mucous plugs may also be implicated in inflammatory stenosis causing obstruction. Microscopic studies of ductal washings and contents found desquamated parenchymal cells, inflammatory cells and albuminous coagulum.[32] Increased masseter muscular tonicity can also lead to stagnation of salivary flow, allowing the ascent of microbes into the duct.[33] These pathologic states are mostly seen in the female population, with a higher predominance within the parotid glands.[34]

Some causes of obstruction can also arise from neoplasm of the duct, salivary gland or surrounding tissue. Several reports have been cited in the literature, exhibiting the development of sialolithiasis via various benign or malignant salivary gland neoplasms as well as the presence of accessory glands.[35,36]

Miscellaneous Factors

A whole host of other causes can lead to inflammation of glandular parenchyma not necessarily related to obstruction of ductal outflow. Several autoimmune diseases affect salivary glands as well as other organ systems, including Sjogrens disease, Systemic Lupus Erythematousus (SLE), sialodochitis fibrinosa and IgG4-related sclerosing disease, whereby the body's tissues are attacked by autoantibodies and T-cells. These respective diseases occur as a component of a larger symptom complex, often involving other organ systems.[37]

For example, Sjogrens syndrome is a chronic inflammatory disease of the exocrine glands, characterized by keratoconjunctivitis and xerostomia. Histologically the salivary glands are infiltrated with lymphocytes eventually causing destruction.[38] There is an increased association of the development of lithiasis in afflicted patients, especially within the parotid glands.[39] In severe Sjogrens syndrome, the possibility of presenting with multiple microliths has been reported.[40] Typically, Sjogrens begins with symptoms of xerostomia and keratoconjunctivitis, but chronic recurrent parotitis is often the heralding symptom. Sialography will often show diffuse sialectasias and strictures of Stenson's duct, while ultrasound examinations will demonstrate multiple small hypoechogenic areas and punctate calcifications. Diagnostic sialoendoscopy reveals minimal vascular supply to the lining of mucosa and strictures of the interrogated ductal system.[41] Therapeutic management addresses the recurrent symptoms secondary to the stricture formation, via dilatation of these strictures and washing out the ductal system under hydrostatic pressure.

Systemic lupus erythematosus is another multisystemic disease affecting multiple locations in the body including skin, joints, lungs and salivary glands. Presenting symptoms typically are recurrent parotitis due to the sialectasis and strictures present within the duct. Endoscopic findings also show minimally vascularized ducts with strictures, due to the associated inflammation and vasculitis inherent with the disease. Therapeutic strategies also revolve around repeated symptomatic relief rather than complete cure.[41]

Juvenile recurrent parotitis is the second most common cause of recurrent inflammation affecting parotid, with multifactorial causes not fully elucidated. The hallmark as the name suggests are recurrent episodic unilateral glandular swelling in children typically starting in the first or second year of life, associated with pain, fever and malaise.[42] The number of recurrences usually grades disease severity, with progressively more glandular parenchyma destroyed with each episode.[43] With the progressive destruction, there is decreased salivary production and transport via the duct, acting as an avenue of intraoral pathogens to ascend causing infection.[44] Sonographic findings include vacuoles, widened Stensen's duct and orifice while sialography indicates sialectasis and endoscopic findings often demonstrate white and atrophic ductal linings.[45] Treatment typically ranges from conservative medical treatment with sialagogues to invasive surgical procedures with total parotidectomy. For patients who experience multiple episodes per year, they can be considered for sialoendoscopic intervention with hydrostatic dilation and washing. The premise for this recommendation is based on the pathogenesis of repeated infections due to the multiple strictures noted in diseased glands. Nahlieli et al. noted marked improvement in symptoms in a report of 26 patients after performing bilateral ductal lavage and dilation with 60 ml of normal saline and subsequent hydrocortisone 100 mg infusion. After 36 months of follow-up the resolution of symptoms was noted to be 92%.[46] In a follow-up report by Shacham et al. further analysis for a total of 70 patients noted resolution of symptoms in 93% of patients after a single treatment.[45]

Radioiodine induced sialadenitis has also been noted in patients that have received therapy for the treatment of residual thyroid tissue.[47] The incidence of disease has been noted to be approximately 18%, primarily affecting parotid glands.[48] A dose and time dependent effect exists in the development of the disease, due to the ability of the striated serous cells to concentrate the iodine and subsequently damage glandular tissue.[49] Symptoms are primarily due to damaged salivary glands including xerostomia, taste alteration and sialadenitis.[50] Imaging studies available include scintigraphy, which allows evaluation of the damage in the salivary gland parenchyma and sialography, which allows evaluation of ductal strictures and acinar anatomy. Diagnostic sialoendoscopy can also aide in the diagnosis, showing an avascular lining of ductal mucosa without any vascular proliferation, multiple mucous plaques and stenosis of the main duct.[51] In 2006, Nahlieli et al. described therapeutic intervention in 15 patients, utilizing either saline hydrostatic pressure or balloon dilation and subsequently followed by 100 mg infusion of hydrocortisone. Postintervention follow-up was between 1 and 4 years, with 100% complete resolution of all symptoms within 12 hours of intervention.[51]

SIALOENDOSCOPY

As noted above, the various disease states encountered in salivary gland pathology make it imperative that the inciting factor is elucidated so appropriate treatment can begin. Even after years of disease, obstruction and inflammation, upon removal of the inciting factor, there is near total recovery of the gland.[52,53] These improvements are described histologically, scintigraphically and functionally, allowing full sparing of the gland.[53-55] Current management techniques have shifted from salivary gland excision to more minimally invasive therapy that includes sialoendoscopy.

Operative Indications

Sialoendoscopy allows for the ability to perform both diagnostic procedures and therapeutic interventions. Diagnostic procedures are indicated if there is a clinical suspicion or concern for physical ductal obstruction and prior test has not revealed a possible source. Once pathology has been determined, therapeutic interventions may be employed to relieve the pathologic cause. The indications for therapeutic sialoendoscopy include the treatment of salivary stones, dilatation and localization of strictures and irrigation of ducts in the treatment of chronic sialadenitis (Table 12.2).[56]

Absolute contraindications to sialoendoscopy include acute sialadenitis and complete distal obliteration of the duct (Table 12.3).[57,58] For acute infection, this is extremely important as with any other surgical intervention.

Table 12.2: Operative indications for sialoendoscopy[56]
Indications
Treatment of salivary stones
Dilatation and localization of strictures
Irrigation of ducts

Table 12.3: Absolute and relative contraindications of sialoendoscopy[57,58]	
Absolute contraindications	*Relative contraindications*
Acute Sialadenitis	Size of sialolith
Complete distal duct obliteration	Small duct diameter

The ductal milieu should be "cooled off" prior to any endoscopic intervention. The risk of complications increases during infected periods including ductal perforation, bleeding and scarring. The restricted maneuverability of the endoscope within the duct in the acutely infected setting, decreases visibility, hampers entry into the ductal ostia and ultimately prevents the utilization of invasive tools via the working channel. With regards to complete distal obstruction, the importance lies in the inability to adequately cannulate the distal duct. With such impedance, an open procedure would be better suited so as to adequately address the distal portion.

Relative contraindications also include the size of the obstructing sialoliths. Commonly, those larger than 10 mm may necessitate an open or combined procedure. A favorably positioned large stone, lodged long axis parallel to the salivary duct, may in fact be efficiently removed endoscopically despite its size (Fig. 12.4). Another relative contraindication restricting endoscopic intervention is small duct diameter.

ENDOSCOPES AND INSTRUMENTATION

Endoscopes

Endoscopic technology has evolved and advances in miniaturization and optical clarity have allowed clinicians to provide improved treatment. There are several different types of scopes available with certain specifications for clinical use.

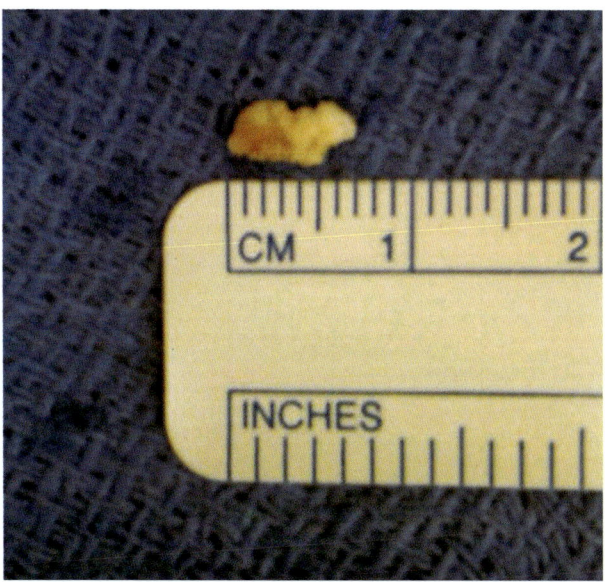

Fig. 12.4: A 7 mm stone retrieved en bloc, note the irregularities of the surface. This stone was oriented with long axis parallel to the duct. Forceps were utilized to retrieve this stone, engaging with the tapered end. This illustrates that size is only a relative contraindication, as an appropriately positioned stone may be retrieved successfully

Flexible Endoscopes

Since 1991, when Katz used a flexible scope to aid in sialolith removal, these scopes have come a long way.[6] The advantage of these scopes is the ability to negotiate tight ductal kinks and bend while being atraumatic to the ductal lining. It also has the added advantage of actually reaching some of the distally positioned stones in the further reaches of the glands. The "maneuverability" is provided with gentle forces applied to the extraluminal portion of the scope. Learning these maneuvering tactics is associated with a steeper learning curve as compared to some of the more rigid scopes. Given the fragility of the housing and scope materials, they tend to have a very short lifespan.[19]

Rigid Endoscopes

Rigid endoscopes compromise maneuverability and size for the clear resolution and crisp optics that the lenses within the system affords (Figs 12.5A and B). On average the scopes tend to have a larger diameter making "maneuvering "limited and at times can cause trauma to the ductal lining.

Semi-Rigid Endoscopes

Semi-rigid endoscopes afford the advantages of the previous two scopes into one device. There are two variations that exist, compact scopes and modular scopes. The compact is primarily a therapeutic device, and houses a working and irrigation channel. The modular endoscopes are primarily a diagnostic scope, but also have the capability to introduce various instruments for intervention. The flexibility and optical clarity that semi-rigid scopes provide, make them a versatile instrument to handle the multitude of scenarios encountered in sialoendoscopy.

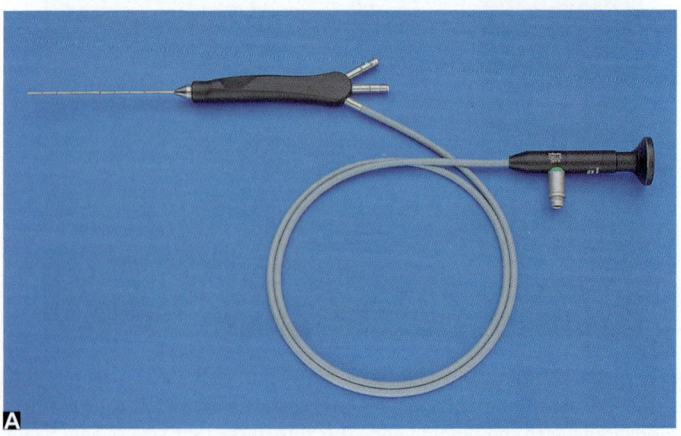

Fig. 12.5A

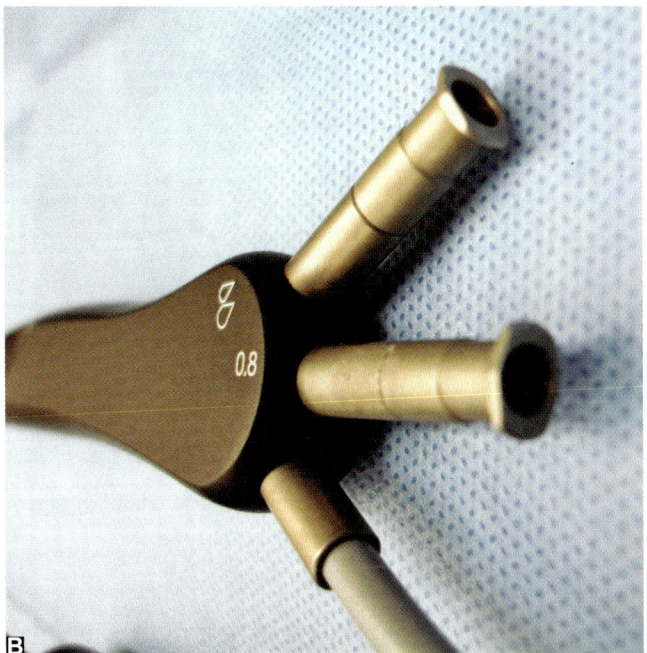

Fig. 12.5B

Figs 12.5A and B: (A) Typical rigid sialoendoscope; (B) Close up of irrigation port and a 0.8 working channel

Source: © 2011 KARL STORZ Endoscopy–America, Inc.

Instrumentation

There are a myriad of instruments available for use with the endoscopes, from initial dilatation and entry into ostium to retrieval and destruction of sialoliths (Fig. 12.6). The following is a brief listing and description of the many instruments utilized during a sialoendoscopic procedure.

Introduction into Ostium

This is considered an important and arguably a difficult aspect of sialo-endoscopy, as without proper identification, exposure and entry into the salivary duct the procedure would not take place. The importance is greatly magnified when considering the potential sequelae of inadequately dilated ostia, including scarring, inadvertent entry into a blind pouch and the increased risk of performing a papillotomy. The first of such devices are conical dilatators/bougies, which as noted below have a conical tapered end, allowing for gentle probing and dilatation (Fig. 12.7). These are typically available in two varieties sharp and blunt tip. The conical tip has pencil like maneuvering which allows for easy and precise control during the use.

Blunt lacrimal probes are typically used in other procedures, but, have the advantage of familiarity with the clinician. They are available in grad-

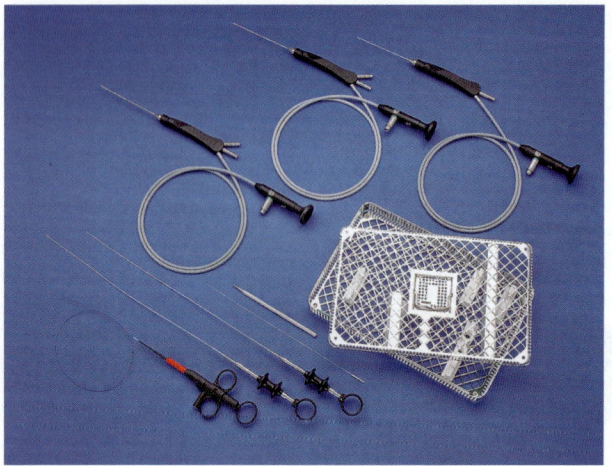

Fig. 12.6: Typical sialoendoscopy set: endoscopes, conical dilator, grasper/forceps and wire basket
Source: © 2011 KARL STORZ Endoscopy–America, Inc.

uated sizes for gentle dilatation. The correct use of the blunt probe allows the clinician to investigate the patency, diameter and direction of the duct. Obtaining this information allows easy maneuvering and decreases the risk of perforation and creating a blind tract.

Other devices and makeshift solutions have been described in the literature. Angiocatheters have been utilized and shown success in maintaining the ostia. The low cost of acquisition and their ubiquity allows for a cheap alternative to maintain patency. The main disadvantages of these products are the lack of expandability and they require an already dilated ostia for insertion.[59] Cardiovascular stents have also been described as a means of accessing and protecting from the repeated manipulation and entry into the respective salivary ostium. These have been described to be left in place for maintenance of ostia and duct patency for up to 30 days.[60] Many times visualizing the papilla can be difficult to aide in this step, methylene blue has been described as a method of increasing success. It

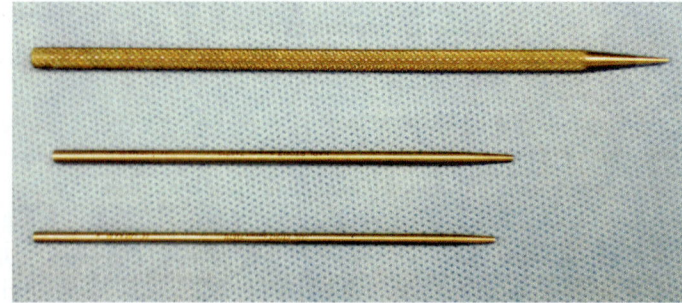

Fig. 12.7: Picture is a conical dilator (above) and bougie dilators (below) for entry into ostium

entails using a cotton-tipped applicator soaked in methylene blue and painting the area of interest. Once applied, the gland is palpated allowing the expression of saliva from the papilla.[61]

Extraction

Forceps are primarily available for the manipulation and retrieval of various debris encountered during an exam. A multitude of tips are available to provide a wide range of function, including scissor tip, biopsy cup and grasping serrated tip. The variety of tips allows a wide range of function, including retrieval of debris/stones, biopsy of suspicious ductal lesions and dilates encountered strictures. The advantage of graspers allows the possibility of addressing impacted stones with minimal space retrograde to it.

Baskets are available in different sizes and typically classified by the number and material type of their wires (Fig. 12.8). The stronger the "wire" material, the more force can be applied while deploying the basket, allowing for the possibility of dilating stenotic areas. The number of wires available is typically important when dealing with smaller stones, as they are easier to retrieve with less risk of dislodging. A major risk to using baskets is the possibility of jamming within the duct while it is deployed retrieving a stone or fragment. When a basket is utilized to retrieve stones or fragments, an important point is to deploy the basket when behind the stone. This strategy allows for maximal maneuvering and prevents the stone from becoming further impacted and moving proximally towards the gland.

Dilatation

Drills are typically used for the purpose of producing holes in encountered stones or creating tracts in occluded ducts. In the case of stones, the drilled holes allow for further intervention with forceps or fragmentation versus extraction. The drill can also be effectively utilized for opening pinpoint ductal strictures.

Balloons are primarily used for the dilatation of strictures and occlusions. There are two varieties available: low-pressure balloons have primarily been used for thin membrane strictures while high-pressure balloons have the ability to dilate denser strictures. Also available are "cutting" balloons, which have small microtome blades, mounted along the length of the balloon, allowing the ability to cut through dense fibrous strictures. Techniques have also been described for utilizing balloons for stone removal, where the balloon is threaded beyond the stone, inflated and slowly withdrawn.[62]

Stents can be used as both an aid for insertion into ducts or as a means of preventing scarring and contracting of the ostium. The stents are often sutured in place to prevent any migration proximally into the gland or extruded into the oral cavity.

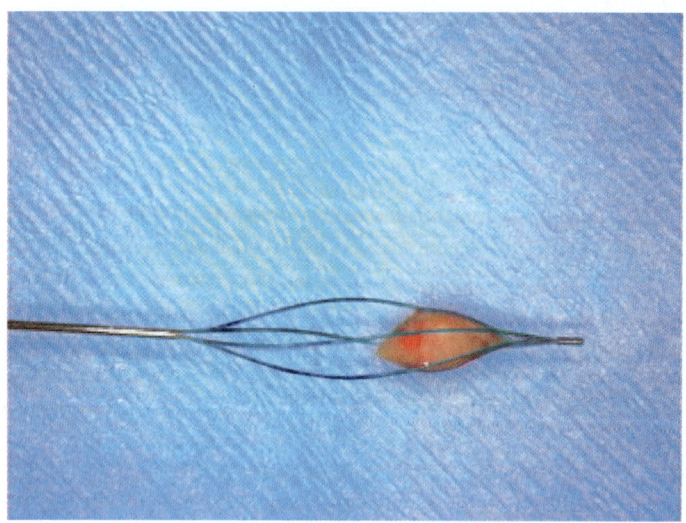

Fig. 12.8: Wire basket with retrieved sialolith
Source: © 2011 KARL STORZ Endoscopy–America, Inc.

Lithotripsy

Lasers, as in other areas of otolaryngology, have also been applied for use in sialoendoscopy. There are various types that are beyond the scope of this chapter but include the Excimer, flash lamp pulsed dye, Alexandrite, Neodymium: yttrium aluminum garnet (YAG), Rhodamine-6G, Holmium:YAG, Erbium:YAG and the frequency doubled Q-switched-double pulse Nd:YAG frequency-doubled double-pulse neodymium (FREDDY) laser. The principle behind these lasers revolves around creating mechanical shock waves on the surface of the calculi as a layer of plasma is formed with each laser pulse.[63] The lasers have an advantage of being able to deliver the energy source via thin fibers, ultimately allowing flexible scopes to accommodate them. The fragments produced by these lasers can be relatively small, allowing removal via irrigation, basket or graspers.[64] Unfortunately, they are susceptible to producing peripheral tissue damage, ductal perforations and abscess formation. Any residual stone fragments may require repeat procedures or lead to secondary stone formation.

The high cost associated with acquiring laser technology, can be a hindrance to some. The Ho:YAG laser, for example, is a popular laser amongst institutions, given the multiple uses shared with other surgical services. The intrinsic properties of this laser and its color absorptive specificity in targeting stones, decreases the amount of damage to surrounding tissue.[65]

The use of extracorporeal lithotripsy is a technique that is well established with a multitude of studies in various subspecialties of medicine and surgery. Marmary et al. first reported its use in salivary gland calculi in 1986.[66] The mechanism behind the technology is the utilization of high frequency shock waves transduced via the surrounding tissue and directed towards the sialolith. Applying this mechanical force causes fragmentation and allows it to be flushed out of the gland. Limitations of the intervention include treatment of sialoliths greater than 2.4 cm, due to the lower limit of electromagnetic focus, otherwise all other stones and ductal locations may be treated.[67] As with any other intervention, complications exist with the most common being pain, glandular swelling, ductal bleeding and cutaneous petechiae. Other possible complications include acute sialadenitis, temporary hearing impairment, temporary tinnitus and tooth filling loss.[68]

In a study by Eggers et al. 38 patients were examined after undergoing extracorporeal shock wave lithotripsy. The average size of calculi was 5.1 mm and was evenly split between submandibular and parotid glands. Contraindications of the procedure were listed as complete distal duct stenosis, pregnancy and presence of a cardiac pacemaker. The overall success rate was 55.3% for all patients, with 68.2% and 37.5% success noted in the parotid and submandibular glands respectively.[69]

Nahlieli et al. described the combination of external lithotripsy and sialoendoscopic techniques for advanced sialolithiasis cases in 94 patients, of which 60 were found in the submandibular gland and 34 in the parotid gland. Lithotripsy was effective in the extrusion of stones in 32% of cases, while endoscopic assistance resulted in success for an additional 29% of cases. The authors theorized that addition of lithotripsy prior to endoscopic intervention allowed the stone to be disconnected from the ductal wall and reduced stone volume.[70]

Operative Procedure

Sialoendoscopy like any other surgical procedure can be broken down into essential steps. With close study and anticipation of what to encounter with each step, it can translate into a successful and efficient procedure. The breakdown can typically be made into several main steps, including preparation and entry into the duct, diagnosis and visualization of pathology, employment of intervention and closure.

Entering the Duct

The operating room should be setup to the surgeon's preferences with regards to location of video monitor, surgical assistant, surgical technician and anesthesia. After prepping and draping the patient, the anesthetic delivery method should be selected. The minimally invasive procedure can be done either under local or general anesthesia. Typically, it is generally recommended the procedure be performed under general anesthesia initially. As the surgeon becomes acquainted with the procedure and tactile feedback of the various devices and instruments, it is possible for local anesthesia to be used. Other indications for general anesthesia include complicated salivary pathology and treating children. If local anesthesia is selected, typically xylometazolin 2% or bupivacaine 3% is used. The easiest method to deliver the anesthetic is to cannulate the papilla of interest and irrigate the ductal system, which tends to be sufficient anesthetic. Other methods include irrigating the anesthetic solution via the working channel of the endoscope. Additional injections to surrounding tissue or specific nerve blocks may be utilized.

Once the anesthesia is established, the exam should interrogate all the papilla for the respective glands, presence of purulence, lack of salivary flow upon "milking" the gland and surrounding erythema. If difficulty is encountered in appropriately identifying the papilla, magnification loupes may be used, simply "milking" the gland or application of methylene blue[61] may help to distinguish the area. Since the average papilla diameter is noted to be around 0.5 mm,[13] it may likely need to be dilated to allow easy entry and manipulation with the endoscope. As previously mentioned above, the use of conical dilators may be used initially (Fig. 12.9) and then serial dilation may occur with the blunt probes.

The blunt probes typically start at diameter 0000 and range up to diameter 8. With each progressive change the papilla hole is decannulated and recannulated with the next largest probe (Fig. 12.10). There is a risk of losing the hole and increased difficulty with recannulation for each subsequent change. Marchal et al. described a method based on the Seldinger technique,[71] whereby a titanium guidewire is introduced into the papilla after cannulation with the 0000 probe. Once the guide wire is situated in the papilla, increasingly larger Marchal bougies are directed to the papilla via the guidewire (Fig. 12.11). With entry of each progressively sized bougie, it is gently turned allowing incremental dilatation. Once the adequate diameter is reached, the last bougie is removed while keeping the guidewire in place. The endoscope is inserted in an all-in-one fashion through the distal end of the guidewire and directed towards the papilla for entry.[72]

Caution must be heeded with forceful dilation, which may tear the duct resulting scarring postoperatively or even more detrimental the formation of a false passage. Scenarios may be encountered where the stricture or obstruction at the papilla will not allow passage of the dilator, in which

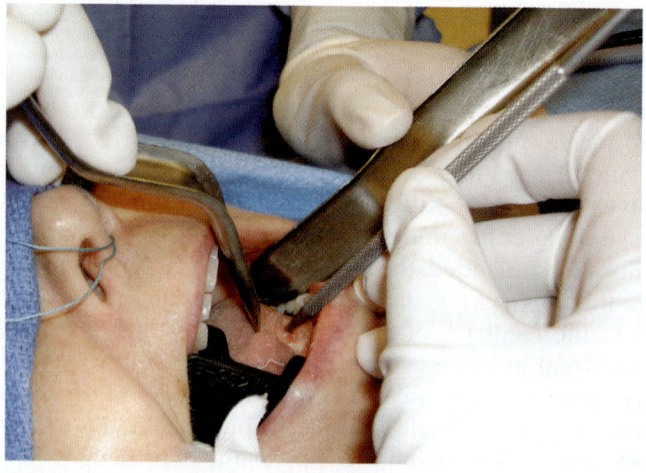

Fig. 12.9: Initial dilation as performed with conical dilator

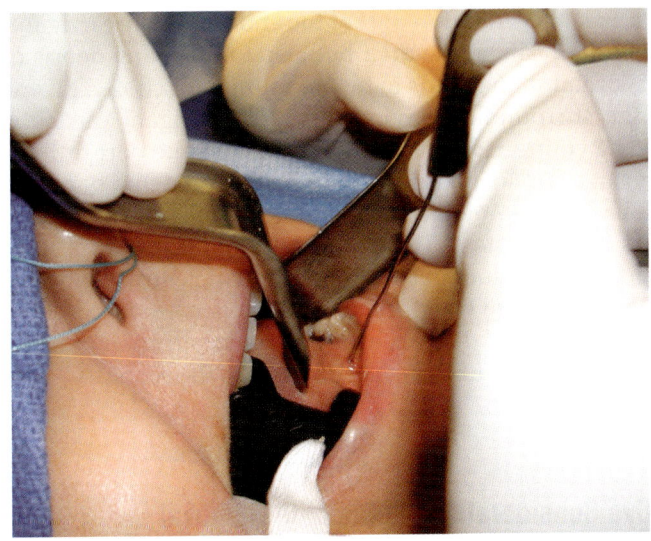

Fig. 12.10: Serial dilation as performed with blunt lacrimal probe

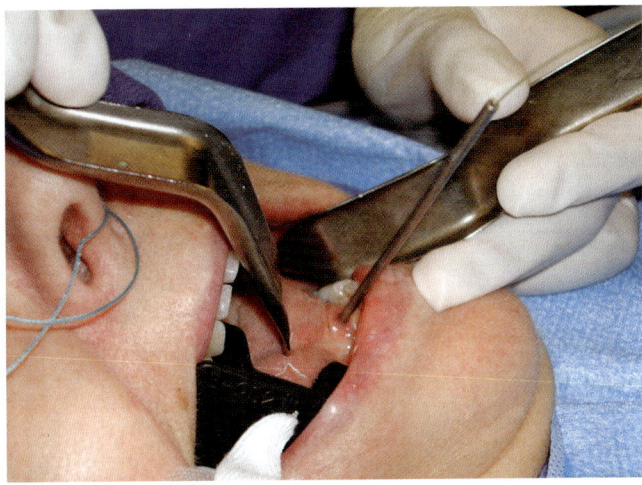

Fig. 12.11: Utilizing the Seldinger technique for dilation of ostium. Shown is bougie being passed over guidewire for gradual dilation of ostia

case it would be advised to carry out a papillotomy or a cut down on the duct. One such method as described by Nahlieli, uses a 0000 probe inserted in the papilla and electrocautery is used to open up the papilla.[62]

Establishing Visualization

Once the scope has entered into duct, it will be noted that the natural tendency of the duct is to collapse upon itself. To prevent this collapse and allow adequate visualization, a constant stream of irrigation should be provided via the irrigation port of the endoscope. The irrigant not only acts to stent the walls of the duct but also to flush any debris or foreign material. Normal saline tends to be the solution of choice, given its isotonicity to the surrounding environment. The irrigant can be delivered via an IV bag connected directly to the endoscopic port or having large volume syringes preloaded supplying a constant delivery of solution.

With an adequate amount of irrigant flow, the endoscope is steered in the salivary ductal system. The clinician should methodically interrogate the ducts for various clues of pathology and efficiently identify the area of concern (Figs 12.12A to C). Once an area is visualized and deemed to be the pathologic cause of disease, appropriate localization of the scope can be made via palpation, utilizing gradations on the scope.

INTERVENTIONS

Operative Considerations in Sialolith Removal

Recently with the improvements in instrumentation, device optics and development of novel techniques, multiple modalities are available in the armamentarium of clinicians in addressing ductal obstruction. The instrumentation described above can be used to attempt stone removal from interrogated ducts, via exertion of force on the stone to cause fragmentation or engaging with the foreign body to manually remove from the duct. An important step in establishing the type of intervention to be employed is determination of the relationship between stone size and duct diameter during the diagnostic step of sialoendoscopy.

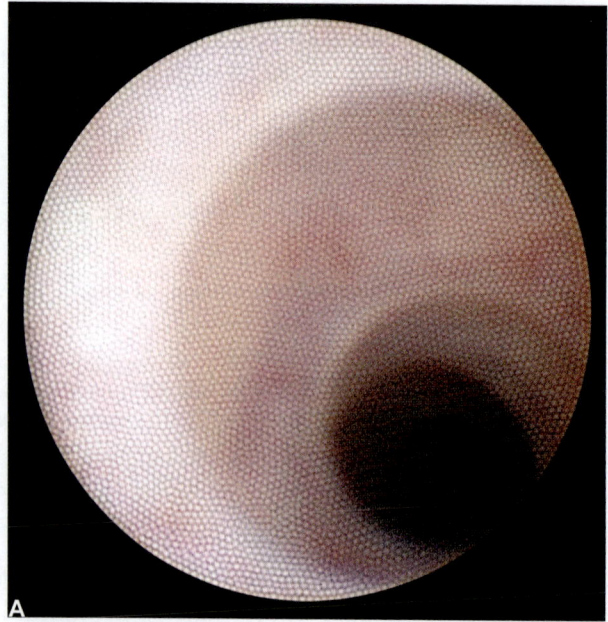

Fig. 12.12A

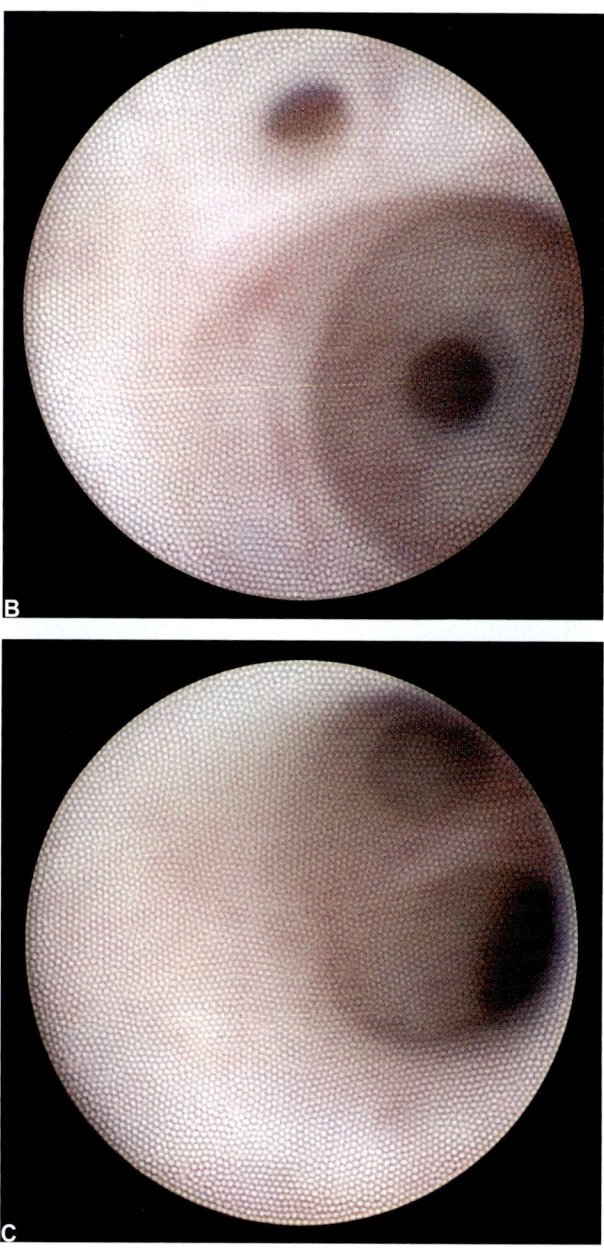

Figs 12.12B and C

Figs 12.12A to C: Intraoperative endoscopic views demonstrating variations in normal anatomy encountered

Stones may be encountered either in the papilla/distal duct, proximal duct/hilum or intraparenchymally, governing the method of stone retrieval.[30] McGurk et al. divides the decision tree depending on the location of stones in respective glands. The authors' partitioning of the gland differed with parotid versus submandibular tissue, given the innate anatomical differences. The algorithm developed included options such as transoral slitting for stones located distally, minimally invasive techniques for stones located throughout the gland, open excision for multiple stones especially found in the parenchyma. In general, for nonimpacted stones less than 7 mm, they may be retrieved with graspers, baskets, or forceps while larger stones may require fragmentation techniques.[21] For stones located in the distal duct/hilum, a transoral duct slitting technique may be employed.[73]

In a review by Nahlieli et al. the efficacy of glandular stone removal was evaluated in 736 glands. The authors proposed an algorithm for stone removal once visualized, it utilizes a combination of endoscopic techniques used in succession until the stone is completely removed. The stepwise progression includes, the removal of the stone in total using forceps or basket, mechanical fragmentation using forceps, intracorporeal laser fragmentation, and combined use of intracorporeal laser lithotripter wire basket and minigrasping forceps. Applying the various endoscopic techniques as described afforded the authors a success rate of 89% for submandibular glands and 86% for parotid glands.[4]

In the largest review to date by Iro et al. the authors reported a comprehensive multi-institutional effort of evaluating their experience in 4,691 patients. The authors used either extracorporeal shock lithotripsy, extraction of stones using wire baskets or microforceps, or gland preserving surgery utilizing intraoral cut downs on respective ducts. It is important to note that the extraction of stones was limited to those, typically less than 5 mm and noted to be mobile within the respective ducts. With those restrictions, the retrieval success rate was noted to be 91.6%.[74]

Luers et al. examined the prognostic factors for successful stone extraction without use of fragmentation and the association with duration of disease. The patients reviewed were treated with either basket or grasping forceps, stone size, stone mobility, shape and location were significant predictors to successful removal. The mean size of endoscopically removed stones were 5 mm, while nonremovable stones were greater than 7 mm and tended to be fixed within the duct. Stone shape was also noted to affect prognosis, with round and oval stones more successfully removed as compared to angulated or irregular shapes. Location was an important factor in removal of sialoliths, it was noted that distal stones found in the main excretory duct had a higher rate of success versus those located proximal to hilum.[75] Stone size was directly correlated with the duration of symptoms, while stone mobility was inversely related to the duration of glandular disease.[76]

▮ Operative Considerations in Ductal Strictures

Ductal strictures, kinks and non-sialolith obstructions are also common findings during endoscopy. It is important to determine the characteristic of the stenosis (inflammatory vs. fibrotic), location within the gland, pathogenesis, total length, number of areas affected and degree of obstruction.

Several techniques have been mentioned in the literature as approaches to deal with these various findings.

Nahlieli et al. reported on 25 salivary gland obstructions (14 parotid glands and 11 submandibular glands) diagnosed with ductal kinks or strictures. The authors used a variety of methods to treat strictures and kinks including hydrostatic infusion of saline, balloon dilatation, forced manipulation, advancement ductoplasty or balloon contouring. With regard to strictures, they reported an 80% success rate with resolution of symptoms during the follow-up period of 8–36 months. All kinks treated experienced complete resolution of symptoms during the 6–24 months follow-up period.[11] Furthermore, intraductal infusion of steroids and use of ductal stents have helped to avoid long-term recurrences.[11,77]

Severe strictures can be treated with either repeated inflation of balloons or utilizing the miniature grasper forceps to mechanically relieve the obstruction. As reported by Nahlieli et al. balloon dilators can be inflated to 3 mm with up to 18 bar of pressure.[3] A case series of 249 salivary strictures, 92% of which involved the parotid gland, reported the success with salivary ductoplasties. Follow-up sialography showed complete elimination in 82% of those treated and a partial elimination in 13% of strictures treated. A long follow-up period is important in these patients as restenosis is very common.[29] Alternatively, it has been described to utilize a miniforcep grasper for the enlargement of strictures. The closed tines of the forcep are inserted into the stricture. Upon engagement with the distal end of the stricture, the tines are opened, mechanically forcing the stricture open.[3,11]

Ardekian et al. described their experience in the treatment of strictures in 87 parotid glands. The authors instituted a 4-step procedure of addressing strictures, which consisted of orifice dilatation, followed by ductal dilation by advancing the endoscope under hydrostatic pressure until the posterior portion of the gland was encountered. The Sialoballoon was then utilized to dilate any strictures that would not resolve with the infused hydrostatic pressure. In the case of difficult stenosis, the endoscope would be manually advanced to manipulate the duct or a manual drill would be utilized. A stent was then placed to prevent in the recreation of strictures. The authors experienced a success rate of 81.7% in the treatment of stenosis using this method. They concluded that in the treatment of simple strictures of inflammatory origin measuring less than half of ductal diameter, a pressurized infusion of saline irrigant can easily stretch to relieve the obstruction. For severe or multiple strictures, a balloon or microdrill should be utilized to relieve the obstruction.[31]

▌Considerations for Endoscopically Assisted Removal of Stones

To address stones that may be impacted, not amenable to utilizing alternative techniques, or located within parenchymal tissue, more advanced procedures may need to be employed. One such technique first described by Nahlieli et al. in 2002, involves the assistance of sialoendoscopes to assist in localization and incision planning for extraductal sialolithotomies. The technique can be performed via intraoral or extraoral incision, with the later solely reserved for parotid sialoliths.[78]

McGurk et al. in 2005 described their technique and experience of endoscopically assisted sialolithiasis retrieval in eight patients afflicted with parotid stones. The procedure involved establishing endoscopic visualization of the stone. Once visualization was achieved, the light source was increased so as to transilluminate the overlying skin and marked (Fig. 12.13). A preauricular incision is made and skin flaps are raised. Using the endoscope light as guidance, an incision was made into the parotid fascia and brought down to the parotid duct. The duct is incised longitudinally, the duct is entered, stone delivered and the duct closed primarily or ligated. Contraindications of the procedure included severe stenosis precluding cannulation of proximal ducts and for stones located greater than 6 mm from the outer skin surface. Postoperative complications included swelling, paresthesia of preauricular skin, infections, postoperative strictures and damage to the ductal system. The patients treated with the aforementioned method experienced complete resolution of symptoms and no long-term complications were reported after a 10-month follow-up.[79]

Marchal in 2007 presented his description for extraction of parotid and submandibular stones utilizing the combined approach. With regards to his parotid technique, he presented 37 patients with a mean follow-up period of 19 months and had 92% improvement in symptoms. While in this submandibular data, 29 patients were followed for an average of 22 months and reported a 69% success in symptomatic relief. The failures reported while addressing the submandibular gland were due to continuous glandular swelling noted postoperatively secondary to premature floor of mouth mucosal closure. The close anatomical relationships between lingual nerve and Wharton's duct must be respected to prevent postoperative morbidity.[80]

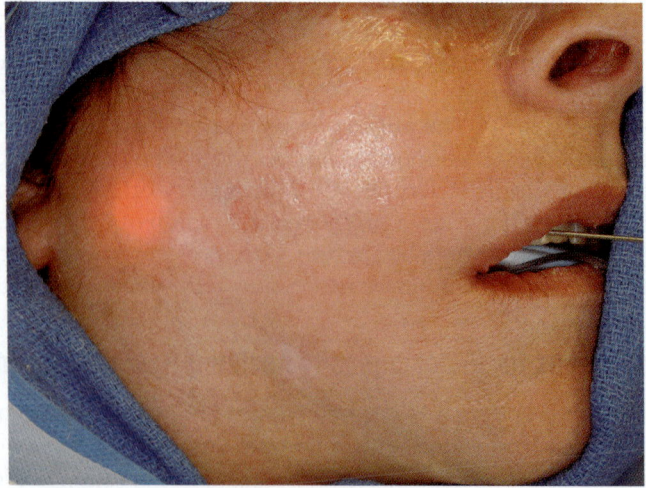

Fig. 12.13: Transillumination of skin overlying parotid gland in preparation of endoscopic assisted stone removal

COMPLICATIONS

The most frequently reported side effect in 80–100% of cases has been a transient swelling of the gland, primarily caused by the instillation of irrigation used for the procedure.[9,10] It is commonly self limiting and resolved within several hours with warm compresses and massages. A case report by Baptista et al. reported a case of massive tongue and floor of mouth swelling secondary to duct lesion or perforation enabling instillation of large amount saline irrigation into surrounding tissue. They subsequently advocated for the use of general anesthetic with adequate airway control for procedures involving stones larger than 4 mm.[81] Other possible complications reported include wire basket block (6%), ductal perforations (0.3–6%), recurrence of symptoms (1–6%), temporal lingual nerve paresthesia (0.5%), ranula (1%), postoperative infections (2%) and ductal strictures (0.3–3.5%) (Table 12.4).[19,10]

Stricture formation postoperatively is often cued by the ongoing symptomology and reduced salivary production. These strictures are often located at or near the orifice, which highlights the importance of adequate maintenance of papilla caliber, and kept well protected during the instrumentation phase of the intervention. Some methods of preventing orifice stricture and stenosis are the implementation of postoperative stents and intraductal irrigation with hydrocortisone.

The risk of perforation is often seen during two different aspects of sialoendoscopy. The first aspect is during the initial instrumentation of the papilla and ductal orifice, which is a result of the separation of the ductal wall from the buccal mucosa. Not only does this require prompt repair, but also it completely obscures and prevents the cannulation of the duct without a papillotomy. The second aspect of the procedure at increased risk for ductal perforation is while maneuvering the endoscope or instrumenting with forceps, baskets, drills and lasers for stone retrieval or stricture dilatation. It is imperative to watch for the sequelae of ductal perforation, which can lead to irrigant extravasation and cause severe swelling of the gland and surrounding tissue.

Ranula formation can be another important complication to be aware of. These are more commonly noted with submandibular sialoendsocopy. The risk of formation is thought to be directly proportional to the extent

Table 12.4: Associated complications of sialoendoscopy[9,10,19]
Transient glandular swelling
Ductal perforations
Temporal lingual nerve paresthesias
Postoperative infections
Wire basket block
Soft tissue swelling (floor of mouth)
Ranula
Ductal strictures

of the procedure. It is diagnosed by the appearance of swelling, often a blue hue, along the floor of the mouth. After review of over 1,500 sialoendoscopy cases, involving submandibular and sublingual instrumentation there was a 2.5% risk of this complication.[82]

CONSIDERATIONS IN PEDIATRIC SIALOENDOSCOPY

Sialoadenitis in the pediatric population is described to occur in about 10% of all cases of recurrent salivary gland swellings.[83] The pathogenesis is still in debate and involves many factors, including autoimmune disorders, genetic factors, ductal obstruction and congenital abnormalities. Juvenile recurrent parotitis, as described previously, is the second most common cause of salivary obstruction. As in adults salivary swelling in the pediatric population can be secondary to ductal obstruction via stenosis and sialolithiasis.[23,84] The diagnosis of salivary obstruction secondary to sialolithiasis is especially difficult in the pediatric population given the limitations of sonography in detecting stones less than 2 mm in diameter, which can be seen in pediatric populations causing obstructive symptoms.[85]

Sialoendoscopy has allowed for direct visualization in the small ductal anatomy found in the pediatric population. Technically, the introduction of endoscopes into these ostia is much more demanding and delicate. Despite size constraints, successful diagnostic and interventional procedures have been well described being undertaken with 1.1 mm and 1.3 mm endoscopes with excellent long-term results.[86] Age of intervention is not a limitation to intervention as reports exist in the literature of procedures on submandibular glands in a 4-month-old patient.[87]

The procedure of diagnostic and therapeutic sialoendoscopy is similar to that described above for adults. For successful visualization, maneuverability and intervention, it becomes crucial that an adequate sized endoscope is selected. Several reports in the literature have successfully used endoscopes of 1.1 mm and 1.3 mm caliber to visualize ductal pathology and adequately intervene.[83,86,87] Despite the smaller caliber of the working channel in the smaller scopes, successful interventions have been employed including laser fragmentation, wire basket stone retrieval, stenotic balloon dilatation.[83,86,87] Martins-Carvalho et al. reported 38 patients undergoing sialoendoscopic intervention with a mean age of 9-years old and a mean follow-up of 24 months. The primary pathology encountered was salivary duct stenosis, reported to be 55% of the population while sialolithiasis was noted 31% of the cases. The majority of the salivary glands treated were parotid glands (60%). They reported an 84% completion rate, whereby stone removal was performed solely by endoscopic means. Sialolithiasis detection during diagnostic interventions was found to be more sensitive than sonography. Of the ten cases of lithiasis diagnosed by endoscopy, only four were detected by sonography. Follow-up showed that 77% of the patients with stenotic ducts had no evidence of recurrence at 24 months.[86]

Typically sialoendoscopic procedures in children occur in the operating room under general anesthesia, providing a controlled setting, decreasing patient intolerability and minimizing discomfort. Konstantinidis et al. examined performing sialoendoscopy under local anesthesia in children with a mean age of 9 years suffering from recurrent parotid swellings with non-lithiasis pathology. The lack of sialolithiasis was preferred as it would require less intervention and require shorter operative time. The procedure described irrigating and flushing out the ductal network under direct visualization and allowing for the infusion of medications. Despite a moderate pain level, the procedure was well tolerated amongst the seven children studied. Successful intervention was noted in six/seven patients with only one patient requiring repeat intervention. Complication rates did not differ with those reported for procedures undertaken with general anesthesia.

CONCLUSION

The treatment of salivary gland pathology has undergone a huge paradigm shift over the past 20 years. In the past, salivary gland pathology was treated with open neck gland excisions. Now utilizing sialoendoscopic techniques has allowed adequate diagnosis and treatment from within. Success rates reported in the literature are similar to previous modalities with substantially less morbidity and retention of salivary function. Given the robust armamentarium available to address the various ductal pathology and the vigorous data associated with minimally invasive techniques, open total gland excision should be reserved when all other measures have been exhausted. This is an exciting time for the field of sialoendoscopy, the progress made in instrumentation miniaturization and optical resolution will surely make even greater strides in patient outcomes.

REFERENCES

1. Amin MA, Bailey BM, Patel SR. Clinical and radiological evidence to support superficial parotidectomy as the treatment of choice for chronic parotid sialadenitis: a retrospective study. Br J Oral Maxillofac Surg. 2001;39(5):348-52.
2. Motamed M, Laugharne D, Bradley PJ. Management of chronic parotitis: a review. J Laryngol Otol. 2003;117(7):521-6.
3. Nahlieli O, Bar T, Shacham R, et al. Management of chronic recurrent parotitis: current therapy. J Oral Maxillofac Surg. 2004;62(9):1150-5.
4. Nahlieli O, Nakar LH, Nazarian Y, et al. Sialoendoscopy: a new approach to salivary gland obstructive pathology. J Am Dent Assoc. 2006;137(10):1394-400.
5. McGurk M, Escudier MP, Thomas BL, et al. A revolution in the management of obstructive salivary gland disease. Dent Update. 2006;33(1):28-30.
6. Katz P. Endoscopy of the salivary glands. Ann Radiol. 1991;34(1-2):110-3.
7. Nahlieli O, Neder A, Baruchin AM. Salivary gland endoscopy: a new technique for diagnosis and treatment of sialolithiasis. J Oral Maxillofac Surg. 1994;52(12):1240-2.
8. Nahlieli O, Baruchin AM. Sialoendoscopy: three years' experience as a diagnostic and treatment modality. J Oral Maxillofac Surg. 1997;55(9):912-8.

9. Nahlieli O, Baruchin AM. Endoscopic technique for the diagnosis and treatment of obstructive salivary gland diseases. J Oral Maxillofac Surg. 1999;57(12):1394-401.

10. Nahlieli O, Baruchin AM. Long-term experience with endoscopic diagnosis and treatment of salivary gland inflammatory diseases. Laryngoscope. 2000;110(6):988-93.

11. Nahlieli O, Shacham R, Yoffe B, et al. Diagnosis and treatment of strictures and kinks in salivary gland ducts. J Oral Maxillofac Surg. 2001;59(5):484-90.

12. Zenk J, Hosemann WG, Iro H. Diameters of the main excretory ducts of the adult human submandibular and parotid gland: a histologic study. Oral Surg Oral Med Oral Pathol Oral Radiol Endod. 1998;85(5):576-80.

13. Zenk J, Zikarsky B, Hosemann WG, et al. The diameter of the Stenon and Wharton ducts. Significance for diagnosis and therapy. HNO. 1998;46(12):980-5.

14. Marchal F, Dulguerov P. Sialolithiasis management: the state of the art. Arch Otolaryngol Head Neck Surg. 2003;129(9):951-6.

15. Triantafyllou A, Harrison JD, Garrett JR. Production of salivary microlithiasis in cats by parasympathectomy: light and electron microscopy. Int J Exp Pathol. 1993;74(1):103-12.

16. Kuttner H. Ueber entzündliche tumoren der submaxillar-speicheldruse. Beitrage zür klinischen chirurgie. 1896;15:815-28.

17. Harrison JD, Triantafyllou A, Garrett JR. The effects of obstruction and secretory stimulation on microlithiasis in salivary glands of cat: light and electron microscopy. Virchows Arch B Cell Pathol Incl Mol Pathol. 1993;64(1):29-35.

18. Epivatianos A, Harrison JD, Dimitriou T. Ultrastructural and histochemical observations on microcalculi in chronic submandibular sialadenitis. J Oral Pathol. 1987;16(10):514-7.

19. Marchal F, Dulguerov P, Becker M, et al. Specificity of parotid sialendoscopy. Laryngoscope. 2001;111(2):264-71.

20. Rauch S. Speichelsteine. Die Speicheldrusen des menschen. Anatomie, Physiologie und Klinische Pathologie. Stuttgart: Georg Thieme; 1959.

21. McGurk M, Escudier MP, Brown JE. Modern management of salivary calculi. Br J Surg. 2005;92(1):107-12.

22. Zenk J, Constantinidis J, Kydles S, et al. Clinical and diagnostic findings of sialolithiasis. HNO. 1999;47(11):963-9.

23. Nahlieli O, Eliav E, Hasson O, et al. Pediatric sialolithiasis. Oral Surg Oral Med Oral Pathol Oral Radiol Endod. 2000;90(6):709-12.

24. Escudier MP. The current status and possible future for lithotripsy of salivary caliculi. Atlas Oral Maxillofac Surg Clin North Am. 1998;6(1):117-32.

25. Marchal F, Kurt AM, Dulguerov P, et al. Retrograde theory in sialolithiasis formation. Arch Otolaryngol Head Neck Surg. 2001;127(1):66-8.

26. Harrison JD, Epivatianos A, Bhatia SN. Role of microliths in the aetiology of chronic submandibular sialadenitis: a clinicopathological investigation of 154 cases. Histopathology. 1997;31(3):237-51.

27. Koutsoukos PG, Sheehan ME, Nancollas GH. Epitaxial considerations in urinary stone formation. II. The oxalate-phosphate system. Invest Urol. 1981;18(5):358-63.

28. Bodner L. Salivary gland calculi: diagnostic imaging and surgical management. Compendium. 1993;14(5):572, 4-6, 8 passim; quiz 86.

29. McGurk M, Brown J. Alternatives for the treatment of salivary duct obstruction. Otolaryngol Clin North Am. 2009;42(6):1073-85.

30. Koch M, Zenk J, Iro H. Algorithms for treatment of salivary gland obstructions. Otolaryngol Clin North Am. 2009;42(6):1173-92.

31. Ardekian L, Shamir D, Trabelsi M, et al. Chronic obstructive parotitis due to strictures of Stenson's duct — our treatment experience with sialoendoscopy. J Oral Maxillofac Surg. 2010;68(1):83-7.

32. Qi S, Liu X, Wang S. Sialoendoscopic and irrigation findings in chronic obstructive parotitis. Laryngoscope. 2005;115(3):541-5.

33. Bernkopf E, Colleselli P, Broia V, et al. Is recurrent parotitis in childhood still an enigma? A pilot experience. Acta Paediatr. 2008;97(4):478-82.

34. Ngu RK, Brown JE, Whaites EJ, et al. Salivary duct strictures: nature and incidence in benign salivary obstruction. Dentomaxillofac Radiol. 2007;36(2):63-7.

35. Giger R, Mhawech P, Marchal F, et al. Mucoepidermoid carcinoma of Stensen's duct: a case report and review of the literature. Head Neck. 2005;27(9):829-33.

36. Koybasioglu A, Ileri F, Gencay S, et al. Submandibular accessory salivary gland causing Warthin's duct obstruction. Head Neck. 2000;22(7):717-21.

37. Koch M, Zenk J, Bozzato A, et al. Sialoscopy in cases of unclear swelling of the major salivary glands. Otolaryngol Head Neck Surg. 2005;133(6):863-8.

38. Moutsopoulos HM. Sjogren's syndrome: autoimmune epithelitis. Clin Immunol Immunopathol. 1994;72(2):162-5.

39. Zenk J, Gottwald F, Bozzato A, et al. Submandibular sialoliths. Stone removal with organ preservation. HNO. 2005;53(3):243-9.

40. Shimizu M, Yoshiura K, Nakayama E, et al. Multiple sialolithiasis in the parotid gland with Sjogren's syndrome and its sonographic findings — report of 3 cases. Oral Surg Oral Med Oral Pathol Oral Radiol Endod. 2005;99(1):85-92.

41. Shacham R, Puterman MB, Ohana N, et al. Endoscopic treatment of salivary glands affected by autoimmune diseases. J Oral Maxillofac Surg. 2011;69(2):476-81.

42. Quenin S, Plouin-Gaudon I, Marchal F, et al. Juvenile recurrent parotitis: sialendoscopic approach. Arch Otolaryngol Head Neck Surg. 2008;134(7):715-9.

43. Galili D, Marmary Y. Juvenile recurrent parotitis: clinicoradiologic follow-up study and the beneficial effect of sialography. Oral Surg Oral Med Oral Pathol. 1986;61(6):550-6.

44. Mandel L, Witek EL. Chronic parotitis: diagnosis and treatment. J Am Dent Assoc. 2001;132(12):1707-11; quiz 27.

45. Shacham R, Droma EB, London D, et al. Long-term experience with endoscopic diagnosis and treatment of juvenile recurrent parotitis. J Oral Maxillofac Surg. 2009;67(1):162-7.

46. Nahlieli O, Shacham R, Shlesinger M, et al. Juvenile recurrent parotitis: a new method of diagnosis and treatment. Pediatrics. 2004;114(1):9-12.

47. Mandel SJ, Mandel L. Persistent sialadenitis after radioactive iodine therapy: report of two cases. J Oral Maxillofac Surg. 1999;57(6):738-41.

48. Kim JW, Han GS, Lee SH, et al. Sialoendoscopic treatment for radioiodine induced sialadenitis. Laryngoscope. 2007;117(1):133-6.

49. Newkirk KA, Ringel MD, Wartofsky L, et al. The role of radioactive iodine in salivary gland dysfunction. Ear Nose Throat J. 2000;79(6):460-8.

50. Blahd WH. Treatment of malignant thyroid disease. Semin Nucl Med. 1979;9(2):95-9.

51. Nahlieli O, Nazarian Y. Sialadenitis following radioiodine therapy—a new diagnostic and treatment modality. Oral Dis. 2006;12(5):476-9.

52. Su YX, Xu JH, Liao GQ, et al. Salivary gland functional recovery after sialendoscopy. Laryngoscope. 2009;119(4):646-52.

53. Makdissi J, Escudier MP, Brown JE, et al. Glandular function after intraoral removal of salivary calculi from the hilum of the submandibular gland. Br J Oral Maxillofac Surg. 2004;42(6):538-41.

54. Yoshimura Y, Morishita T, Sugihara T. Salivary gland function after sialolithiasis: scintigraphic examination of submandibular glands with 99mTc-pertechnetate. J Oral Maxillofac Surg. 1989;47(7):704-10.

55. Marchal F, Kurt AM, Dulguerov P, et al. Histopathology of submandibular glands removed for sialolithiasis. Ann Otol Rhinol Laryngol. 2001;110(5 Pt 1):464-9.

56. Geisthoff UW. Basic sialendoscopy techniques. Otolaryngol Clin North Am. 2009;42(6):1029-52.

57. Nahlieli O, Iro H, McGurk M. Minimal invasive methods and procedures for the treatment of salivary gland sialolithiasis. In: Nahlieli O, Iro H, McGurk M (Eds). Modern Management Preserving the Salivary Glands. Herzeliya (Israel): Isradon; 2007. pp. 136-76.

58. Capaccio P, Torretta S, Ottavian F, et al. Modern management of obstructive salivary diseases. Acta Otorhinolaryngol Ital. 2007;27(4):161-72.

59. Papadaki ME, McCain JP, Kim K, et al. Interventional sialoendoscopy: early clinical results. J Oral Maxillofac Surg. 2008;66(5):954-62.

60. Papadaki M, Kaban L, Kwolek C, et al. Arterial stents for access and protection of the parotid and submandibular ducts during sialoendoscopy. J Oral Maxillofac Surg. 2007;65(9):1865-8.

61. Luers JC, Vent J, Beutner D. Methylene blue for easy and safe detection of salivary duct papilla in sialendoscopy. Otolaryngol Head Neck Surg. 2008;139(3):466-7.

62. Nahlieli O, Shacham R, Bar T, et al. Endoscopic mechanical retrieval of sialoliths. Oral Surg Oral Med Oral Pathol Oral Radiol Endod. 2003;95(4):396-402.

63. Mulvaney WP, Beck CW. The laser beam in urology. J Urol. 1968;99(1):112-5.

64. Raif J, Vardi M, Nahlieli O, et al. An Er:YAG laser endoscopic fiber delivery system for lithotripsy of salivary stones. Lasers Surg Med. 2006;38(6):580-7.

65. Siedek V, Betz CS, Hecht V, et al. Laser induced fragmentation of salivary stones: an in vitro comparison of two different, clinically approved laser systems. Lasers Surg Med. 2008;40(4):257-64.

66. Marmary Y. A novel and non-invasive method for the removal of salivary gland stones. Int J Oral Maxillofac Surg. 1986;15(5):585-7.

67. Lustmann J, Regev E, Melamed Y. Sialolithiasis. A survey on 245 patients and a review of the literature. Int J Oral Maxillofac Surg. 1990;19(3):135-8.

68. Capaccio P, Torretta S, Pignataro L. Extracorporeal lithotripsy techniques for salivary stones. Otolaryngol Clin North Am. 2009;42(6):1139-59.

69. Eggers G, Chilla R. Ultrasound guided lithotripsy of salivary calculi using an electromagnetic lithotriptor. Int J Oral Maxillofac Surg. 2005;34(8):890-4.

70. Nahlieli O, Shacham R, Zaguri A. Combined external lithotripsy and endoscopic techniques for advanced sialolithiasis cases. J Oral Maxillofac Surg. 2010;68(2):347-53.

71. Seldinger SI. Catheter replacement of the needle in percutaneous arteriography; a new technique. Acta radiol. 1953;39(5):368-76.

72. Chossegros C, Guyot L, Richard O, et al. A technical improvement in sialendoscopy to enter the salivary ducts. Laryngoscope. 2006;116(5):842-4.

73. Zenk J, Constantinidis J, Al-Kadah B, et al. Transoral removal of submandibular stones. Arch Otolaryngol Head Neck Surg. 2001;127(4):432-6.

74. Iro H, Zenk J, Escudier MP, et al. Outcome of minimally invasive management of salivary calculi in 4,691 patients. Laryngoscope. 2009;119(2):263-8.

75. Luers JC, Grosheva M, Stenner M, et al. Sialoendoscopy: prognostic factors for endoscopic removal of salivary stones. Arch Otolaryngol Head Neck Surg. 2011;137(4):325-9.

76. Luers JC, Grosheva M, Reifferscheid V, et al. Sialendoscopy for sialolithiasis: Early treatment, better outcome. Head Neck. 2011 11.

77. Koch M, Iro H, Zenk J. Role of sialoscopy in the treatment of Stensen's duct strictures. Ann Otol Rhinol Laryngol. 2008;117(4):271-8.

78. Nahlieli O, London D, Zagury A, et al. Combined approach to impacted parotid stones. J Oral Maxillofac Surg. 2002;60(12):1418-23.

79. McGurk M, MacBean AD, Fan KF, et al. Endoscopically assisted operative retrieval of parotid stones. Br J Oral Maxillofac Surg. 2006;44(2):157-60.

80. Marchal F. A combined endoscopic and external approach for extraction of large stones with preservation of parotid and submandibular glands. Laryngoscope. 2007;117(2):373-7.

81. Baptista P, Gimeno CV, Salvinelli F, et al. Acute upper airway obstruction caused by massive oedema of the tongue: unusual complication of sialoendoscopy. J Laryngol Otol. 2009;123(12):1402-3.

82. Nahlieli O. Advanced sialoendoscopy techniques, rare findings, and complications. Otolaryngol Clin North Am. 2009;42(6):1053-72.

83. Jabbour N, Tibesar R, Lander T, et al. Sialendoscopy in children. Int J Pediatr Otorhinolaryngol. 2010;74(4):347-50.

84. Faure F, Froehlich P, Marchal F. Paediatric sialendoscopy. Curr Opin Otolaryngol Head Neck Surg. 2008;16(1):60-3.

85. Rinast E, Gmelin E, Hollands-Thorn B. Digital subtraction sialography, conventional sialography, high-resolution ultrasonography and computed tomography in the diagnosis of salivary gland diseases. Eur J Radiol. 1989;9(4):224-30.

86. Martins-Carvalho C, Plouin-Gaudon I, Quenin S, et al. Pediatric sialendoscopy: a 5-year experience at a single institution. Arch Otolaryngol Head Neck Surg. 2010;136(1):33-6.

87. Capaccio P, Gaini LM, Pagani D, et al. Videosialoendoscopic assessment of bilateral atresia of the Wharton's duct orifice in an infant. J Pediatr Surg. 2007;42(9):E5-7.

Chapter

13

ROBOTIC SURGERY IN THE HEAD AND NECK

Niels Kokot, Gregory S Weinstein, Bert W O'Malley Jr

INTRODUCTION

The concept of robots appears to have originated with Aristotle, while the Czech playwright Karel Ĉapek first introduced the term robot in his 1921 play "Rossum's Universal Robots."[1] Surgical robotic technology emerged from advances in industrial, military and aerospace technology. The field of medical robotics began in 1985 when the PUMA 560 was used to perform a stereotactic brain biopsy.[2] The PROBOT was developed in 1988 to perform a transurethral resection of the prostate.[3,4] In 1992, the ROBODOC was introduced as a milling device to assist in total hip arthroplasty.[5] However, clinical application of these early robots was limited. Computer Motion, Inc. was founded in 1989, and in 1994 the Federal Drug Administration (FDA) cleared the voice controlled endoscope holder, AESOP®, for clinical use. The same company later developed ZEUS® for gastrointestinal, cardiac and urologic use in 1998. Intuitive Surgical, Inc. (Mountain View, CA) was founded in 1995 and developed the da Vinci® Surgical System. In 1998, the first mitral valve procedure and robot assisted coronary artery bypass graft were performed in live patients.[6,7] These early procedures led to more widespread use, and the FDA cleared the da Vinci® Surgical System for general laparoscopic use in 2000. Computer Motion, Inc. was eventually acquired by Intuitive Surgical, Inc. in 2003, and the da Vinci® Surgical System is currently the most widely used surgical robot. The FDA has cleared the da Vinci® Surgical System for use in urological surgical procedures, general laparoscopic surgical procedures, gynecological laparoscopic surgical procedures, general thoracoscopic surgical procedures, thoracoscopically assisted cardiotomy procedures, and most recently in December 2009 transoral otolaryngology surgical procedures restricted to benign and malignant tumors classified as T1 and T2. The da Vinci® Surgical System is approved for adult and pediatric indications except transoral otolaryngology procedures.

The da Vinci® Surgical System has four components: the surgeon console, the patient side cart, the Endowrist® instruments and the vision system (Figs 13.1A to C). To operate the da Vinci® Surgical System, the surgeon sits at a console that is adjusted to comfort while viewing a high definition, three-dimensional image inside the patient's body. The console is fitted with a glove-like apparatus that translates the surgeon's hand, wrist and finger movements into real time movements of the surgical instruments. The patient side cart is positioned next to the patient and utilizes four robotic arms to carry out the surgeon's actions, with one arm holding the camera and the other arms holding the instruments. There are a variety of Endowrist® instruments such as graspers, forceps, scissors, retractors and several cautery devices. Each instrument has seven degrees of freedom: three translational (up and down, left and right, forward and backward), three rotational (roll, yaw and pitch), and one grip (cutting, grasping, etc.). The tip of each instrument allows 90 degrees of articulation. When inserted into the patient, the Endowrist® instruments mimic the surgeon's hands operating in the patient. The da Vinci Surgical System has the additional benefit of motion scaling and tremor reduction, such that large movements by the surgeon are translated into fine movements of the robotic instruments without tremor. The vision system is equipped

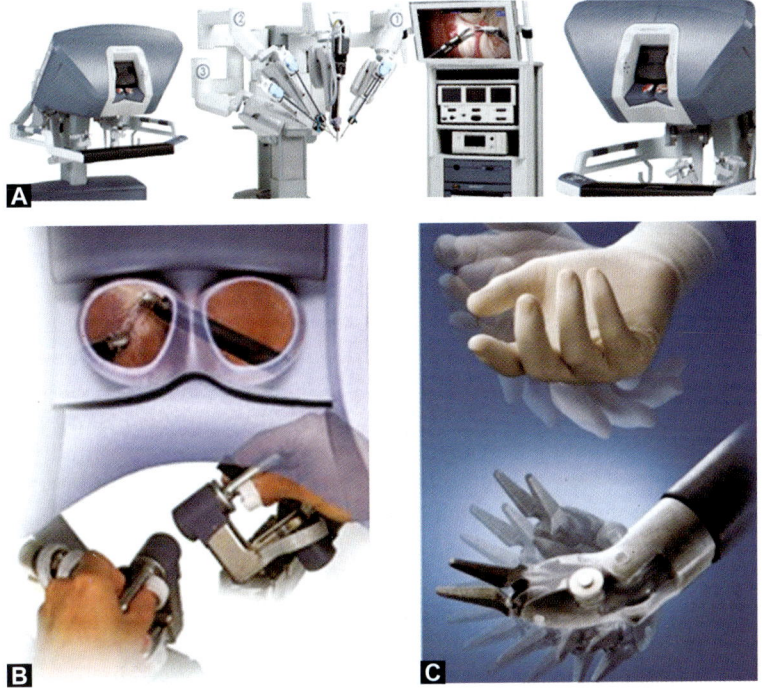

Figs 13.1A to C: The da Vinci Surgical System®. (A) Surgeon console, patient side cart, and vision system; (B) Surgeon console demonstrating three-dimensional view and control of robotic instrumentation; (C) Endowrist® instruments demonstrating degrees of freedom
Adapted from: www.intuitivesurgical.com

with a high definition, dual lens endoscope with two three-chip cameras that are integrated to provide the surgeon with a three-dimensional view of the operative field. Both a zero degree and 30 degree endoscope with either 12 mm or 8 mm diameter are available. These components are integrated such that the robot is controlled in a master-slave fashion to carry out the actions of the operating surgeon. The surgeon is provided with a feeling of standing inside the patient's mouth and operating with his hands.

The da Vinci® Surgical System has gained the most widespread use in the fields of urology, general surgery, cardiothoracic surgery and gynecology. Current applications include valve replacement, coronary artery bypass grafting, atrial fibrillation ablation and correction of congenital anomalies. Studies showed fewer blood transfusions, shorter hospital stays, faster recovery of preoperative functional ability and improved quality of life when comparing robot-assisted procedures with sternotomy.[8] In general surgery, a number of procedures have been reported including cholecystectomy, Nissen fundoplication, Heller myotomy, bowel resection and anastomosis, splenectomy and pancreatectomy.[9] In gynecology, surgeons have performed hysterectomies, myomectomies, sacrocolpopexy, adnexectomy, tubal reanastomoses with a shorter hospital stay and less blood loss when compared with open surgery.[10] Advantages of robotic surgery over traditional laparoscopic surgery include improved three-dimensional visualization, greater precision, improved dexterity with wristed instruments and better ergonomics while operating from the surgeon's console. Lack of haptic feedback, time of setup and cost have been cited as disadvantages of robotic technology.

Until recently robot-assisted radical prostatectomy has been the most commonly performed robotic procedure. In 2010 robotic-assisted hysterectomy surpassed prostatectomy as the most commonly performed robotic operation with 110,000 hysterectomies compared to 98,000 prostatectomies performed robotically.[11] Nonetheless, roughly 80% of radical prostatectomies are performed in the United States with robotic assistance.[12] When compared with open radical prostatectomy, robot-assisted radical prostatectomy has been shown to have less blood loss and lower rates of blood transfusion, lower rate of positive surgical margins, and higher rates of potency and urinary continence when performed in high volume centers.[13] Due to the potential benefits of robot-assisted prostatectomy, many centers have seen a large increase in patient demand for this procedure.

RATIONALE FOR TRANSORAL ROBOTIC SURGERY

Traditional treatment of aerodigestive tract carcinomas includes open approaches that allow direct visualization of the tumor to achieve wide surgical margins, as well as control of the great vessels in the neck. For many tumors, this necessitates a lip splitting mandibulotomy with either regional or free flap reconstruction. This approach requires long operative times, increased blood loss, and most patients require a tracheostomy and feeding tube. Patients undergo prolonged rehabilitation with variable recovery of speech and swallowing function that is further impaired by adjuvant radiation or chemoradiation.

The morbidity associated with radical surgery led oncologists to explore nonsurgical organ preserving treatment for head and neck carcinomas. The VA larynx trial paved the way for organ preservation protocols by proving equivalent survival with laryngeal preservation in patients treated with chemotherapy and radiation compared to total laryngectomy followed by radiation.[14] The VA trial, funded in part by Bristol Myers Squibb, the manufacturers of cisplatin, was the last major trial to include a surgical arm.[15] Oropharyngeal cancer protocols evaluating chemoradiation versus radiation alone, all of which lacked a surgical arm, indicated modest improvements in survival by the addition of chemotherapy, but with significant treatment related morbidity.[16] In addition, the demographic of patients with oropharyngeal squamous cell carcinoma (OPSCC) has changed, with human papilloma virus (HPV) playing an increasing role in the etiology of OPSCC. HPV induced OPSCC has proven to be chemoradiation sensitive with improved survival when compared with non-HPV induced carcinomas.[17] Although almost all of the randomized chemoradiation protocols for oropharyngeal carcinoma have led to an acceptance of these non-surgical approaches as a standard of care when compared to radiation alone, at the last evaluation of the national cancer database surgery has remained the primary treatment in advanced oropharyngeal cancer for about 30% of all patients in the United States.[18,19]

While organ preservation therapy is favored in many centers, it is not without morbidity to the patient, with 35 of 101 (34.6%) long-term surviving oropharygneal cancer patients treated in RTOG trials, experiencing severe late toxicity which was defined as "as chronic grade 3 to 4 pharyngeal/laryngeal toxicity (RTOG/European Organisation for the Research and Treatment of Cancer late toxicity scoring system) and/or requirement for a feeding tube > or = 2 years after registration and/or potential treatment-related death (e.g. pneumonia) within 3 years."[20] Given the morbidity associated with either traditional open surgery or organ preservation chemoradiation, there was certainly a need for head and neck surgeons to develop minimally invasive techniques that offer local control equal to standard therapy while preserving speech and swallowing function. Transoral laser microsurgery (TLM) was initially introduced in the 1970s for treatment of laryngeal papillomas, and was later championed by Steiner in Germany as a means of treating laryngeal carcinoma and achieving excellent local control while preserving speech and swallowing function.[21] TLM for laryngeal carcinoma gained popularity, but transoral approaches were slow to develop as an alternative to open surgery or chemoradiation as the primary treatment of OPSCC. Steiner's group reported 85% 5-year local control and 73% recurrence-free survival in advanced staged base of tongue squamous carcinoma treated with TLM, neck dissection and adjuvant therapy as indicated. Functional outcomes were excellent with 92% normalcy of diet, and no patients had a tracheostomy or gastrostomy tube.[22] In the United States, only a few centers have reported their results of TLM for OPSCC. Recently, Haughey et al. reported combined data collected from three institutions over a ten-year period in patients with advanced stage OPSCC treated with TLM, neck dissection and adjuvant therapy as indicated. They achieved three-year 97% local control, 86% overall survival, 88% disease-specific survival and 82% disease-free survival. Eighty seven percent of patients had normal swallowing or only episodic dysphagia.[23]

While the reported oncologic and functional outcomes of TLM for treatment of OPSCC have been excellent, the limitations of TLM have prevented it from gaining popularity beyond selected tertiary centers. Access to the oropharynx is limited by laryngoscopes and retractors that are used in conjunction with the operating microscope such that the view of the operative field is restricted by the "line of sight" of the microscope. Coupled with rigid instrumentation and single handed surgery, operating "around corners" in the oropharynx is difficult with TLM and requires repeated adjustment of instrumentation to achieve optimal visualization. Furthermore, TLM approaches critical neurovascular anatomy from inside-out in a way that may be unfamiliar to many surgeons. Robotic technology offers a potential to overcome the limitations of TLM with enhanced three-dimensional imaging, wristed instrumentation and angled telescopes. This technology may allow improved dexterity and precision to achieve access to the oropharynx when compared to standard technology.

DEVELOPMENT AND FEASIBILITY OF TRANSORAL ROBOTIC SURGERY

Initial research utilizing the da Vinci® Surgical System in the field of otolaryngology — head and neck surgery — focused on endorobotic neck surgery, performing salivary gland excision, and neck dissection in a porcine and cadaver model.[24,25] The concept of TORS was established at the University of Pennsylvania and developed in a systematic fashion, leading to the first widespread clinical application of robotic technology in otolaryngology. In 2005, Hockstein et al. first demonstrated the feasibility of utilizing the da Vinci® Surgical System in an airway mannequin and human cadaver models for transoral laryngopharyngeal dissections.[26,27] The investigators discovered that the key to achieving adequate exposure, which would allow access of the robotic instruments, was utilization of standard mouthgags such as those used in tonsillectomy rather than traditional laryngoscopes. Weinstein et al. successfully performed a supraglottic laryngectomy in a canine model noting minimal blood loss, excellent visualization, shorter operative time than traditional transoral laser resection and multiplaner transection utilizing instruments that mimic normal hand movements. In addition, they noted the ability to perform caudal to cranial transection, which was seen to be advantageous over traditional transoral laser resection which is limited by "line of site", no caudal to cranial resection possible and no axial plane resection possible.[28] Once the feasibility of TORS was established, safety trials were conducted, and in 2005, the first prospective human trial utilizing the da Vinci® Surgical System for TORS was initiated.[29,30]

Initial reports from the University of Pennsylvania documented successful completion of TORS supraglottic laryngectomy and base of tongue resections, achieving negative surgical margins with minimal bleeding and minimal morbidity.[31,32] Weinstein et al. described the new procedure — TORS radical tonsillectomy — in their first series of 27 patients with tonsillar squamous cell carcinoma.[33] Their technique modifies the transoral lateral oropharyngectomy described by Holsinger et al. and allows an en bloc resection of the tumor.[34] Twenty one patients had T1-T2 tumors, while six patients were staged T3. Negative surgical margins were achieved in 93% of patients, and 26 patients underwent staged modified radical neck dissection. One patient had a planned tracheostomy but was later decannulated, while another patient underwent an unplanned tracheostomy for exacerbation of sleep apnea. Complications were minimal. Two patients avoided adjuvant radiotherapy, while 33% of patients underwent adjuvant radiotherapy alone, and 56% of patients underwent adjuvant chemoradiation therapy. All patients had a gastrostomy tube placed, although all but one patient had the gastrostomy tube removed at last follow-up. The authors concluded that TORS allows excellent access for resection of carcinoma of the tonsil with acceptable acute morbidity.

Through their initial work, the investigators at the University of Pennsylvania established the optimal room setup, patient and robot positioning, and instrumentation that are used in TORS (Figs 13.2 to 13.4). Their standardized approach was taught to a group of surgeons who then went out to establish a TORS program in their home institutions with similar success. Genden et al. reported their first series of 20 patients undergoing TORS for aerodigestive tract malignancies.[35] They successfully completed TORS in 18 patients with T1 and T2 tumors of the oropharynx and larynx, achieving negative margins in all cases. Intraoral reconstruction with musculomucosal flaps was performed in eight patients. There were no complications and all patients resumed oral intake within a mean of 1.4 days. The investigators noticed a dramatic decrease in the surgical setup and operative time over the course of the study. The decrease in setup time was also noticed by other investigators.[36] Boudreaux et al. reported successful TORS in 29 out of 36 patients with mostly T1 and T2 malignancies of the head and neck.[37] They found that factors associated with successful TORS resection included lower T-stage and edentulism. Nine patients were gastrostomy tube dependent. Factors associated with gastrostomy-tube dependence were advanced age, tumor location in the larynx, higher T-stage and lower preoperative MD Anderson Dysphagia Inventory score. Moore et al. successfully completed TORS with negative margins in 45 patients with predominantly T1 and T2 tumors of the tonsil and tongue base.[38] Thirty one percent and forty nine percent of patients

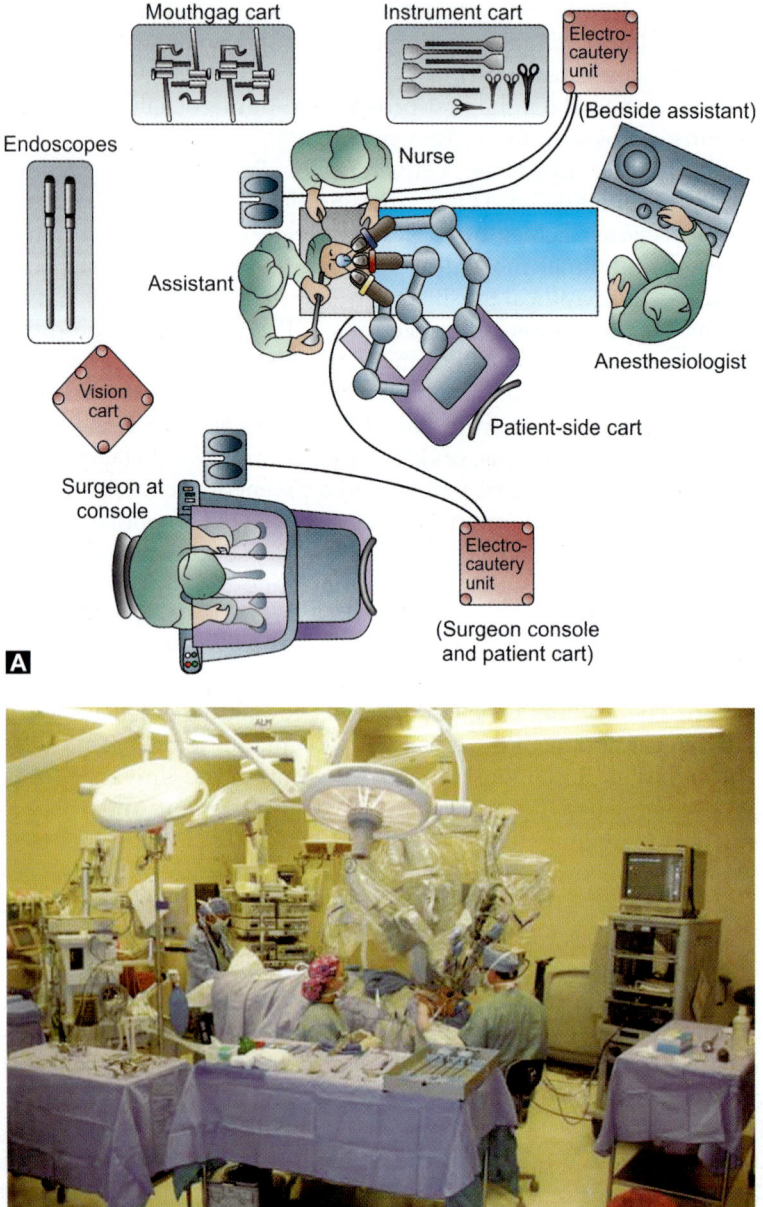

Figs 13.2A and B: Operating room setup for TORS. (A) Diagram; (B) Intraoperative photograph

Adapted from: da Vinci Transoral Surgery Procedure Guide, Intuitive Surgical, Inc.

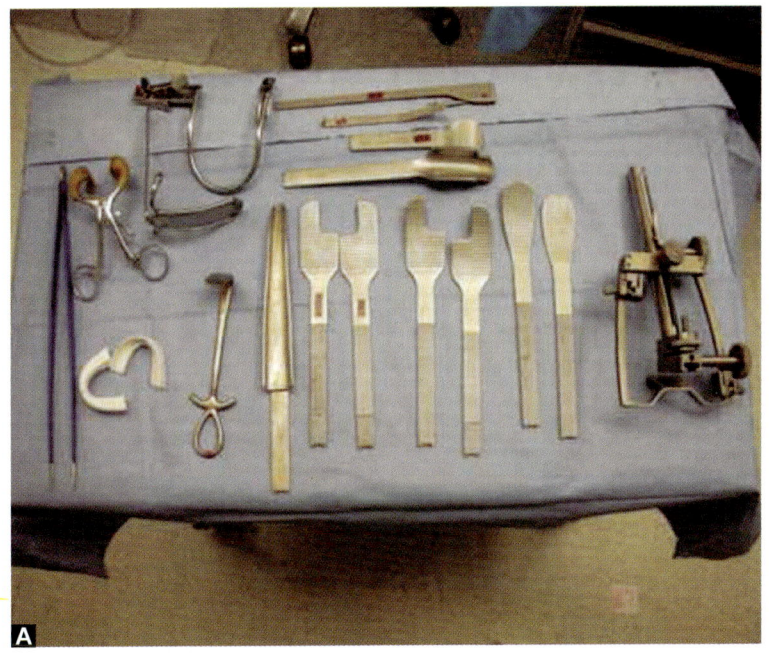

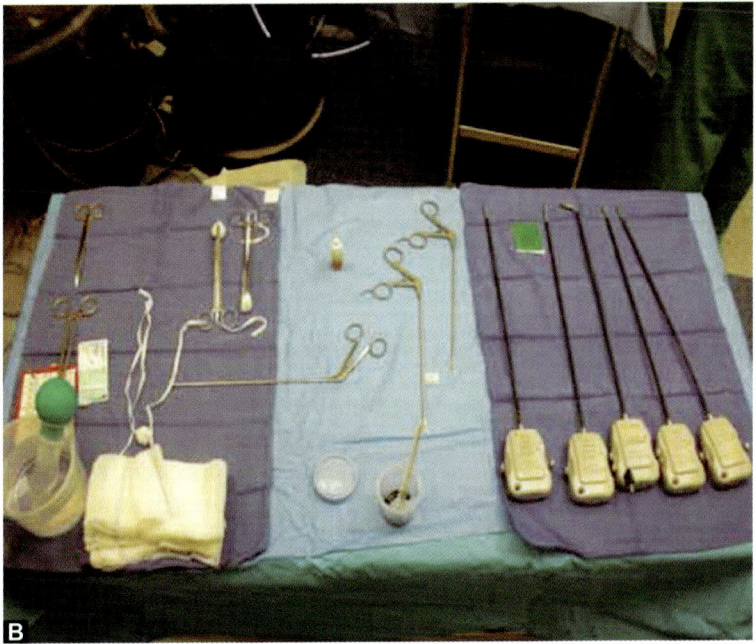

Figs 13.3A and B: Mouth gags and surgical instruments used in TORS
Adapted from: da Vinci Transoral Surgery Procedure Guide, Intuitive Surgical, Inc.

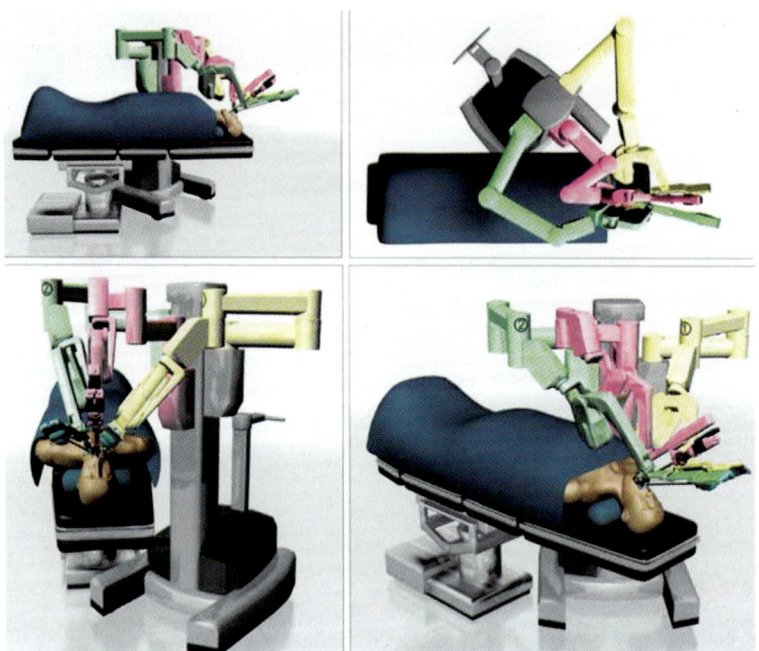

Fig. 13.4: Patient positioning and system setup for TORS
Adapted from: da Vinci Transoral Surgery Procedure Guide, Intuitive Surgical, Inc.

had a tracheostomy and feeding tube placed respectively, although all patients had the tubes removed. The authors performed a concomitant neck dissection in 43 patients. While they found an obvious communication between the pharynx and neck in 40% of patients, only 6.7% of patients developed a salivary fistula. All resolved with conservative treatment (Figs 13.5A to C).

ONCOLOGIC AND FUNCTIONAL OUTCOME

The data from these institutions established the feasibility and safety of TORS as a minimally invasive treatment alternative for malignancies of the head and neck. This resulted in TORS being approved by the FDA in 2009 for transoral otolaryngology surgical procedures in adults restricted to benign and malignant tumors classified as T1 and T2. Advanced T-stage tumors were not approved since these studies only had a small number of advanced-stage tumors. While these initial studies reported their oncologic outcomes, the follow-up was short due to the relative infancy of the procedure. However, the oncologic data for TORS is beginning to mature, and longer term follow-up data is being reported.

The University of Pennsylvania reported the results of 47 consecutive patients with advanced-stage OPSCC and a minimum of 18 months follow-up who were treated with primary TORS, staged neck dissection, and adjuvant radiation or chemoradiation as indicated.[39] Seventy

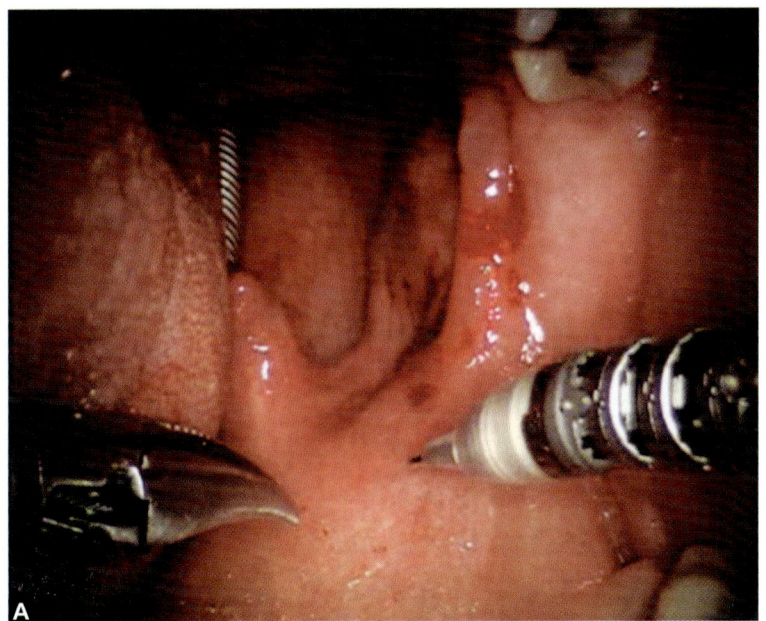

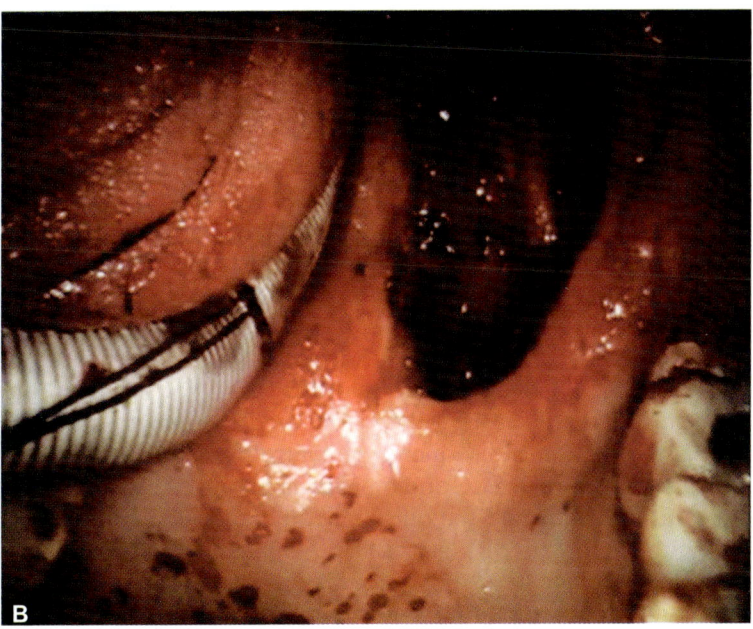

Figs 13.5A and B

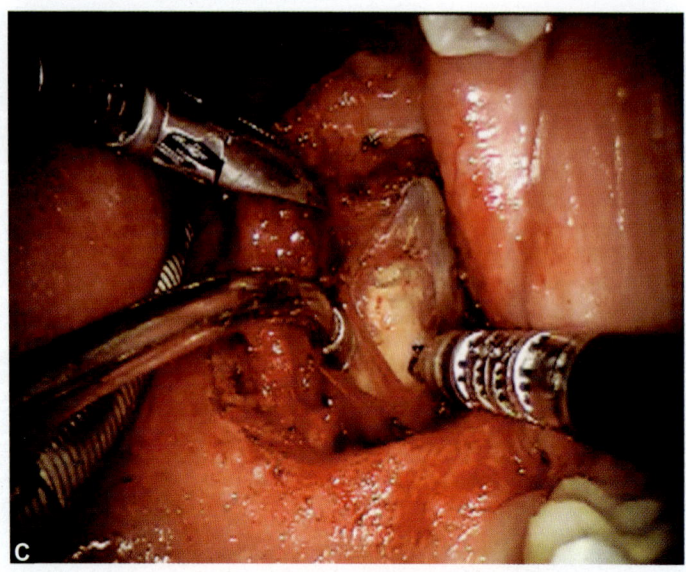

Fig. 13.5C

Figs 13.5A to C: Intraoperative photos of TORS radical tonsillectomy for T1 squamous cell carcinoma of the tonsil. (A) Tumor arising from the right tonsil; (B) Dissection in the parapharyngeal space fat; (C) Postoperative defect left to heal by secondary intention
Adapted from: Photos provided by Niels Kokot, MD

seven percent of patients had T1 and T2 tumors, while fifty one percent of patients had N1 disease, and forty nine percent of patients had N2 disease. Negative margins were achieved in 98% of patients. Five patients avoided radiotherapy altogether, while 13 patients received radiotherapy only, two patients received chemotherapy only and 27 patients received concurrent chemoradiation. Local control and regional control were 98% and 96% respectively. Actuarial 1-year and 2-year overall survival was 96% and 82% respectively. Actuarial disease-specific survival at 1-year and 2-years was 98% and 90% respectively. Disease-free survival was 96% at 1-year and 79% at 2 years. When compared to similar organ preservation chemoradiation trials, oncologic control was similar.[40,41] With the changing landscape of OPSCC and more tumors caused by HPV infection, the same authors analyzed the oncologic outcomes of a cohort of TORS patients with respect to HPV status.[42] In 50 patients treated with TORS, staged neck dissection, and adjuvant radiation or chemoradiation as indicated, 37 patients (74%) had HPV-positive tumors and 13 patients (26%) had HPV-negative tumors. There was no statistical difference between the two groups with respect to the margin status, presence of cervical metastases, recurrence and survival curves. Many HPV-induced tumors are presenting with smaller tumors at the primary site, but with advanced-stage neck disease. To determine the rates of regional recurrence in their patients, the authors examined 31 patients, all with negative margin TORS who underwent selective neck dissection and adjuvant therapy, and found only one regional recurrence. Examination of the pathological specimens in the neck showed that 33% and 43% of the clinical N0 and N1 patients respectively were pathologically upstaged, while four of the 14 clinical N1 patients had negative pathological necks. Pathological staging of the necks allowed the authors to selectively administer adjuvant therapy, and to de-intensify therapy in some cases.[43]

The University of Alabama-Birmingham (UAB) and the Mayo Clinic pooled their data to report their 2-year survival analysis in a cohort of 89 patients with carcinoma of the oral cavity, oropharynx and supraglottic larynx.[44] Seventy nine percent of patients were stage T1 and T2, and negative margins were achieved in all patients. Seventy six percent of patients underwent staged or concomitant neck dissection. Of the patients who underwent TORS as primary treatment, 63% received adjuvant radiation therapy, and 48% had chemotherapy either before or after surgical treatment. Two-year recurrence-free survival in patients who underwent TORS as primary treatment was 89.3%. Genden et al. reported 18-month survival data in 30 patients with head and neck squamous cell carcinoma, the majority of which were OPSCC.[45] All patients underwent TORS, concomitant neck dissection and adjuvant therapy as indicated. Because all patients were pathologically staged, adjuvant therapy was de-intensified in four patients while it was escalated in five patients. Eighteen-month locoregional control, distant control, disease-free survival and overall-survival rates were 91%, 93%, 78%, and 90% respectively. Comparison with a matched group of patients undergoing primary chemoradiation showed no statistically significant survival differences.

In addition to excellent oncologic outcomes, patients treated with TORS have shown excellent functional outcomes with longer follow-up. The University of Pennsylvania reported a 2.4% (one patient) gastrostomy tube dependency rate at a minimum of 1-year follow-up, while the rate of feeding tube dependency in the combined UAB and Mayo Clinic as well as the Mt. Sinai study was 0%.[39,44] In addition to gastrostomy tube dependency rate, quality of life data is now available in patients undergoing TORS. Leonhardt et al. found that in 38 patients with OPSCC undergoing TORS, staged neck dissection and adjuvant therapy, declines in the eating and diet domains on the Performance Status Scale that were seen at 6 months returned to baseline at 12 months.[46] Declines in the speech domain remained significantly decreased at 6 months and 12 months. Patients receiving adjuvant chemoradiation had significantly lower diet domain scores at 6 months and 12 months compared to those who underwent surgery only. Hurtuk et al. used the Head and Neck Cancer Inventory to show that speech, aesthetics, attitude and overall quality of life remained in the high domain at 12 months, while the eating domain dropped to the intermediate level at 12 months in 18 out of 64 patients who underwent TORS and adjuvant therapy for HNSCC at all sites.[47] Genden et al. compared TORS patients to a similar cohort of patients treated with primary chemoradiation and found that all TORS patients returned to baseline in the eating, speech and diet domains on the Performance Status

Scale for Head and Neck, as well as the Functional Oral Intake Score. In contrast, patients treated with chemoradiation had a lower than baseline diet score and lower Functional Oral Intake Score.[45]

Since its inception, TORS has proven to be a safe and efficacious, minimally invasive means of achieving an en bloc resection of head and neck malignancies. Functional outcomes have been excellent, and as the data matures, the oncologic outcomes appear to be equivalent to those achieved with standard open surgery or organ preservation chemoradiation protocols. By surgically staging patients with TORS and neck dissection, adjuvant therapy can be tailored to the individual patient and de-intensified in some cases of low risk disease. TORS offers the potential to maximize oncologic control while maximizing functional outcomes. This approach is in stark contrast to chemoradiation protocols in which all patients receive identical therapy. More studies are necessary to validate long-term outcomes.

FUTURE APPLICATIONS OF TRANSORAL ROBOTIC SURGERY

Transoral robotic surgery (TORS) has been applied most commonly to treat oropharyngeal malignancies, and to a lesser extent malignancies of the supraglottic larynx. In the glottic larynx, application of TORS has been limited due to the bulky nature of current instrumentation. As TORS expands to more centers, there will be a greater need for finer, more flexible instrumentation that will be useful in treating both malignant and benign pathology of the glottic larynx.

Surgery of the anterior and middle skull base has traditionally relied on open approaches that dismantle the craniofacial skeleton to gain access. Advances in endoscopic sinus surgery have made many skull base lesions accessible without facial incisions, but current technology is limited by two-dimensional visualization and rigid instrumentation. Robotic technology has the potential to offer distinct advantages due to three-dimensional visualization and wristed instruments. To date, application of robotic technology has been limited primarily to the laboratory, although, case reports in human patients are emerging. Using a standard TORS approach, the group at the University of Pennsylvania has been able to perform cadaveric dissections of the upper cervical spine, clivus, sella region and infratemporal fossa. Robotic technology was beneficial in providing exposure, dissection of the carotid artery, jugular vein, and lower cranial nerves, as well as in achieving dural closure, but there remains a lack of robotic technology necessary for removal of bony structures, and this work must be done by the bedside assistant. A novel approach, C-TORS, places the instrument arms of the robot through cervical ports while the camera is placed transorally, and this improves visualization of the sella region.[48-50] Other novel approaches to the skull base include placing a suprahyoid port as well as placing the camera arm transnasally, while the instrument arms are placed through maxillary antrostomies.[51,52] Skull base applications in human patients have been described to remove parapharyngeal space tumors, to perform an odontoidectomy for basilar invagination and to perform nasopharyngectomy for recurrent nasopharyngeal carcinoma.[53-56] As new robotic technology emerges to accommodate the needs of the head and neck surgeon, applications in endoscopic skull base surgery are certain to expand.

While the defect created with TORS is usually left to heal by secondary intention, there may be some patients who would benefit from free flap reconstruction of their defect. In many instances, a lip splitting mandibulotomy is required to inset the free flap for oropharyngeal defects, thereby negating the benefits of transoral surgery. Mukhija et al. described the first two cases of free flaps inset via TORS, and noted that they were able to avoid an otherwise necessary mandibulotomy in both patients and a tracheostomy in one.[57] Selber reported a series of five patients with robotically assisted reconstruction of oropharyngeal defects, including one arterial anastomosis that was sewn using the 8 mm robotic microforceps. He noted the advantages of tremor reduction and motion scaling in performing the microvascular anastomosis, but felt the optics of the endoscope and the lack of haptic feedback were limitations in performing microvascular surgery.[58]

One area of otolaryngology that has a large potential to benefit from TORS is the treatment of obstructive sleep apnea (OSA). Up to 20 million adults in the United States suffer from some degree of OSA and the resultant effect on health and quality of life. Many surgical interventions designed to address OSA have been developed, but procedures that address the role of tongue base hypertrophy have either been ineffective or they carry the morbidity associated with open surgery. TORS can potentially address the role of tongue base hypertrophy in OSA in minimally invasive fashion with improved efficacy and minimal morbidity. Vicini et al. were the first authors to report their experience using TORS to address the tongue base in treating OSA and were encouraged by their results.[59] In their follow-up study, they reported 20 patients with 10-month follow-up who underwent a TORS tongue base reduction and showed mean reduction of the apnea-hypopnea index by 24.6 ± 22.2 SD, while the Epworth Sleepiness Scale improved by 5.9 ± 4.4.[60] All patients had a temporary tracheostomy and complications were minimal. While defining success in treating OSA can be challenging, early results support the role for TORS in managing OSA, and this may prove to be a field amenable to expanded application of TORS.

ROBOTIC ASSISTED THYROIDECTOMY

Surgery remains the standard of care for diagnosis and treatment of thyroid neoplasms. The approach to thyroid surgery has changed over the last 10 years, with an increase in the number of minimally invasive techniques performed. The video assisted thyroidectomy described and popularized by Miccoli utilizes endoscopes through a small cervical incision, and has been shown to be as safe as standard open surgery with improved pain and cosmesis.[61,62] Remote access techniques have been developed, primarily in Asia, where the population is aggressively screened for thyroid disease and where a cervical incision carries a social stigma. A variety of endoscopic transcervical, transaxillary and breast approaches, with or without CO_2 insufflation, have been described, but these approaches carry the same limitations of two-dimensional visualization and rigid instrumentation.[63]

Dr. Chung and his group at Yonsei University in Seoul, South Korea have applied the da Vinci® Surgical System to the unilateral gasless, transaxillary technique, using a single incision in the axilla with or without an additional parasternal incision to gain remote access to the thyroid bed (Figs 13.6 and 13.7). Their initial reports in over 300 patients demonstrated the feasibility and safety of the technique in patients undergoing subtotal or total thyroidectomy with central compartment lymph node dissection for thyroid malignancies.[64-66] Recently, a multicenter study led by Dr. Chung reported 1043 consecutive unilateral transaxillary robotic assisted thyroidectomy (RAT) for well-differentiated thyroid carcinoma. Of these patients, 677 patients had a subtotal thyroidectomy performed, while only 366 patients received a total thyroidectomy. Nine hundred and forty patients had a central compartment neck dissection, and 46 patients underwent a lateral neck dissection. The mean tumor size was 0.8 cm, and the mean number of central compartment lymph nodes retrieved was 5.1 ± 3.8. The mean operative time and console time were 132.4 minutes and 63.9 minutes, respectively. Transient hypocalcemia was the most common complication, occurring in 18.4% of patients, whereas transient hoarseness occurred in 4.3% of patients. Only five patients had a permanent recurrent laryngeal nerve injury. The authors did note three tracheal injuries and three transient brachial plexus neuropathies resulting from the

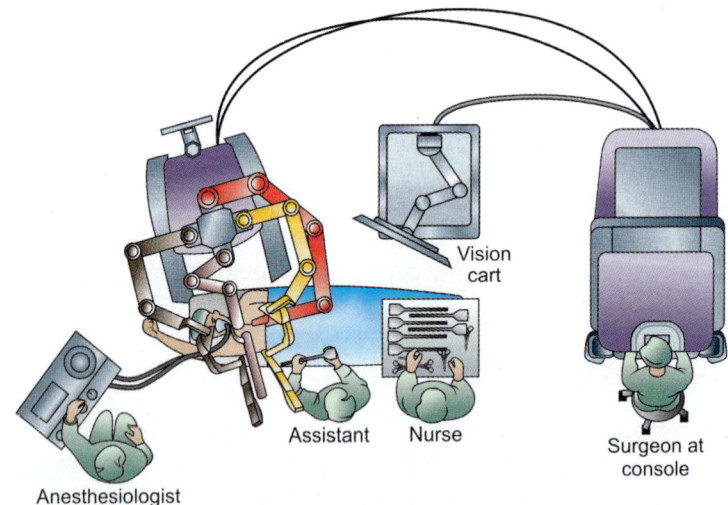

Vision cart

Assistant Nurse

Surgeon at console

Anesthesiologist

Fig. 13.6: Room setup for transaxillary robotic assisted thyroidectomy
Adapted from: da Vinci Transaxillary thyroidectomy procedure guide, Intuitive Surgical, Inc.

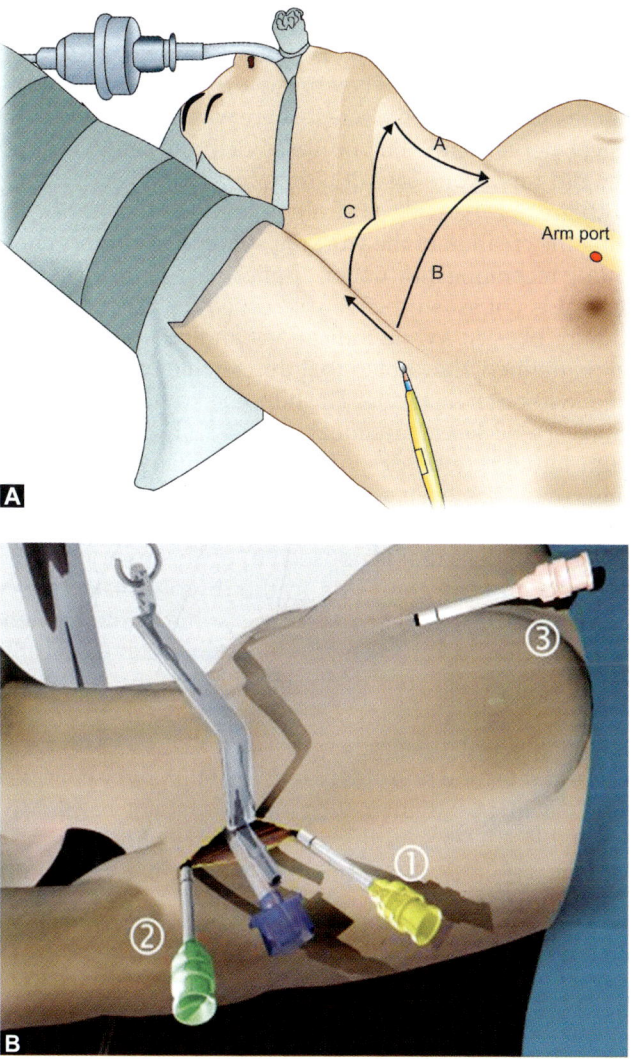

Figs 13.7A and B: Transaxillary robotic assisted thyroidectomy. (A) Incision and area of dissection needed for exposure; (B) Positioning of retractor and cannulas

Adapted from: da Vinci Transaxillary thyroidectomy procedure guide, Intuitive Surgical, Inc.

arm positioning. They did not report oncologic outcomes in their patients. The authors concluded that their technique is safe for treatment of low risk, well-differentiated thyroid carcinoma with morbidity that is similar to conventional or endoscopic thyroidectomy.

These reports generated considerable interest in the United States, and a number of U.S. thyroid surgeons have adopted this technique.[-67-71] Kuppersmith and Holsinger reported their first 31 patients undergoing RAT using the Chung technique. Eleven patients received a total thyroidectomy, and the authors subjectively noted that contralateral recur rent laryngeal nerve and parathyroid dissection was more challenging, and that it was difficult to remove all of the contralateral thyroid tissue in two patients. Only three patients had a malignancy, and no patient had a central compartment neck dissection. They noted a trend toward improvement in operative times after the first ten cases. There was one case of transient recurrent laryngeal nerve injury but no cases of postoperative hypocalcemia. The authors did report one case of temporary radial nerve injury, and two patients with greater than 500 cc of blood loss due to anterior jugular vein injury during the creation of the working space. The authors cited concerns that the Chung technique may not be applicable to the United States patient population that is not as aggressively screened for thyroid disease and has a higher rate of obesity. While indications and contraindications for RAT are not clearly defined, they noted that thin female patients with a less than 3 cm nodule, without a history of Hashimoto's thyroiditis, and who desire the avoidance of a neck scar, are ideal patients[70] (Table 13.1).

Although initial reports describing transaxillary RAT in the U.S. are encouraging, there has been some hesitation in accepting the technique due to new complications such as brachial plexopathy, tracheal injury and excessive blood loss that is not seen in open surgery. In addition, the length of dissection from the axilla to the thyroid makes this approach far from "minimally invasive." To address some of the challenges faced with transaxillary RAT, Terris et al. developed the robotic facelift thyroidectomy.[72,73] This approach places the incision in the postauricular skin crease with extension to the occipital hairline, and a fixed retractor system maintains the exposure during the procedure (Figs 13.8A and B). Sixteen lobectomies and one total thyroidectomy (through two separate incisions) were performed in 14 patients, all on an outpatient basis. Mean operative time was 154.9 ± 23.8 minutes. There were two seromas, one transient case of vocal fold dysfunction, but no cases of hypoparathyroidism

Table 13.1: Criteria for robotic assisted thyroidectomy
Patient Selection Criteria
1. Motivated patient desiring absence of cervical scar
2. Non-morbidly obese
3. American Society of Anesthesiologist class 1 or 2
4. Absence of previous neck surgery
Disease Criteria
1. Anticipated unilateral surgery (enlarging benign thyroid nodule or follicular neoplasm)
2. Dominant nodule no bigger than 4 cm
3. Absence of clinically apparent thyroiditis
4. Absence of lymphadenopathy, substernal extension, or extrathyroidal extension
Adapted from: Terris DJ, Singer MC, Seybt MW. Robotic facelift thyroidectomy: patient selection and technical considerations. Surg Laparosc Endosc Percutan Tech. 2011;21(4):237-42.

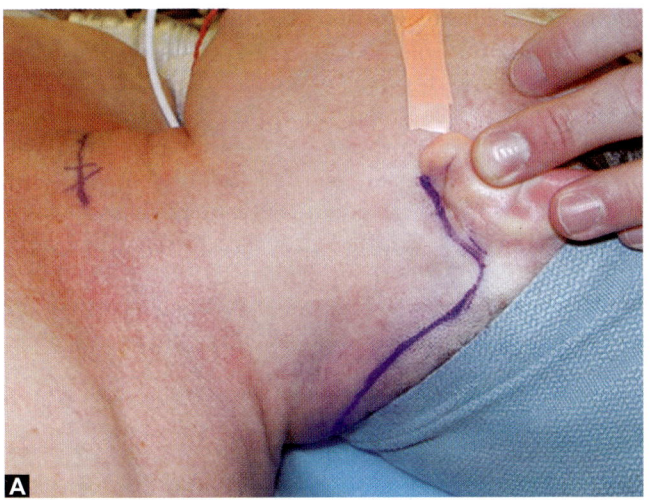

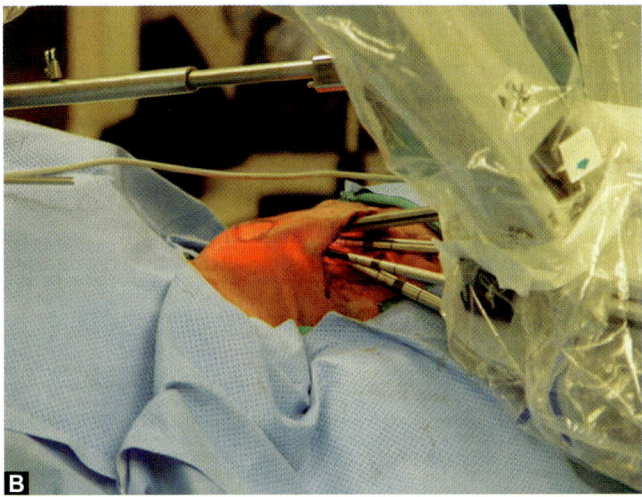

Figs 13.8A and B: Robotic facelift thyroidectomy. (A) Incision; (B) Positioning of robotic arms
Adapted from: Terris DJ, Singer MC, Seybt MW. Robotic facelift thyroidectomy: patient selection and technical considerations. Surg Laparosc Endosc Percutan Tech. 2011;21(4):237-42.

in those patients having a completion thyroidectomy or total thyroidectomy. All patients complained of transient periauricular hypesthesia. The authors found this technique to be advantageous over transaxillary RAT due to the straightforward patient positioning without risk of brachial plexopathy, shorter length of dissection, ability to stimulate the recurrent laryngeal nerve and the ability to perform the procedure in slightly obese patients due to the ease of raising the skin flaps. The major disadvantage they noted was the temporary hypesthesia in the great auricular nerve distribution.

Although RAT is established as a viable remote access approach to thyroidectomy in Asia, the technique has not been fully adopted in the

US. Indications for RAT are emerging, but more experience will be necessary to clearly define the role of RAT in treating thyroid disease. Novel transoral robotic assisted approaches to the thyroid have been reported and may have a clinical role in the future.[74] As US surgeons become more experienced with RAT, use of robotic technology may expand to include management of cervical metastases. The feasibility of performing modified radical neck dissection for lateral neck metastases in thyroid carcinoma was reported by Dr. Chung's group in Korea. They performed 33 neck dissections with a mean operative time of 280.8 ± 40.6 minutes. They retrieved a mean of 27.7 ± 11.0 lymph nodes from levels IIA-V. There were no major nerve injuries, and three cases of minor chyle leak occurred. This study offers promise that remote access to treat cervical metastases is possible in selective patients.

CONCLUSION

Transoral robotic surgery is an exciting innovation in the management of head and neck carcinoma that offers a minimally invasive approach to achieve an en bloc resection, maximizing oncologic control while preserving function. By surgically staging patients, TORS may allow for de-intensification of adjuvant therapy. The use of robotic technology in the management of thyroid disease is evolving, and new remote access approaches are emerging. As robotic technology improves to meet the needs of the head and neck surgeon and our experience expands, advances in areas such as robotic skull base surgery and endorobotic management of the neck are certain to continue.

REFERENCES

1. *Capek K. R. U. R. Rossum's Universal Robots. 3. vyd. ed. Praha: Aventinum; 1921.
2. Kwoh YS, Hou J, Jonckheere EA, et al. A robot with improved absolute positioning accuracy for CT guided stereotactic brain surgery. IEEE Trans Biomed Eng. 1988;35(2):153-60.
3. Davies BL, Hibberd RD, Coptcoat MJ, et al. A surgeon robot prostatectomy—a laboratory evaluation. J Med Eng Technol. 1989;13(6):273-7.
4. Davies BL, Hibberd RD, Ng WS, et al. The development of a surgeon robot for prostatectomies. Proc Inst Mech Eng. 1991;205(1):35-8.
5. Bargar WL, Bauer A, Borner M. Primary and revision total hip replacement using the Robodoc system. Clin Orthop Relat Res. 1998(354):82-91.
6. Carpentier A, Loulmet D, Aupecle B, et al. Computer assisted open heart surgery. First case operated on with success. C R Acad Sci III. 1998;321(5):437-42.
7. Mohr FW, Falk V, Diegeler A, et al. Computer-enhanced coronary artery bypass surgery. J Thorac Cardiovasc Surg. 1999;117(6):1212-4.
8. Rodriguez E, Chitwood WR. Robotics in cardiac surgery. Scand J Surg. 2009;98(2):120-4.

9. Maeso S, Reza M, Mayol JA, et al. Efficacy of the Da Vinci surgical system in abdominal surgery compared with that of laparoscopy: a systematic review and meta-analysis. Ann Surg. 2010;252(2):254-62.

10. Reza M, Maeso S, Blasco JA, et al. Meta-analysis of observational studies on the safety and effectiveness of robotic gynaecological surgery. Br J Surg. 2010;97(12):1772-83.

11. Available from: http://investor.intuitivesurgical.com. [Accessed Dec, 2011]

12. Sooriakumaran P, John M, Wiklund P, et al. Learning curve for robotic assisted laparoscopic prostatectomy: a multi-institutional study of 3794 patients. Minerva Urol Nefrol. 2011;63(3):191-8.

13. Coelho RF, Rocco B, Patel MB, et al. Retropubic, laparoscopic, and robot-assisted radical prostatectomy: a critical review of outcomes reported by high-volume centers. J Endourol. 2010;24(12):2003-15.

14. Induction chemotherapy plus radiation compared with surgery plus radiation in patients with advanced laryngeal cancer. The Department of Veterans Affairs Laryngeal Cancer Study Group. N Engl J Med. 1991;324(24):1685-90.

15. Wilson JA. Does pharma fund the pipers? - Scottish Intercollegiate Guidelines Network (SIGN) guidelines 90 - diagnosis and management of head and neck cancer, October 2006. Clin Oncol (R Coll Radiol). 2008;20(9):661-3.

16. Calais G, Alfonsi M, Bardet E, et al. Randomized trial of radiation therapy versus concomitant chemotherapy and radiation therapy for advanced-stage oropharynx carcinoma. J Natl Cancer Inst. 1999;91(24):2081-6.

17. Ang KK, Harris J, Wheeler R, et al. Human papilloma virus and survival of patients with oropharyngeal cancer. N Engl J Med. 2010;363(1):24-35.

18. Forastiere AA, Trotti A. Radiotherapy and concurrent chemotherapy: a strategy that improves locoregional control and survival in oropharyngeal cancer. J Natl Cancer Inst. 1999;91(24):2065-6.

19. Chen AY, Schrag N, Hao Y, et al. Changes in treatment of advanced oropharyngeal cancer, 1985-2001. Laryngoscope. 2007;117(1):16-21.

20. Machtay M, Rosenthal DI, Hershock D, et al. Organ preservation therapy using induction plus concurrent chemoradiation for advanced resectable oropharyngeal carcinoma: a University of Pennsylvania Phase II Trial. J Clin Oncol. 2002;20(19):3964-71.

21. Steiner W, Ambrosch P. Endoscopic laser surgery of the upper aerodigestive tract: with special emphasis on cancer surgery. New York: Stuttgart Thieme; 2000.

22. Steiner W, Fierek O, Ambrosch P, et al. Transoral laser microsurgery for squamous cell carcinoma of the base of the tongue. Arch Otolaryngol Head Neck Surg. 2003;129(1):36-43.

23. Haughey BH, Hinni ML, Salassa JR, et al. Transoral laser microsurgery as primary treatment for advanced-stage oropharyngeal cancer: a United States multicenter study. Head Neck. 2011;33(12):1683-94.

24. Haus BM, Kambham N, Le D, et al. Surgical robotic applications in otolaryngology. Laryngoscope. 2003;113(7):1139-44.

25. Terris DJ, Haus BM, Gourin CG. Endoscopic neck surgery: resection of the submandibular gland in a cadaver model. Laryngoscope. 2004;114(3):407-10.

26. Hockstein NG, Nolan JP, O'Malley BW, et al. Robotic microlaryngeal surgery: a technical feasibility study using the Da Vinci surgical robot and an airway mannequin. Laryngoscope. 2005;115(5):780-5.

27. Hockstein NG, Nolan JP, O'Malley BW, et al. Robot-assisted pharyngeal and laryngeal microsurgery: results of robotic cadaver dissections. Laryngoscope. 2005;115(6):1003-8.

28. Weinstein GS, O'Malley BW, Hockstein NG. Transoral robotic surgery: supraglottic laryngectomy in a canine model. Laryngoscope. 2005;115(7):1315-9.

29. Hockstein NG, O'Malley BW, Weinstein GS. Assessment of intraoperative safety in transoral robotic surgery. Laryngoscope. 2006;116(2):165-8.

30. Hockstein NG, Weinstein GS, O'Malley BW. Maintenance of hemostasis in transoral robotic surgery. ORL J Otorhinolaryngol Relat Spec. 2005;67(4):220-4.

31. O'Malley BW, Weinstein GS, Snyder W, et al. Transoral robotic surgery (TORS) for base of tongue neoplasms. Laryngoscope. 2006;116(8):1465-72.

32. Weinstein GS, O'Malley BW, Snyder W, et al. Transoral robotic surgery: supraglottic partial laryngectomy. Ann Otol Rhinol Laryngol. 2007;116(1):19-23.

33. Weinstein GS, O'Malley BW, Snyder W, et al. Transoral robotic surgery: radical tonsillectomy. Arch Otolaryngol Head Neck Surg. 2007;133(12):1220-6.

34. Holsinger FC, McWhorter AJ, Menard M, et al. Transoral lateral oropharyngectomy for squamous cell carcinoma of the tonsillar region: I. Technique, complications, and functional results. Arch Otolaryngol Head Neck Surg. 2005;131(7):583-91.

35. Genden EM, Desai S, Sung CK. Transoral robotic surgery for the management of head and neck cancer: a preliminary experience. Head Neck. 2009;31(3):283-9.

36. Hurtuk A, Agrawal A, Old M, et al. Outcomes of transoral robotic surgery: a preliminary clinical experience. Otolaryngol Head Neck Surg Aug. 2011;145(2):248-53.

37. Boudreaux BA, Rosenthal EL, Magnuson JS, et al. Robot-assisted surgery for upper aerodigestive tract neoplasms. Arch Otolaryngol Head Neck Surg. 2009;135(4):397-401.

38. Moore EJ, Olsen KD, Kasperbauer JL. Transoral robotic surgery for oropharyngeal squamous cell carcinoma: a prospective study of feasibility and functional outcomes. Laryngoscope. 2009;119(11):2156-64.

39. Weinstein GS, O'Malley BW, Cohen MA, et al. Transoral robotic surgery for advanced oropharyngeal carcinoma. Arch Otolaryngol Head Neck Surg. 2010;136(11):1079-85.

40. de Arruda FF, Puri DR, Zhung J, et al. Intensity-modulated radiation therapy for the treatment of oropharyngeal carcinoma: the Memorial Sloan-Kettering Cancer Center experience. Int J Radiat Oncol Biol Phys. 2006;64(2):363-73.

41. Lawson JD, Otto K, Chen A, et al. Concurrent platinum-based chemotherapy and simultaneous modulated accelerated radiation therapy for locally advanced squamous cell carcinoma of the tongue base. Head Neck. 2008;30(3):327-35.

42. Cohen MA, Weinstein GS, O'Malley BW, et al. Transoral robotic surgery and human papillomavirus status: oncologic results. Head Neck. Dec 6. Epub ahead of print.

43. Weinstein GS, Quon H, O'Malley BW, et al. Selective neck dissection and deintensified postoperative radiation and chemotherapy for oropharyngeal cancer: a subset analysis of the University of Pennsylvania transoral robotic surgery trial. Laryngoscope Sep;120(9):1749-55.

44. White HN, Moore EJ, Rosenthal EL, et al. Transoral robotic-assisted surgery for head and neck squamous cell carcinoma: one- and 2-year survival analysis. Arch Otolaryngol Head Neck Surg. 2010;136(12):1248-52.

45. Genden EM, Kotz T, Tong CC, et al. Transoral robotic resection and reconstruction for head and neck cancer. Laryngoscope. 2011;121(8):1668-74.

46. Leonhardt FD, Quon H, Abrahao M, et al. Transoral robotic surgery for oropharyngeal carcinoma and its impact on patient-reported quality of life and function. Head Neck. 2011.

47. Hurtuk AM, Marcinow A, Agrawal A, et al. Quality-of-life outcomes in transoral robotic surgery. Otolaryngol Head Neck Surg. 2011.

48. Lee JY, O'Malley BW, Newman JG, et al. Transoral robotic surgery of the skull base: a cadaver and feasibility study. ORL J Otorhinolaryngol Relat Spec. 2010;72(4):181-7.

49. Lee JY, O'Malley BW, Newman JG, et al. Transoral robotic surgery of craniocervical junction and atlantoaxial spine: a cadaveric study. J Neurosurg Spine. Jan;12(1):13-8.

50. O'Malley BW, Weinstein GS. Robotic skull base surgery: preclinical investigations to human clinical application. Arch Otolaryngol Head Neck Surg. 2007;133(12):1215-9.

51. Hanna EY, Holsinger C, DeMonte F, et al. Robotic endoscopic surgery of the skull base: a novel surgical approach. Arch Otolaryngol Head Neck Surg. 2007;133(12):1209-14.

52. McCool RR, Warren FM, Wiggins RH, et al. Robotic surgery of the infratemporal fossa utilizing novel suprahyoid port. Laryngoscope. 2010;120(9):1738-43.

53. O'Malley BW, Quon H, Leonhardt FD, et al. Transoral robotic surgery for parapharyngeal space tumors. ORL J Otorhinolaryngol Relat Spec. 2010;72(6):332-6.

54. Lee JY, Lega B, Bhowmick D, et al. Da Vinci Robot-assisted transoral odontoidectomy for basilar invagination. ORL J Otorhinolaryngol Relat Spec. 2010;72(2):91-5.

55. Yin Tsang RK, Ho WK, Wei WI. Combined transnasal endoscopic and transoral robotic resection of recurrent nasopharyngeal carcinoma. Head Neck. 2011.

56. Wei WI, Ho WK. Transoral robotic resection of recurrent nasopharyngeal carcinoma. Laryngoscope. 2010;120(10):2011-4.

57. Mukhija VK, Sung CK, Desai SC, et al. Transoral robotic assisted free flap reconstruction. Otolaryngol Head Neck Surg. 2009;140(1):124-5.

58. Selber JC. Transoral robotic reconstruction of oropharyngeal defects: a case series. Plast Reconstr Surg. 2010;126(6):1978-87.

59. Vicini C, Dallan I, Canzi P, et al. Transoral robotic tongue base resection in obstructive sleep apnoea-hypopnoea syndrome: a preliminary report. ORL J Otorhinolaryngol Relat Spec. 2010;72(1):22-7.
60. Vicini C, Dallan I, Canzi P, et al. Transoral robotic surgery of the tongue base in obstructive sleep Apnea-Hypopnea syndrome: anatomic considerations and clinical experience. Head Neck. Mar 11.
61. Miccoli P, Berti P, Materazzi G, et al. Minimally invasive video-assisted thyroidectomy: five years of experience. J Am Coll Surg. 2004;199(2):243-8.
62. Radford PD, Ferguson MS, Magill JC, et al. Meta-analysis of minimally invasive video-assisted thyroidectomy. Laryngoscope. 2011;121(8):1675-81.
63. Linos D. Minimally invasive thyroidectomy: a comprehensive appraisal of existing techniques. Surgery. 2011;150(1):17-24.
64. Kang SW, Jeong JJ, Nam KH, et al. Robot-assisted endoscopic thyroidectomy for thyroid malignancies using a gasless transaxillary approach. J Am Coll Surg. 2009;209(2):e1-7.
65. Kang SW, Jeong JJ, Yun JS, et al. Robot-assisted endoscopic surgery for thyroid cancer: experience with the first 100 patients. Surg Endosc. 2009;23(11):2399-406.
66. Kang SW, Lee SC, Lee SH, et al. Robotic thyroid surgery using a gasless, transaxillary approach and the da Vinci S system: the operative outcomes of 338 consecutive patients. Surgery. 2009;146(6):1048-55.
67. Lewis CM, Chung WY, Holsinger FC. Feasibility and surgical approach of transaxillary robotic thyroidectomy without CO(2) insufflation. Head Neck. 2010;32(1):121-6.
68. Landry CS, Grubbs EG, Morris GS, et al. Robot assisted transaxillary surgery (RATS) for the removal of thyroid and parathyroid glands. Surgery. 2011;149(4):549-55.
69. Berber E, Heiden K, Akyildiz H, et al. Robotic transaxillary thyroidectomy: report of 2 cases and description of the technique. Surg Laparosc Endosc Percutan Tech. 2010;20(2):e60-3.
70. Kuppersmith RB, Holsinger FC. Robotic thyroid surgery: an initial experience with North American patients. Laryngoscope. 2010;121(3):521-6.
71. Lobe TE, Wright SK, Irish MS. Novel uses of surgical robotics in head and neck surgery. J Laparoendosc Adv Surg Tech A. 2005;15(6):647-52.
72. Terris DJ, Singer MC, Seybt MW. Robotic facelift thyroidectomy: II. Clinical feasibility and safety. Laryngoscope. 2011;121(8):1636-41.
73. Singer MC, Seybt MW, Terris DJ. Robotic facelift thyroidectomy: I. Preclinical simulation and morphometric assessment. Laryngoscope. 2011;121(8):1631-5.
74. Richmon JD, Pattani KM, Benhidjeb T, et al. Transoral robotic-assisted thyroidectomy: a preclinical feasibility study in 2 cadavers. Head Neck. 2011;33(3):330-3.

Chapter

14

MANAGEMENT OF ACUTE TRAUMA TO THE OPTIC NERVE

Thomas Kühnel

INTRODUCTION

Approximately 5% of closed head injuries are associated with optic nerve damage, which may result in permanent loss of vision. The key features involved in a traumatic optic nerve lesion remain a topic of controversial debate. Because the pathophysiology of damage to the optic nerve due to blunt trauma is understood only in part, treatment proposals tend to be guided by similar situations in general traumatology. The present chapter discusses the problems posed by diagnosis and by currently available therapy.

In the main, three treatment approaches are described in the literature: corticosteroids in varying dosages, surgical decompression of the intracanalicular portion of the optic nerve, and expectant management to establish whether the clinical situation resolves spontaneously. While various combinations of these approaches have been discussed, no treatment regimen is supported by a sufficient body of data. The time window within which treatment, especially surgical intervention, is to be recommended has yet to be defined. Is corticosteroid administration helpful or in fact counter-productive? Is decompression of the bony optic canal sufficient on its own or is optic nerve sheath fenestration necessary?

In the context of the management of a traumatic optic nerve lesion, there is one fundamental methodological problem that hinders the advance of knowledge: in evidence-based medicine research findings become more robust if the number of cases increases and if the description of the patients studied is as precise as possible in terms of the main outcome measure. Control groups should be definable in detail. Collectively, these prerequisites are difficult to achieve in rare medical conditions. Additionally, if the main outcome measure fails to be described in a relevant number of cases and the control group cannot be matched in any meaningful way, then it is only with very great difficulty that a viable result can be achieved using the methods of evidence-based medicine.

Although serious efforts have been undertaken,[1] all attempts to resolve this methodological quandary have come to nothing.

Nonetheless, using the literature on the subject, I shall endeavor to formulate a recommendation for the procedure to be adopted in traumatic optic neuropathy (TON).

SPECIAL ANATOMICAL FEATURES OF IMPORTANCE FOR OPTIC NERVE DAMAGE

The intraocular portion of the optic nerve is approximately 1 mm long. Avulsion injuries occur here only following very serious direct trauma to the orbit, and for such injuries no further treatment is possible. It is more common in this segment of the optic nerve to encounter nutritive disturbances caused by damage to the ciliary arteries.[2]

In its 25–30 mm long intraorbital segment the optic nerve takes a sinuous course, and displays a degree of laxity that allows free movement of the globe. Injuries in this territory are caused either by the penetrating impact of bone fragments and foreign-body impingement or as a result of intraorbital pressure increases in the setting of an orbital compartment syndrome.

The optic nerve is most vulnerable in its 6–8 mm long intracanalicular portion. At the entrance to the optic canal, the optic nerve is surrounded by the fibrous annulus of Zinn. If nerve decompression is the intended objective, then fenestration of the annulus is recommended because the narrowest section of the optic canal is located at this point. The optic nerve is an outgrowth from the diencephalon and forms part of the white matter of the brain. It is therefore ensheathed along its course by all three layers of the meninges with varying degrees of tightness. The optic canal itself is lined with periosteum which is continuous with the dura mater at the cerebral end, and with the periorbita and the dural sheath of the optic nerve at the orbital end. Since division of the dura occurs at this point, it might be possible when performing optic nerve sheath fenestration to leave the inner layer intact and thus to spare the subarachnoid space. In fact this is hardly ever achieved and surgical planning must anticipate the possibility of cerebrospinal fluid (CSF) leakage.[3]

The pia mater invests the optic nerve closely and accompanies it from the optic chiasm to the point of entry into the globe. The dura mater is continuous with the periosteal lining.

The arachnoid mater also accompanies the optic nerve along its entire length. In the intracanalicular segment, however, the sheaths are tightly adherent with each other, and the subarachnoid fluid spaces are therefore constricted. Bony deformations of the sphenoid wings are therefore transferred directly to the optic nerve because it can take no evasive path.[3]

The ophthalmic artery enters the dural sheath medially to the optic nerve in 40% of cases, centrally beneath the nerve in 35% of cases, and laterally beneath the nerve in 25% of cases. In 85–90% of cases the artery travels inferolaterally to the nerve as it passes through the bony canal, whereas in the remaining 10–15% it travels medially to the nerve and is thus potentially at risk during decompression surgery. If the artery were to be severed, then eyesight would in all probability be lost.[4]

Inside the optic canal, the optic nerve is supplied via the vascular plexus of the pia mater, which is fed by the ophthalmic artery.

In terms of surgical technique, the pathway followed by the optic nerve through the posterior ethmoid and the sphenoidal sinus is an important factor: endonasal endoscopic optic nerve decompression can only be considered if adequate pneumatization has occurred to expose the nerve in the sphenoidal sinus. As is also the case in functional endoscopic ethmoid surgery, careful attention must be paid to spheno-ethmoidal (Onodi) cells which enclose the optic nerve in the posterior ethmoid in 10–15% of cases.

EPIDEMIOLOGY AND ETIOLOGY

The commonest causes of TON are motor vehicle accidents (increasingly also including bicycle accidents), assault and falls. Young men are predominantly affected and there is initial loss of consciousness in 50% of cases. Where it occurs, loss of vision already develops in most cases directly subsequent to trauma.[5] In this process, a blunt blow to the cranial bones is transmitted to the optic canal and thence to the optic nerve which it firmly encloses. The present chapter takes this form of indirect blunt trauma as its starting point. Direct intraorbital or intraocular injuries to the optic nerve are generally the consequence of a sharp, penetrating injury, for example, due to stabbing or gunshot wounds. Interruptions to the continuity of the optic nerve sustained in this way are irreversible and no treatment is possible. Such injuries are distinct from indirect damage to the optic nerve in its orbital course caused by increased pressure in the orbital compartment. If the pressure within the orbit exceeds the perfusion pressure of the ciliary arteries, in particular, the result is an ischemic disturbance that may be reversible if treated early enough. Traumatic optic neuropathies are noted in up to one-fifth of serious frontobasal injuries.[6] Mid-facial fractures are associated with monocular blindness in 1.2% of cases.[7] Acute loss of visual acuity has been reported in 1.7% of patients with head injuries with ocular involvement.[2] In half of cases the loss of visual acuity remains permanent.[8]

One classification of injuries in terms of pathophysiology and injury pattern (Table 14.1) dates back to Frank B. Walsh and offers a guide to the implications for treatment.[9] The pathological mechanism underlying TON can be formulated briefly as follows: trauma causes arterial compression or spasm, and this leads to ischemia, which in turn entails intraneural edema and necrosis of the optic nerve. If we subscribe to this simple, mechanistic view, then damage to the optic nerve in its bony casing in the optic canal is an inexorable sequence of events and states that can only be interrupted if the prevailing conditions are altered. It is therefore plausible to call for measures that will reduce swelling or create space.[10]

Table 14.1: Classification of traumatic optic neuropathy by pathomechanism

Radiological diagnosis possible	Direct trauma	Radiological diagnosis generally not possible	Indirect trauma
	Penetrating foreign objects		Interruption of axonal transport
	Fractures of the optic canal		Ischemia
	Hematoma		Modified CSF transport
	Compression caused by bone fragments		
	Primary lesion		**Secondary lesion**
	Optic nerve concussion		Swelling and edema of the nerve
	Hemorrhages in the nerve, dural or sheath spaces		Softening (infarction) due to vascular spasm or thrombosis
	Tears in the nerve or chiasm		
	Contusion necrosis		

Alongside indirect damage to the optic nerve in its canal caused by pressure waves, other mechanisms of injury to the peripheral visual pathway must also be considered. For example, an intraconal retrobulbar hematoma caused by compression of the ciliary arteries that are arranged around the optic nerve may result in ischemic damage to the nerve and thus in loss of vision. By comparison with TON, retrobulbar hematomas and bulbar rupture are more common causes of visual loss. The trauma mechanism plays a more important role than the fracture pattern in determining the nature and extent of damage.[2]

DIAGNOSIS

Polytrauma patients are generally in a situation that does not permit precise ophthalmological diagnosis. Two-thirds of injured patients with TON are unconscious, a fact which means that no psychophysical findings can be elicited. The timing of visual impairment therefore cannot be determined with the precision required to give an estimate of the prognosis. Objective procedures that render the patient's cooperation nonessential provide a decision-making aid in establishing which therapy is indicated, but are too imprecise to allow scientific appraisal of treatment procedures in TON.

As a basis for establishing whether surgical intervention is indicated, the usefulness of electrophysiological diagnostic techniques [visual evoked potentials (VEP) and the electroretinogram] is undisputed.

However, the only prognostic criterion for which there is a broad consensus in the literature is the patient's initial visual function. Already at the scene of the accident, therefore, the person administering first aid should perform a basic test of visual function. Subsequent decision-making is greatly facilitated merely by the straightforward indication that visual function—assessed separately for each eye—was present or abolished immediately after the accident.

An ophthalmologist must always be included in the diagnostic process. The following set of examinations (adapted from reference no. 3) can be used as a starting point for the clinical diagnosis:

- Computed tomography (CT), 1 mm slices, multiplanar reconstruction in the setting of head injury diagnosis
- Preliminary intraocular pressure measurement to disclose any orbital pressure increase and any perforating injury to the eyeball
- The swinging flashlight test to identify a relative afferent pupillary defect (RAPD)
- Ophthalmometry (with a Hertel exophthalmometer) to detect unilateral eyeball protrusion in a right-left comparison
- Funduscopy: the pupil and retina are typically normal during the initial weeks after trauma. Optic nerve atrophy ensues only 3–4 weeks later. However, circulatory disturbances may possibly be detected earlier
- Determination of visual acuity, color vision (red is the first quality to be lost) and visual field perimetry if the patient is able to cooperate
- Flashlight VEP examination if the patient is unconscious

Where internal carotid artery (ICA) aneurysms are suspected or in the event of an ICA-cavernous sinus fistula, magnetic resonance imaging (MRI) angiography or conventional angiography is required.

The best functional tests to conduct in the clinic are visual acuity and visual field perimetry. Wherever possible, these tests should be repeated over time and the results meticulously documented. Testing for ocular motility and pupillary reactions is also an indispensable element in ophthalmological diagnosis.

In reality, however, a psychophysical examination of this kind is precluded in the majority of patients with TON. Almost invariably trauma will have resulted in considerable eyelid swelling or even in head injury that necessitates management in intensive care.

The swinging flashlight test is a standard diagnostic procedure that in many cases, assuming adequate experience, yields helpful information concerning optic nerve damage in particular. The test is used to detect a RAPD. 'Relative' means that it is only when both sides are compared that a weaker pupillary reaction can be detected in the eye that is presumed to be damaged. Of course, both eyes may be equally affected, in which case the swinging flashlight test will not yield any meaningful result. Injury or pre-existing disturbance of the refractive media of the eye, however, does not trigger any RAPD, making this test extremely useful specifically in the trauma setting.

The pupillary reflexes of both eyes are tested and compared in a dimly lit room. Using as bright a lamp as possible, both eyes are illuminated simultaneously from below. There should be no major anisocoria and the pupils must show an adequate reaction to light. In the present context, the commonly encountered phenomenon of opiate-induced miosis constitutes a major limitation. A light is shone on one eye and, after 2–3 seconds, is moved swiftly across to the other eye, before being shifted back again after a further 2–3 seconds. To be sure of the test result, the change sequence should be repeated 4–5 times. If one pupil shows a weaker reaction than the other, then this is a pathological finding. If pupillary constriction is absent or if there is actually pupillary dilation ('pupillary escape'), then a RAPD has been demonstrated and the suspicion of optic nerve injury is corroborated.

■ Visual Evoked Potentials

In patients with multiple injuries, it is generally the case that the techniques described up to this point, do not yield sufficiently reliable information concerning the state of the optic nerve. However, in order to be able to establish the indication for such far-reaching measures as pharmacotherapy with high-dose steroids or surgery involving the orbital apex, an assessment of optic nerve function is called for that is as reliable as possible, not least for medicolegal reasons. VEP recording provides information about the function of the visual pathway even in the unconscious patient whose eyelids are closed.[11,12] Of the two procedures practiced in a standard diagnostic work-up, the pattern stimulus VEP can be discounted because it would require the cooperation of the patient. With the flash VEP the retina is stimulated with light flashes, and the response of the visual pathway is described by averaging the potentials. Half-field VEPs should be recorded where chiasmal lesions are suspected. Today, portable devices are available, meaning that the investigation (which takes about 15 minutes) can also be performed in the Accident and Emergency Department or the Intensive Care Unit. However, the procedure has a number of substantial limitations. It may be that VEPs can no longer be elicited in cases where pronounced media turbidity is present. If one neuron is damaged, then all downstream neurons also yield abnormal findings (cone dystrophy causes changes in VEPs, even if no optic nerve damage is present).[13,14] High inter-individual variability in response to the stimulus is typical, even where inter-ocular asymmetry is minimal. Ischemic disorders cause only minor changes in VEP latency, and the curve recording may be characterized by morphological changes and reduced amplitude. In comatose patients, there are changes in both latency and amplitude.[15] The interpretation of such findings demands a high level of expertise and, as a prerequisite for the recording, standardized conditions which are extremely difficult to achieve given the patients and the setting in question. Refraction errors and pharmacological factors alter the amplitude and latency of the signal and have to be taken into account. Topographical localization of the lesion in the afferent visual system is practically impossible with VEPs.[16]

In summary, the preservation or abolition of VEPs enables conclusions to be drawn concerning the functional capacity of the optic nerve and of the visual pathway beyond. However, given the manifold sources of error, caution should be exercised over the uncritical use of VEP findings in establishing which treatment is indicated.

Direct injuries, whether caused by penetrating objects, optic canal fractures, hematomas or compression of dislocated bone fragments, may be amenable to CT diagnosis. Thin-slice CT with multiplanar reconstruction is the recommended technique. MRI findings can be helpful, especially in avulsion injuries and optic nerve sheath hematomas, axonal injury and ischemia. These conditions are usually the result of indirect trauma and are difficult to diagnose. However, MRI should not be performed until the presence of metallic foreign objects has been excluded, as these might cause additional damage in the orbit inside the powerful magnetic field of the MRI scanner. Multiplanar reconstructed 3D constructive interference in steady state (CISS) sequences, coronal T2-weighted images, short-tau inversion recovery (STIR) and diffusion-weighted (DW) sequences are recommended. It is noteworthy and important for the diagnosis that there is no direct correlation between the extent of a fracture and the severity of nerve damage.[9,17]

Although a key instrument in establishing which treatment might be indicated, CT diagnosis is not able with sufficient reliability to reveal fractures where there is no dislocation. Similarly, optic nerve sheath hematomas or swelling cannot be reliably detected or excluded by MRI. Diagnostic uncertainty therefore remains, and this should also be remembered when interpreting clinical studies. Nevertheless CT diagnosis is a key component in surgical planning because it permits determination of the length of the optic nerve segment that can be reached via a transnasal-transethmoidal approach. Furthermore, it provides an estimate of relationship to the ICA, and possibly also the abducens nerve. In this respect the imaging procedure is analogous to that used in functional paranasal sinus surgery.

INDICATION, TIMING OF INTERVENTION

There can be no doubt that impending loss of vision is a highly dramatic situation in which every effort is worthwhile to save the eye. Even in such a situation, however, careful weighing of the risks and potential benefits of therapy is preferable to therapeutic activism. It is essential to try and exclude those pathologies where any therapy at all is pointless. In all other cases a single-minded course will be followed to select a treatment, even though there may be only a slim chance of saving some part of the patient's eyesight.

Good consensus exists that surgical decompression should be performed on a generous scale in an orbital compartment syndrome. Lateral canthotomy with cantholysis, even under local anesthesia, can be performed as emergency surgery while the patient is still in the trauma room. Outward rotation of the lower eyelid signals the correct performance of the procedure. In the subsequent clinical course, the endonasal technique of orbital decompression is the 'gold standard' and is a routine procedure in the hands of the experienced paranasal sinus surgeon. Standard ethmoidectomy is followed by opening of the orbit. The orbital lamina of the ethmoid bone (lamina papyracea) is removed and an incision is made into the periorbita. This alteration in the volume of the orbit results in decompression but may also cause a shift in the optical axis and hence lead to postoperative squint. In such circumstances, squint-correction surgery would later become necessary.

The prognosis for visual function depends predominantly on visual acuity after the trauma event.[5] If the dynamics of the injury can be reconstructed, then the indication for treatment may be established as follows:

In cases where vision is instantaneously lost (optic nerve concussion, primary compression necrosis, tearing of the optic nerve or chiasm), surgery should be discounted. In optic nerve concussion surgery is unnecessary because the nerve will recover spontaneously; in the other pathologies the eye is lost. Where loss of vision is delayed, the situation is different: intervention appears to offer promise of success if swelling of the nerve leads to hypoxemia.[9]

Surgical measures should be considered in the event of secondary blindness, intracanalicular injury, dislocated bone fragments, and increased pressure in the orbit (orbital compartment syndrome).

Unfortunately, however, reliable details concerning the evolution of the visual disturbance are generally unobtainable.

It is repeatedly stated in the literature that intervention should take place within 8 hours in order to afford any prospect of a successful outcome.[8] In contrast, there have been published reports of cases in which eyesight has also been regained after much longer intervals.[18] This discrepancy has been discussed below.

CONSERVATIVE THERAPY

Expectant Management

A number of authors believe that the correct approach consists of no specific therapy and instead allowing the condition to take its spontaneous course. 40–60% of patients experience some improvement in vision even without therapy.[19] Since it has been impossible to demonstrate the efficacy or superiority of treatment with steroids or surgery compared with expectant management, it can be argued that the risks attendant upon therapy should be avoided.[1]

Such an attitude is at odds with the medical professional's need to act in some way in a desperate situation. This is certainly an irrational, yet understandable and probably even common motivation to embark upon therapy. In order to create a rational basis for treatment decisions in cases where the sight of an eye is vitally threatened, there is a need for clear, easy-to-follow arguments. In a meta-analysis of the literature available up to 1996, Cook et al. concluded that treatment with steroids and surgery was superior to expectant management. However, they did concede that methodological problems rendered any definitive conclusion impossible and they referred to the then still incomplete international study on this topic.[19] In that study a bias has to be borne in mind concerning the interval between trauma and inclusion in the study (Table 14.2).[20] Later publications see no advantage for steroid therapy; instead they point out its risks and they counsel in favor of expectant observation.

Pharmacological Therapy, Steroids, Dosage and the Literature

Corticosteroids have been used in the management of traumatic optic neuropathies for 40 years.[1] The results obtained in central nervous system damage in animal studies were transposed to the visual pathway because the optic nerve, like the spinal cord, is part of the brain.[21] Corticosteroids were assumed to exert a neuroprotective effect due to their antioxidant action and to inhibit the lipid peroxidation induced by free radicals. Because of its milder pharmacological interactions and its effective inhibition of the inflammatory cascade, methylprednisolone is preferred over other representatives of the corticosteroid class.

Clinical recommendations regarding steroid therapy are based largely on the National Acute Spinal Cord Injury Study (NASCIS II and III).[1,22] This study also sets out the recommendation that therapy should be initiated within an 8-hour window. However, the results and in particular the extent to which they can be extrapolated to TON are the subject of ongoing controversy. For example, a significant difference was found for motor but not for sensory fibers. Moreover, NASCIS has been criticized for a lack of methodological clarity (randomization, post hoc analysis of a small subgroup for the actual claim regarding the early treatment of spinal cord injury), and this limits the validity of its conclusions.[1,23-25]

Another publication that provides a critical assessment of corticosteroid therapy merits consideration here. The double-blind, randomized, placebo-controlled study on the efficacy of mega-dose therapy with methylprednisolone in head injury patients in terms of survival

	Table 14.2: List of biases that are relevant when considering the evolution of traumatic optic neuropathy	
1.	Selection bias due to small sample size
2.	Imprecise details concerning time interval between trauma and inclusion in the study
3.	Different methods of measuring visual function and visual field
4.	Patients included in the surgical optic nerve decompression group only after conservative therapy has failed
5.	Patients undergoing surgery have more severe injury
6.	Patients with optic canal fractures and dislocated bone fragments are not studied in groups of their own

[Corticosteroid Randomization After Significant Head Injury (CRASH) study][26] was originally intended to recruit 20,000 patients. After 10,008 patients the study was halted by the ethics committee because it was found that survival at the 6-month follow-up was worse in the active treatment group than in the placebo group. These results need to be taken into account specifically with TON patients who commonly present with head injury.

In a randomized, double-blind, prospective study Entezari et al. compared the effect of high-dose steroid therapy (250 mg methylprednisolone intravenously every 6 hours for 3 days, followed by 1 mg prednisolone/kg bodyweight for 14 days) with placebo in 31 patients with unilateral indirect TON. All patients were included in the study within 7 days after trauma. As it has been remarked elsewhere, herein perhaps lies a problem that is typical of the studies on this subject: the time that elapsed between injury and the start of treatment ranged from 6 hours to 168 hours. The effect of spontaneous remissions may have impacted one group or the other to a varying extent. Furthermore, patients with no perception of light were included in the same way as others whose vision was largely preserved. Leaving these methodological pitfalls to one side, the authors were unable to detect any significant difference between the treatment groups.[27]

In a review published by the Cochrane Collaboration, Yu-Wai-Man and Griffiths[28] have concluded that there are no convincing data to demonstrate the superiority of steroid therapy compared with simple observation of the clinical course. However, scrutiny of 247 articles failed to reveal any that might have satisfied the formal criteria set by the reviewers. Despite this, a number of case report studies were discussed, including that by Cook et al. cited elsewhere in this chapter. All these studies are criticized for methodological shortcomings.

In the intensive care patient, in particular, the side-effects of high-dose or mega-dose steroid therapy (Table 14.3) must be taken into account. Apart from gastrointestinal complications, a diabetogenic effect and steroid psychosis, their immunocompromising effect entailing the threat of nosocomial infections is a risk that must be taken seriously.

It is currently not possible to tell whether therapy with nerve growth factor has any importance. Initial reports have shown positive effects but they are characterized by the same methodological problems as earlier studies with other treatment modalities.[29]

Table 14.3: Steroid dose classification (methylprednisolone as initial daily dose)

Low-dose	< 100 mg
Moderate dose	100–499 mg
High-dose	500–1,999 mg
Very high-dose	2,000–5,399 mg
Mega-dose	> 5,400 mg

Surgery: Endonasal, Transorbital or Neurosurgical Pterional Decompression

The first optic nerve decompression procedures were described by Sewall, Dandy and Pringle during the 1930s. The frontotemporal approach became standard during the two World Wars, with the transtemporal, transorbital, transfrontal intra- and extradural, transnasal and transethmosphenoidal approaches being developed only later.[8,30]

Compared with the transcranial approach, the transethmoidal approach offers the advantages of rapid wound healing, the olfactory bulb is spared, operative stress is less (a major factor in patients with multiple injuries and requiring intensive care), and it leaves no scarring. Provided that the optic nerve can be adequately exposed in the ethmoid bone and sphenoidal sinus, that there are no contraindications, and that no other neurosurgical procedure renders the transcranial approach necessary anyway, the endoscopic, transnasal-transethmoidal approach has become virtually standard for decompression surgery. Decompression for an orbital compartment syndrome can be performed by the same route.[3]

In the hands of an experienced surgeon the procedure may be considered safe and low in risk. Apart from the typical risks associated with endonasal paranasal sinus surgery, the following must be mentioned when obtaining consent: injury to the ophthalmic artery, injury to portions of the nerve resulting from sheath fenestration, CSF leakage and meningitis.

If the path of the optic nerve lies outside the sphenoidal sinus or if the roof of its canal is fractured, the neurosurgical temporal approach is selected. After dissection of the temporalis muscle, circumscribed (pterional) trepanation is performed. Once the dura is lifted, the nerve can be unroofed and revealed along its entire extraorbital course. This approach too is characterized by relatively minimal trauma and rapid recovery by the patient. Disturbances of masticatory function may occur.

The transorbital approach was described even earlier than the transethmoidal route but in the recent past it has fallen out of widespread use. Current publications describing transorbital approaches to the anterior cranial base might establish a new route to the orbital apex in our present context.[31]

In the Cochrane Review of the surgical management of TON, as with the review of steroid therapy, the reviewers conclude that there is no compelling evidence in the literature for the efficacy of decompression surgery.[28] Over against this, however, there are case reports which permit no other conclusion than that decompression of the optic nerve has resulted in the restoration of eyesight in individual cases.

RESULTS, CASE REPORTS

One simple message can be distilled from the data available in the literature: there is no evidence of significant differences between treatment methods.[5] Consequently, no unequivocal treatment recommendation can be made on the basis of current medical research. If we accept the methods of knowledge acquisition as they are applied in evidence-based medicine in particular, then it is to be feared that a decision cannot be reached concerning the best treatment for indirect TON.[1]

Probably the most important publication on TON (Levin et al. The treatment of traumatic optic neuropathy: the International Optic Nerve Trauma Study) was planned as an international, randomized two-arm treatment study.[5] Two years after it started the project had to be abandoned because it proved impossible to recruit sufficient numbers of patients meeting the predefined criteria. It was continued as an observational cohort study and has yielded the most systematically compiled results, the most important of which are:

- Initial visual function is a strong predictor of outcome. This claim has also been advanced by a number of other authors[7,32]
- No advantage can be demonstrated for the administration of 'megadose therapy' with methylprednisolone equivalents of more than 5,400 mg compared with lower dosage levels
- The timing of treatment initiation is not of overriding importance
- Diagnostic findings obtained by CT do not permit conclusions to be drawn concerning visual acuity achieved subsequently
- Neither steroids nor decompression surgery are superior to expectant management

However, the authors concede that the data analysis highlights a number of uncertainties. For example, the group of patients who underwent surgery was found to include a greater number of severe clinical courses. Steroid therapy was initiated before the indication for surgery was established. Serious bias was introduced by patients who underwent surgery only after conservative therapy (expectant management or steroids) had failed. In this manner there was already a measure of patient selection in that patients with a poorer prognosis were assigned to the surgery group. It is possible that optic canal fractures, which resulted more often in the surgical option being chosen, are a further source of bias because they are probably associated with a poorer outcome than cases without fracture (Table 14.2).

There are a large number of case reports which all share certain features in common: it is impossible to define uniform inclusion criteria, baseline circumstances at the start of treatment are rarely comparable, and the study endpoints are almost routinely poorly defined. Probably the most difficult aspect of study design is to measure baseline visual acuity as the most important prognostic criterion. All authors are agreed that the inclusion of patients with undefined visual function leads to distortion of results irrespective of treatment.[5,18,33] A further important aspect concerns the timing of the start of treatment. The earlier treatment begins, whether it be conservative or surgical, the greater the likelihood of patients whose eyesight would have recovered spontaneously anyway being assigned to a treatment group and so giving a false-positive result.

Findings from experimental animal studies in rats subjected to standardized crush injury to the optic nerve can of course be transposed to humans to only a limited extent. Nevertheless, they help to identify fundamental mechanisms in the pathophysiology. In one study[34] no difference was found between the various methylprednisolone regimens and controls in terms of axon loss, while in another study[35] there was a significant dose-dependent reduction in axon counts as the steroid dose increased.

SUMMARY

High-dose or mega-dose therapy should be abandoned in the treatment of TON. Whether lower doses have a positive effect remains to be proven. A neurotoxic effect of corticosteroids in TON has been demonstrated in animal experiments.

There are patients who benefit from surgical decompression, but it is unclear how these can be selected in advance prior to surgery. One possible group might comprise those patients with optic nerve sheath hematoma and declining visual function. In addition, decompression surgery is recommended only in patients with delayed onset of loss of visual acuity or in those who display no improvement in visual acuity after 4 days. Some residual visual function is a prerequisite in every case. There is no general recommendation for surgery.

▮ Dilemma

To date it has not been possible to demonstrate superiority for any of the known treatment modalities. In fact, proof of efficacy is still awaited for any therapy at all.[1]

The data show that the method of comparing one procedure with another or with simple expectant management yields no result. This is due to two factors: firstly, TON is a rare condition, and secondly, the baseline circumstances are routinely heterogeneous. It is difficult to make a clear-cut diagnosis and in the past it has been impossible to define standard inclusion and exclusion criteria that would have made it possible to conduct a study with a high evidence level. Published case series regularly lack a suitable control group, a feature that is essential, however, in order to clarify the superiority of a given treatment compared with the spontaneous clinical course.[1]

The question is therefore raised whether an answer is impossible because no differences exist between treatment methods or whether the methodological tool is unsuitable to shed light on the special situation of TON.

If we now attempt to approach the problem on an individual case basis, another possibility for knowledge acquisition emerges. Let us abandon the search for generally applicable rules for the superiority of one treatment form over another or over placebo using a group of patients with characteristics that are to be verified before the start of the study. For this individual case of TON, let us abandon the rules of evidence-based medicine and try an approach that is used in many branches of the natural sciences. If we base this approach on plausible assumptions and test whether under precisely defined conditions our expectations of a treatment are fulfilled, then a hypothesis can be developed. We can hold firmly to this hypothesis until the opposite is proven. With such rare conditions as TON, it is perhaps possible with this approach to find a way out of the methodological dilemma. The process can be clearly demonstrated by taking an example from the published literature.

In a case report Chen et al.[33] describe the clinical course in a patient with TON who underwent endonasal decompression surgery after conservative therapy had failed. The reported baseline findings were: RAPD in the left eye, preserved perception of light, multiple fractures of the orbit with fragments in the superior and inferior orbital fissure, and optic nerve impingement by bone fragments.

Starting on Day 2 after trauma methylprednisolone pulsed therapy was given for 48 hours. Because the clinical situation did not improve, surgery to fenestrate the optic nerve sheaths and periorbita close to the orbital apex was performed on Day 4 after trauma. The hematoma in the orbital apex was removed and canal debridement was performed.

After one week visual acuity had increased to 6/36; within 2 months visual acuity improved to 6/9, and a normal visual field was restored.

The assumption that forms the basis for establishing which treatment is indicated is simple and plausible: the optic nerve is mechanically compressed in its canalicular course by the fragments of bone. Administration of corticosteroids does not bring about any change in the initial situation.

The hypothesis is that debridement and removal of the hematoma relieves the pressure on the nerve as a prerequisite for its regeneration.

Since decompression ushered in regeneration after a period of 4 days during which there had been no improvement in visual acuity, the hypothesis is supported in as much as the close temporal relationship between measure and effect also renders a causal relationship highly probable. The more pronounced the change in the outcome variable (visual acuity and visual field) over time at the point of intervention, the more reliable the assumption of a causal relationship. The following recommendation may therefore be formulated: in cases of TON with bony compression of the optic nerve in its canalicular course and with optic nerve sheath hematoma and preserved perception of light, decompression surgery with sheath fenestration should be performed. And this can be done even after a latency period of 4 days.

Every case report with similar baseline circumstances and a similar outcome strengthens the hypothesis and thus has a higher value than in the approach advocated by evidence-based medicine. The prerequisite is consistent documentation of the initial situation and of its evolution over time. Visual acuity is determined at time points 2, 3 and 5 and no change is detected. Further determinations postoperatively at time points 7, 9 and 12 highlight the improvement.

Since other patterns of visual acuity over time are conceivable, special attention must be paid to the dynamics of visual acuity.

If ophthalmological findings were to be collected only twice, for example, at time points 2 and 12, it might be conjectured that surgery had been the decisive factor in the improvement of visual acuity.

If progress is to be achieved with this approach, patterns of findings must be described as precisely as possible and related to a particular treatment form. If with a sufficiently large number of individual cases it is possible to separate irrelevant from relevant findings, then an attempt can be made to formulate a rule for situations that are similar.

REFERENCES

1. Yu-Wai-Man P, Griffiths PG. Steroids for traumatic optic neuropathy. The Cochrane Database Syst Rev. 2007;(4):1-12.
2. Magarakis M, Mundinger GS, Kelamis JA, et al. Ocular injury, visual impairment, and blindness associated with facial fractures: A systematic literature review. Plast Reconstr Surg. 2011.
3. Luxenberger W, Stammberger H, Jebeles JA, et al. Endoscopic optic nerve decompression: the Graz experience. Laryngoscope. 1998;108(6):873-82.
4. Lanz Tvon, Wachsmuth W. Praktische Anatomie. Berlin, Göttingen, Heidelberg: Springer-Verlag; 1979.
5. evin LA, Beck RW, Joseph MP, et al. The treatment of traumatic optic neuropathy: the International Optic Nerve Trauma Study. Ophthalmology. 1999;106(7):1268-77.
6. Wang DH, Zheng CQ, Qian J, et al. Endoscopic optic nerve decompression for the treatment of traumatic optic nerve neuropathy. ORL J Otorhinolaryngol Relat Spec. 2008;70(2):130-3.
7. Ansari MH. Blindness after facial fractures: a 19-year retrospective study. J Oral Maxillofac Surg. 2005;63:229-37.
8. Steinsapir KD, Goldberg RA. Traumatic optic neuropathy. Surv Ophthalmol. 1994;38(6):487-518.
9. alsh FB. Pathological-clinical correlations: I. Indirect trauma to the optic nerves and chiasm. II. Certain cerebral involvements associated with defective blood supply. Invest Ophthalmol. 1966;5(5):433-49.
10. Gellrich NC. Kontroversen und aktueller Stand der Therapie von Sehnervenschäden in der kraniofazialen Traumatologie und Chirurgie[Controversies and current status of therapy of optic nerve damage in craniofacial traumatology and surgery]. Mund Kiefer Gesichtschir. 1999;3:176-94.
11. Mahapatra AK. Visual evoked potentials in optic nerve injury--does it merit to be mentioned? Indian J Ophthalmol. 1991;39(1):20-1.
12. Cornelius CP, Altenmuller E, Ehrenfeld M. Blitzevozierte visuelle Potenziale (BVEP) bei Patienten mit kraniofazialen Frakturen [Flash-evoked visual potentials in patients with craniofacial fractures]. Fortschr Kiefer Gesichtschir. 1991;36:158-62.

13. Bach M, Kellner U. Elektrophysiologische Diagnostik in der Ophthalmologie [Electrophysiological diagnosis in ophthalmology]. Ophthalmologe. 2000;97(12):898-920.

14. Odom JV, Bach M, Barber C, et al. Visual evoked potentials standard (2004). Doc Ophthalmol. 2004;108(2):115-23.

15. Cerovski B, Sikic J, Petrovic J. The role of visual evoked potentials in the diagnosis of optic nerve injury as a result of mild head trauma. Coll Antropol. 2001;25(Suppl):47-55.

16. Maurer K, Lang N, Eckert J. Visuell evozierte Potentiale (VEP). Praxis der evozierten Potentiale: SEP, AEP, MEP, VEP. 2nd edition. Darmstadt: Steinkopff; 2005. pp. 227-76.

17. Becker M, Masterson K, Delavelle J, et al. Imaging of the optic nerve. Eur J Radiol. 2010;74(2):299-313.

18. Thakar A, Mahapatra AK, Tandon DA. Delayed optic nerve decompression for indirect optic nerve injury. Laryngoscope. 2003;113(1):112-9.

19. Cook MW, Levin LA, Joseph MP, et al. Traumatic optic neuropathy. A meta-analysis. Arch Otolaryngol Head Neck Surg. 1996;122(4):389-92.

20. Steinsapir KD, Goldberg RA. Traumatic optic neuropathy: an evolving understanding. Am J Ophthalmol. 2011;151(6):928-33.

21. Anderson RL, Panje WR, Gross CE. Optic nerve blindness following blunt forehead trauma. Ophthalmology. 1982;89(5):445-55.

22. Young W. NASCIS. National Acute Spinal Cord Injury Study. J Neurotrauma 1990;7(3):113-4.

23. Hurlbert RJ. Methylprednisolone for acute spinal cord injury: an inappropriate standard of care. J Neurosurg. 2000;93(1 Suppl):1-7.

24. Coleman WP, Benzel D, Cahill DW, et al. A critical appraisal of the reporting of the National Acute Spinal Cord Injury Studies (II and III) of methylprednisolone in acute spinal cord injury. J Spinal Disord. 2000;13(3):185-99.

25. Sayer FT, Kronvall E, Nilsson OG. Methylprednisolone treatment in acute spinal cord injury: the myth challenged through a structured analysis of published literature. Spine J. 2006;6(3):335-43.

26. Edwards P, Arango M, Balica L, et al. Final results of MRC CRASH, a randomised placebo-controlled trial of intravenous corticosteroid in adults with head injury-outcomes at 6 months. Lancet. 2005;365(9475):1957-9.

27. Entezari M, Rajavi Z, Sedighi N, et al. High-dose intravenous methylprednisolone in recent traumatic optic neuropathy; a randomized double-masked placebo-controlled clinical trial. Graefes Arch Clin Exp Ophthalmol. 2007;245(9):1267-71.

28. Yu-Wai-Man P, Griffiths PG. Surgery for traumatic optic neuropathy (Review). Cochrane Database Syst Rev. 2011;(1):CD006032.

29. Zhong Y, Shen X, Liu X, et al. The early effect of nerve growth factor in the management of serious optic nerve contusion. Clin Exp Optom. 2010;93(6):466-70.

30. Li KK, Meara JG, Joseph MP. Reversal of blindness after facial fracture repair by prompt optic nerve decompression. J Oral Maxillofac Surg. 1997;55(6):648-50.

31. Moe KS, Bergeron CM, Ellenbogen RG. Transorbital neuroendoscopic surgery. Neurosurgery. 2010;67(3 Suppl Operative):ons16-28.

32. Chen C, Selva D, Floreani S, et al. Endoscopic optic nerve decompression for traumatic optic neuropathy: an alternative. Otolaryngol Head and Neck Surg. 2006;135(1):155-7.

33. Dickersin K, Manheimer E, Li T. Surgery for nonarteritic anterior ischemic optic neuropathy. Cochrane Database Syst Rev. 2006;(4):1-10.

34. Ohlsson M, Westerlund U, Langmoen IA, et al. Methylprednisolone treatment does not influence axonal regeneration or degeneration following optic nerve injury in the adult rat. J Neuroophthalmol. 2004;24(1):11-8.

35. Steinsapir KD, Goldberg RA, Sinha S, et al. Methylprednisolone exacerbates axonal loss following optic nerve trauma in rats. Restor Neurol Neurosci. 2000;17(4):157-63.

Chapter

15

FUNCTIONAL RHINOPLASTY

Fazil Apaydin

INTRODUCTION

Rhinoplasty is accepted as the most challenging operation in facial plastic surgery. One of the main reasons for that is to keep a balance between form and function. This is a virtual balance which is apt to change from surgeon to surgeon. However, in recent years, many prominent surgeons are prone to go for "functional rhinoplasty". In this article, the main idea is to give you some insight what this term really means.

In a normal functioning nose, there are four valves: septal valve (nasal septum), turbinal valve (inferior turbinates), internal valve and external valve.[1] In functional rhinoplasty, all of these valves should be adressed in order to obtain the best chance for better breathing through the nose.

▌ I. Septal Surgery

Septal surgery is by far one of the most frequent reasons to operate on nasal obstruction. It can be both congenital or acquired. Many attempts have been done to classify septal deformities.[2,3] I have been using SL classification which I have designed 13 years ago (Tables 15.1 and 15.2). This simple classification helps one to describe the pathology, to make pre- and postoperative comparisons much easier. In order to facilitate record-keeping for septal surgery, a mapping system was also prepared by me (Fig. 15.1). In this article, the surgical techniques for septal deviation will be briefly explained.

Surgical Methods in the Management of Deviated Nasal Septum

1. *Submucous resection*: Submucous resection (SMR) has been described by Killian in 1904.[4] The L-strut is left in place while the rest of the nasal septum is removed. Although the disadvantages of saddling, septal perforation, mucosal atrophy and septal flapping have been

Table 15.1: SL classification used to record pathologic conditions of the nasal septum and the lateral nasal wall

S: Septum nasi
0: No evidence of septal deformity
1: Septal deviation confined to the vestibulum nasi
2: Septal deviation confined to the nasal valve area
3: Septal deviation confined to the attic
4: Septal deviation confined to the anterior turbinate area
5: Septal deviation confined to the posterior turbinate area
X: The minimum requirements to assess the septal deviation cannot be met.
L: Lateral nasal wall
n: No evidence of pathology confined to lateral nasal wall
p(s): Polyp (Polyposis nasi)
c: Concha bullosa
h: Inferior turbinate hypertrophy
t: Tumor
r: Rhinitis
x: The minimum requirements to assess the septal deviation cannot be met.
o: Other_____
(L): Left nasal passage (R): Right nasal passage

Table 15.2: Examples to the use of SL classification (1st level of data recording)

SL Classification	Explanation
$S_{2,3}L_{n\,(R)} + S_1L_{h\,(L)}$	Septal deviation confined to the nasal valve region and attic, no pathology confined to the lateral wall on the right side. Septal deviation confined to the vestibulum nasi and hypertrophy of the inferior turbinate on the left side.
$S_{1-3}\,L_{n\,(R)} + S_0L_{ps\,(L)}$	Septal deviation confined to the vestibulum nasi, nasal valve area and anterior turbinate area on the right side. No septal pathology, but polyposis nasi on the left side.
When more than one area is involved and if these are consecutive areas, a hyphen is placed between the lowest and the highest number, if different areas are involved, they are separated by commas.	

mentioned,[5] this technique is still widely used today because it is easier to perform and teach. Besides, the increasing popularity of external rhinoplasty in the past two decades obviated the need for grafts obtained from the septal cartilage. However, the straightened cartilage and bone pieces are usually reinserted between the mucoperichondrial flaps to prevent complications mentioned above (Fig. 15.2).

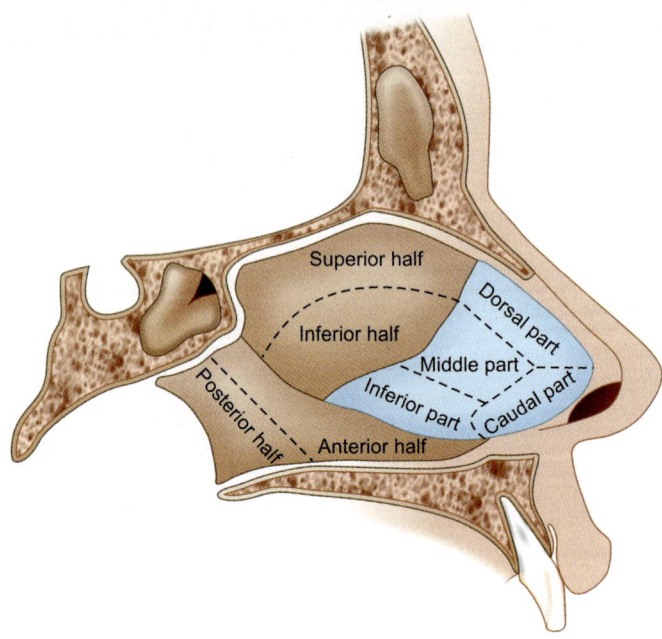

Fig. 15.1: The nasal septum is divided into different sections to facilitate recording on the patient's chart after septal surgery

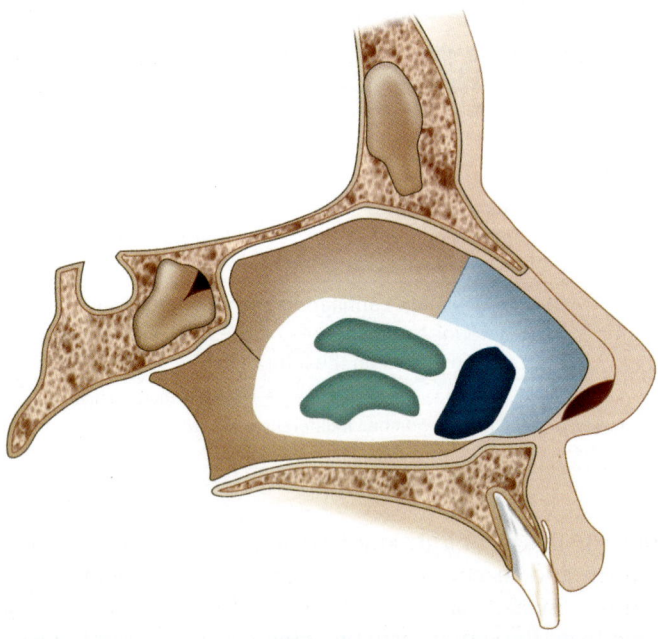

Fig. 15.2: After submucous resection (SMR), the resected and reshaped cartilage (green) and bone (blue) fragments are inserted between the mucoperichondrial flaps to get rid of the complications of SMR

2. *Septoplasty:* After the introduction of this technique in 1959 by Cottle,[6] this technique gained popularity all over the world, because it became a very helpful solution against the disadvantages of SMR, because most of the cartilaginous septum was preserved in place and straightening the septum could be achieved by small maneuvers over the cartilage such as cross-hatching. It is still applied by many surgeons, although it is less often used when septal reconstruction is combined with rhinoplasty.

3. *Limited septoplasty:* After the introduction of endoscope in nasal surgery, limited septoplasty became more popular.[7] In recent years, the developments in powered instrumentation led the surgeons to use it in limited septoplasty as well.[8] In my daily practice, I realized that this technique is performed more by functional endoscopic sinus surgeons than facial plastic surgeons. I use this technique rarely, with a headlight and a loupe, without the need for an endoscope.

4. *L-strut reinforcement techniques:* The L-strut is the main carrier of the nasal pyramid. The previous techniques described before are more often used in daily routine. When it comes to crooked noses and traumatic noses, L-strut reinforcement techniques and subtotal reconstruction techniques are more often used. In my hands, these techniques are the most popular ones in dealing with crooked noses.

   a. Dorsal segment: The deviated dorsal segment can be corrected by splinting it with two spreader grafts from both sides[9] (Figs 15.3A to F). Depending on the individual case, the concave side can be cross-hatched to break the cartilage memory or thicker spreader grafts can also overcome the deviation. I used to insert the spreader grafts via an external approach. Then I found out that it could also be applied under endonasal approach although it is a little bit more difficult. In cases when the middle vault is not separated, precise pockets on both sides of the dorsal segment are created and spreader grafts are placed in these pockets. When the deviation is closer to the key area, longer bony-cartilaginous splinting grafts can be used (Fig. 15.4).

   b. Caudal segment: The deviated caudal septum can usually be corrected by changing its attachment to anterior nasal spine, either by swinging-door technique[10,11] or trimming the surplus of cartilage causing bending. Unfortunately, there are times that these maneuvers are not enough and the caudal septum is still crooked. In these cases, caudal batten grafts (Figs 15.5A to C) or caudal septal extension grafts[12] are usually used to straighten the caudal septum. In revision cases, in cases where the caudal segment is lacking or cannot be used, a caudal septal replacement graft[13] should be used (Figs 15.6A to G).

   c. Dorsal and caudal segment: In severely crooked noses, the combination of the abovementioned two techniques should be used. Another viable alternative in my mind is to use L-strut graft out of cartilage and/or bone.[14,15] Although it can increase the thickness at the caudal border as in the previous technique, usually this does not create a problem (Figs 15.7A to C).

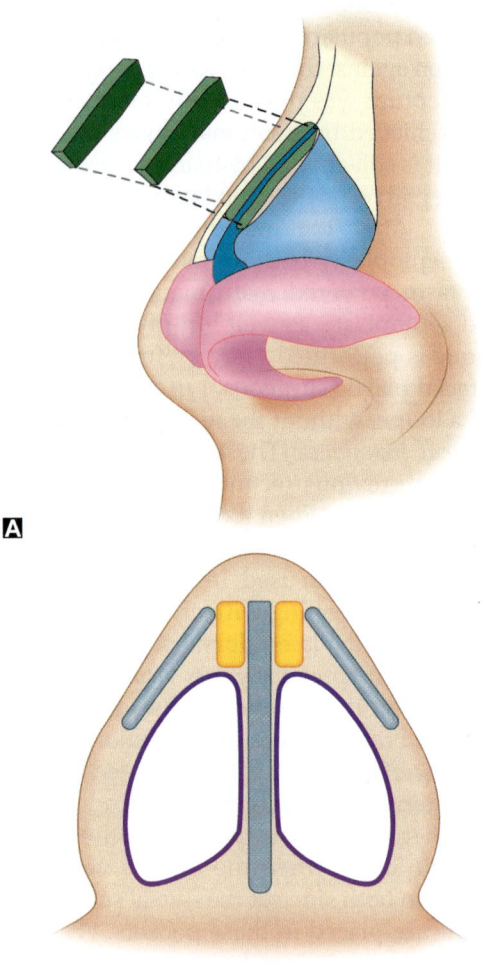

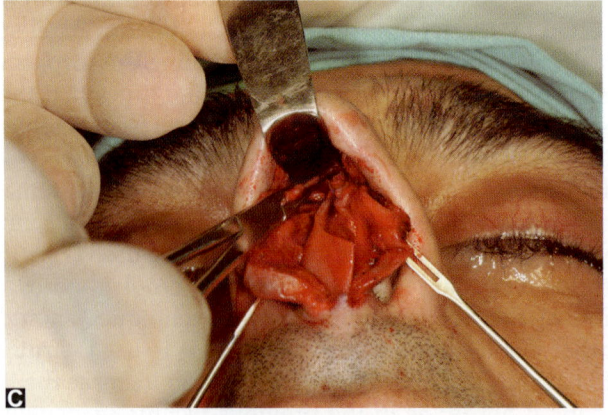

Figs 15.3A to C

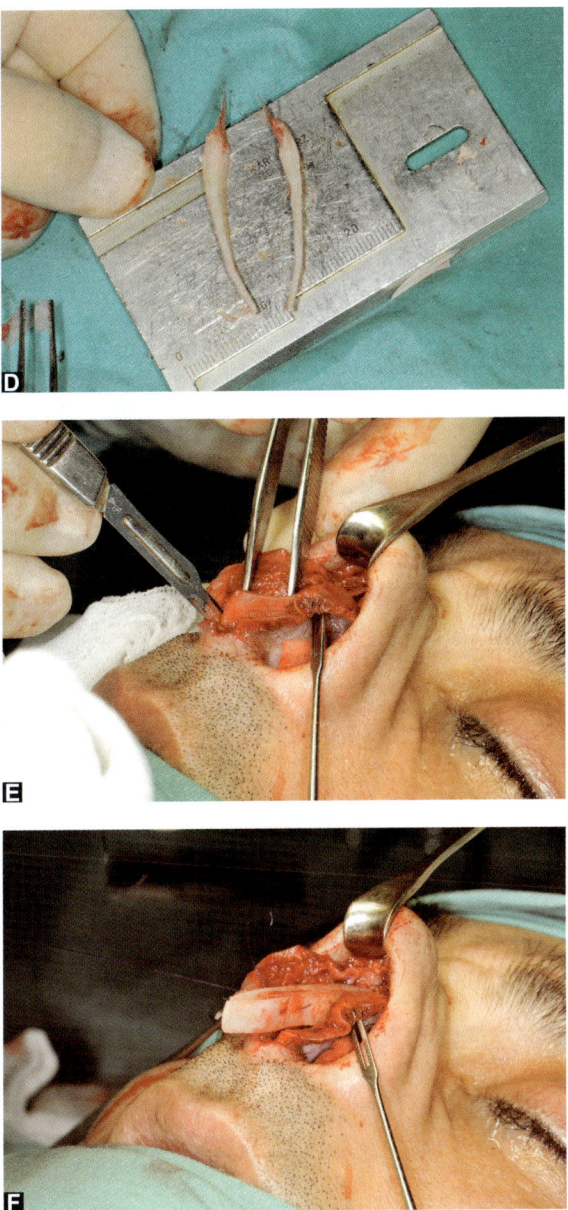

Figs 15.3D to F

Figs 15.3A to F: (A) This drawing illustrates how the spreader grafts are placed to the middle vault; (B) The spreader grafts should be on both sides of the nasal septum and widen the middle vault by lateralizing the upper lateral cartilages (ULCs); (C) After hump removal, the dorsally deviated nasal septum can be identified much easier; (D) Splinting spreader grafts sculptured from bony-cartilaginous septum. It is not always easy to obtain straight and/or longer cartilages. In this case, concave grafts can be used as splinting spreader grafts; (E) Cross-hatching on the concave side of the dorsal segment is done to break the memory of the septal cartilage; (F) Splinting spreader grafts are sutured by 4-0 PDS to keep the dorsal segment straight

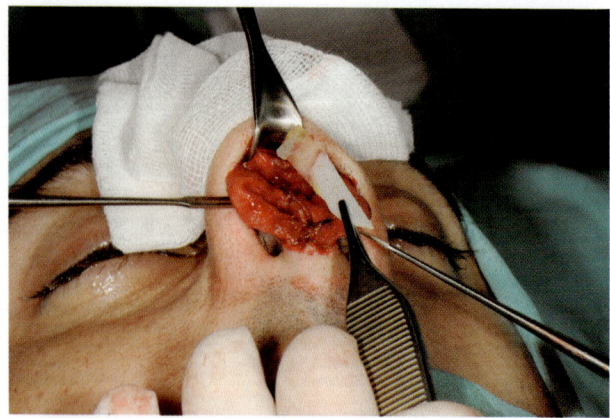

Fig. 15.4: In cases of high septal deviation, a bony-cartilaginous splinting spreader graft is very useful, as the thinner cephalic bony part does not only support the deviated septum, but also does not cause open roof either

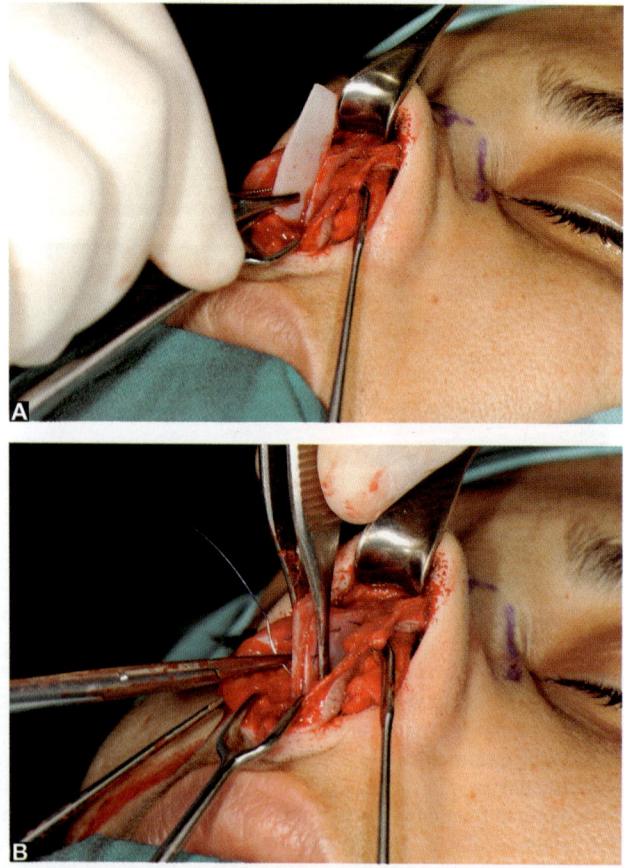

Figs 15.5A and B

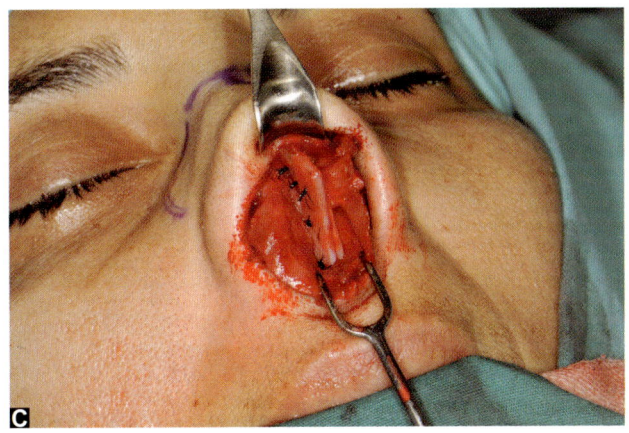

Fig. 15.5C

Figs 15.5A to C: (A) A caudal batten graft is used to support and straighten the caudal segment of the cartilaginous septum; (B) The graft is fixed to the caudal end by 4-0 PDS sutures; (C) View of the graft sutured in place from the other side

5. *Subtotal septal reconstruction techniques:*
   a. One piece L-strut: In severely traumatic noses, the nasal septum can be fractured from many places which can make correction of the nasal septum by keeping the L-strut in place. Even in most of these cases, a big piece of cartilage and/or bone can be obtained. This big piece is sutured to a piece of cartilage at the key area and to the anterior nasal spine.[14] In revision cases, the sixth costal cartilage is used to sculpture a one-piece L-strut[15] (Figs 15.8A to F).

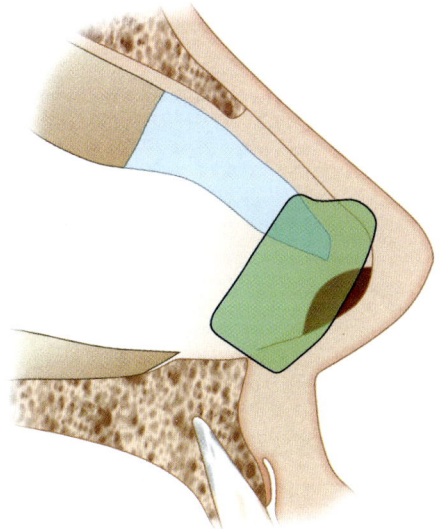

Fig. 15.6A

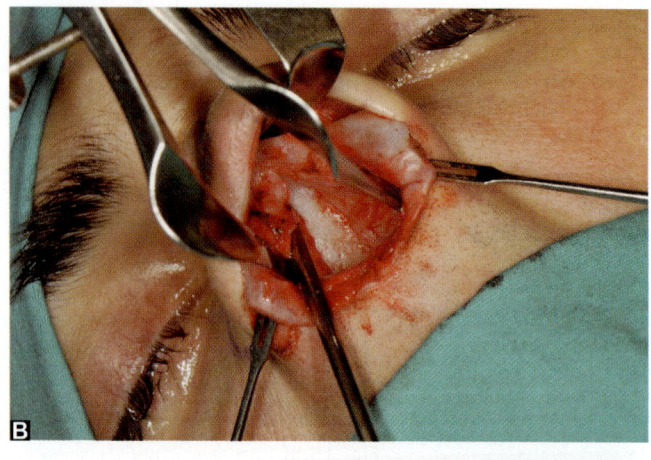

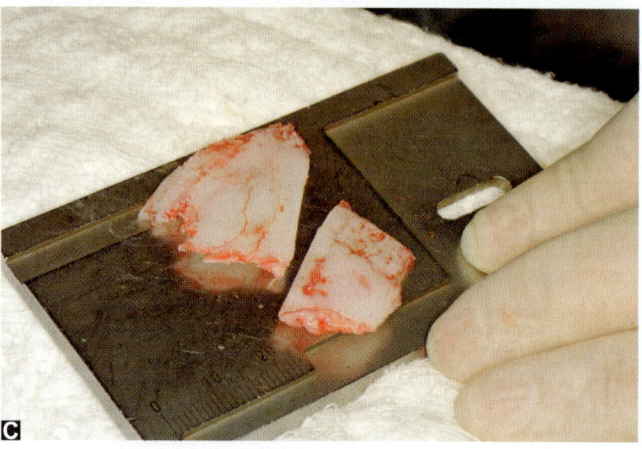

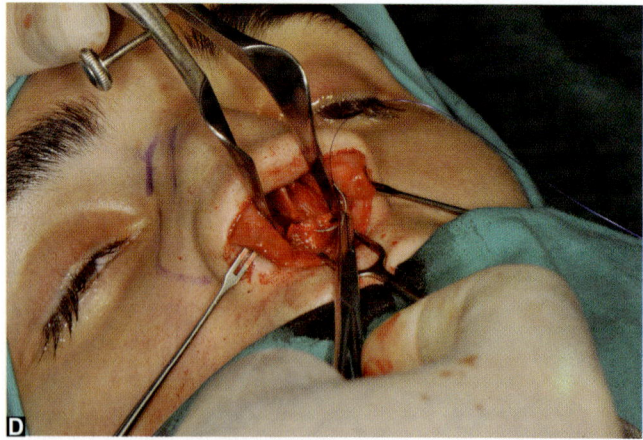

Figs 15.6B to D

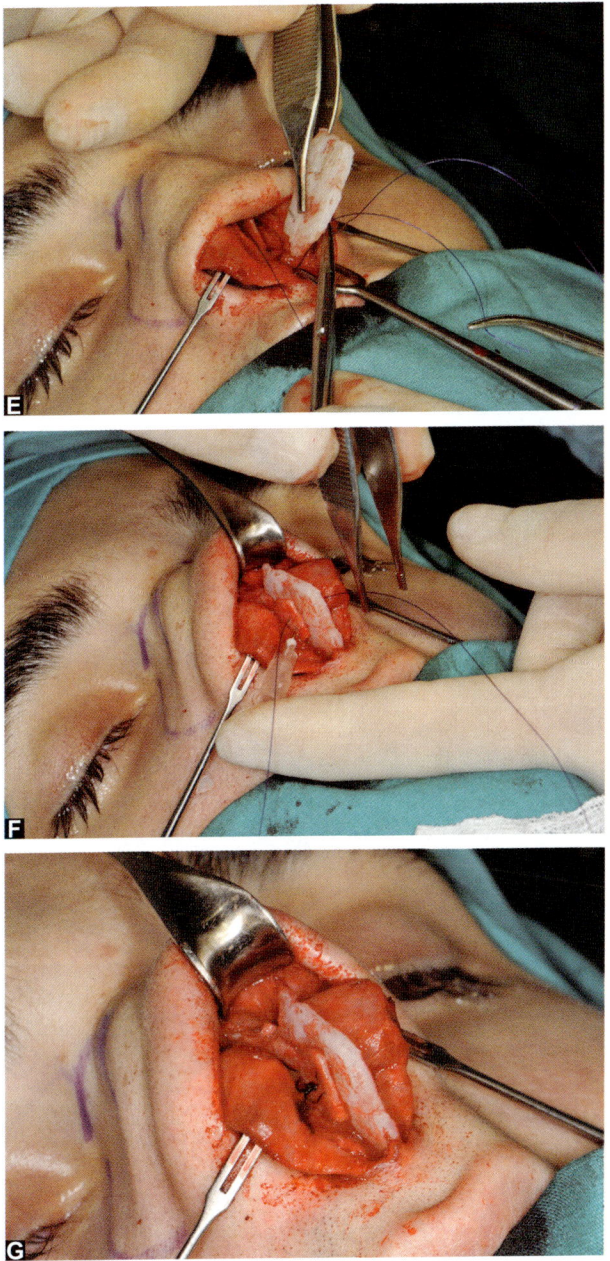

Figs 15.6E to G

Figs 15.6A to G: (A) Caudal septal replacement graft is sutured to the anterior nasal spine and to the dorsal segment; (B) Two vertical fractures can be seen on the caudal segment; (C) Two big pieces of straight cartilage could be harvested in this case; (D) The first suture is passed from the anterior nasal spine; (E) The second suture is put to the postero-inferior part of the graft; (F) It is connected to the dorsal segment by using a small needle for stabilization; (G) Multiple 4-0 PDS sutures are used for fixation

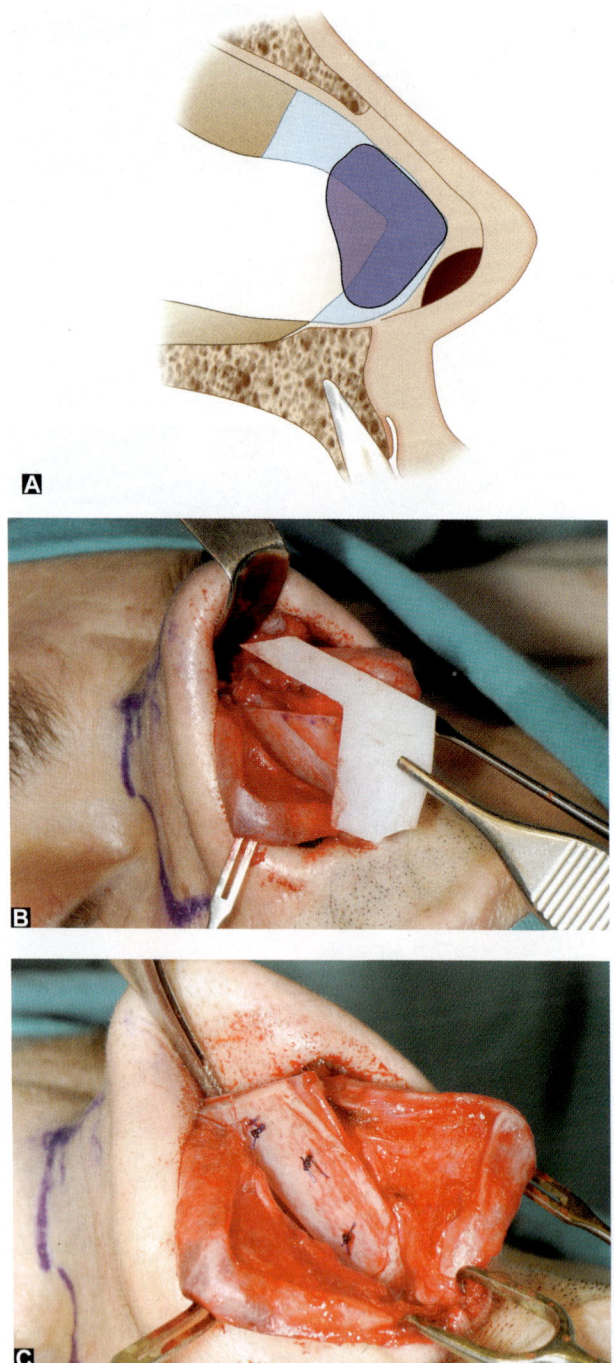

Figs 15.7A to C: (A) L-strut graft is used when both the dorsal and caudal segments are crooked and after the cross-hatching of these segments; (B) It can be carved from septal cartilage according to the need; (C) It is fixed to dorsal and caudal segments by using multiple PDS sutures

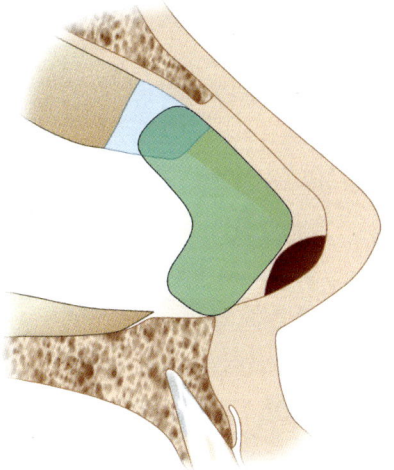

A

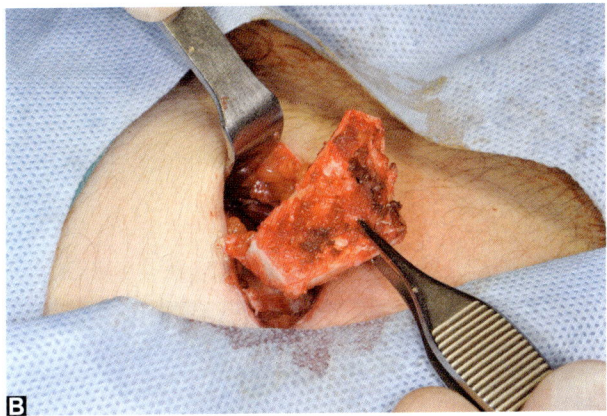

B

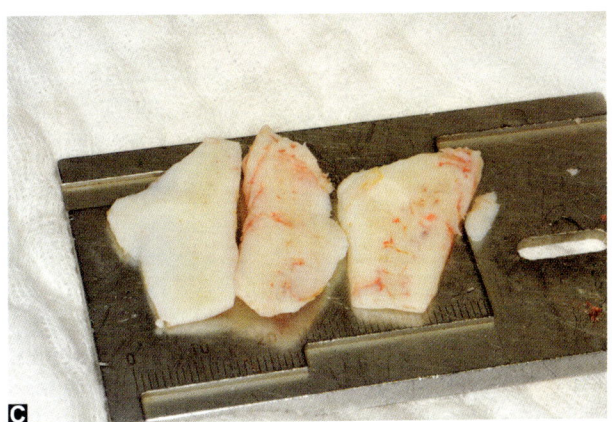

C

Figs 15.8A to C

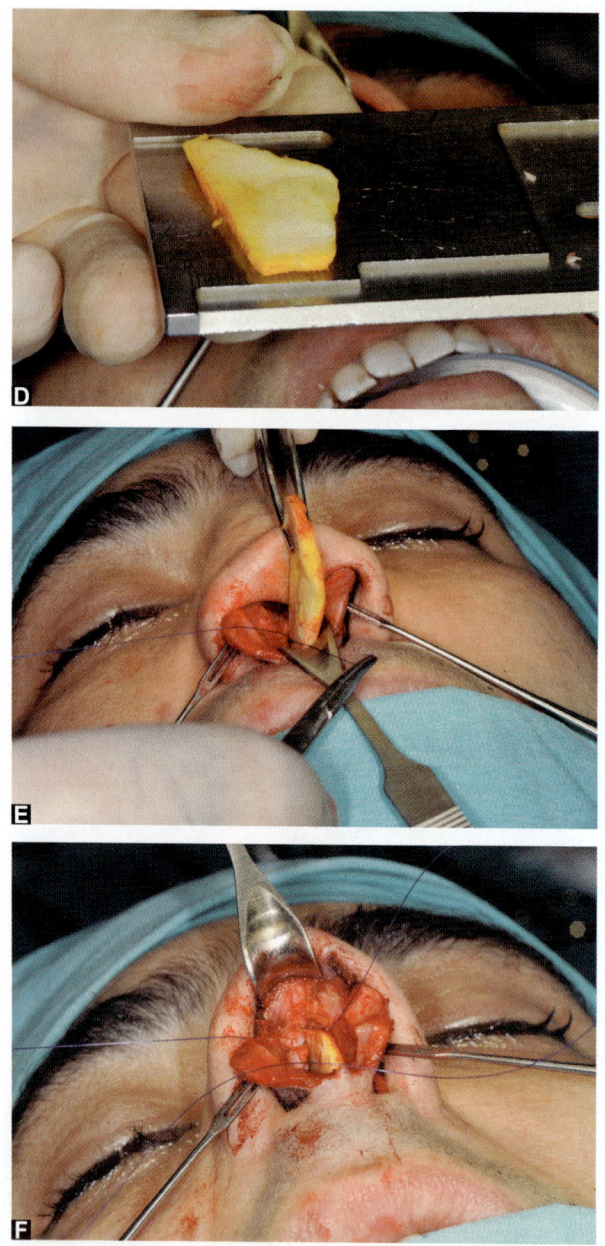

Figs 15.8D to F

Figs 15.8A to F: (A) This drawing illustrates subtotal reconstruction of the nasal septum by using a one piece graft, if possible from the septal cartilage, otherwise from conchal or costal cartilage; (B) In my opinion, the sixth rib is more suitable for one piece reconstruction of the nasal septum when there is no septal cartilage available; (C) The middle third of the sixth rib is sculptured carefully; (D) It is soaked at least for half an hour into a mixture of saline and IV antibiotic; (E) It is first fixed to the anterior nasal spine by PDS sutures; (F) Then it is sutured to the remaining cartilage at the key area

b. Two-piece L-strut: If a big piece in the shape of an L-strut cannot be obtained, two different pieces can be used to replace dorsal and caudal segment. The dorsal segment is first fixed to the key area by 4-0 PDS sutures, then the caudal segment is fixed on the anterior nasal spine either by opening a groove on it or by using multiple PDS sutures. Then these two pieces can be sutured on each other to form an L-strut[16] (Fig. 15.9). The power of this technique lies in its versatility to change rotation and projection. In revision cases where there is no septal cartilage available, grafts obtained from costal cartilages can be used. Within the last 2 years, I started using a very versatile technique called "split technique" to obtain grafts of different sizes and thickness from the costal cartilages (Figs 15.10A to C). This original technique, described by Tastan, has been used by the author for 4 years with successful results.[17] In this technique, the costal cartilage is cut oblique to the logitudinal axis. By doing so, the implants include an intact outer and inner cortex which in theory could resist the forces causing warping. A short-term follow-up of 2 years showed no warping or significant warping in a limited number of my patients.

c. Multiple pieces: In severely traumatic noses, multiple fractures can prevent us to obtain one-piece or two-piece L-strut. In this situation, the cartilaginous and bony septum is removed, cut from the fractured lines, straightened, and sutured to each other.[18] These fragments can be sutured on an ethmoid lamina or more recently on a perforated PDS sheet as a straightening scaffold.[19] This big piece can then be reinserted between the mucoperichondrial flaps and fixed on to the key area and anterior nasal spine. I used to use this technique in the past, but I use it very rarely now, because the abovementioned techniques are usually sufficient to solve most of the problems.

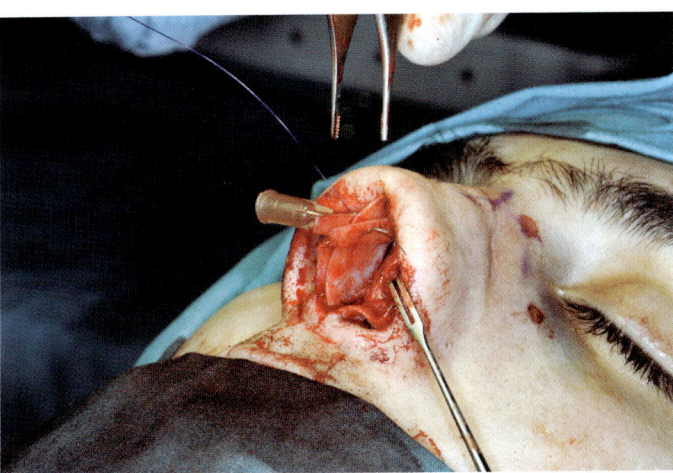

Fig. 15.9: The combination of two spreader grafts and a caudal septal replacement graft is a very powerful and versatile procedure. It is possible to adjust the rotation and projection at the same time by this technique

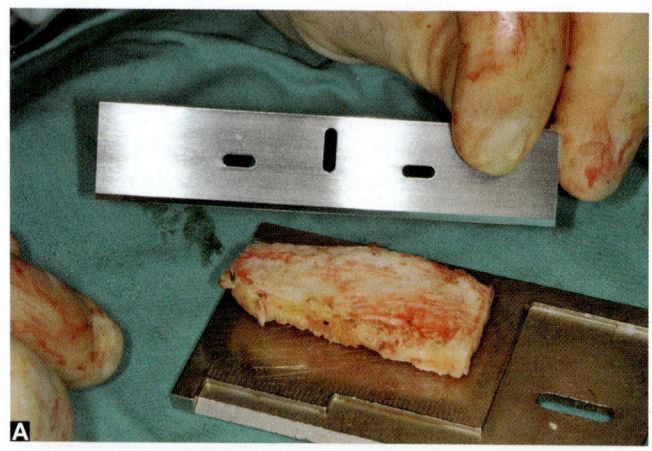

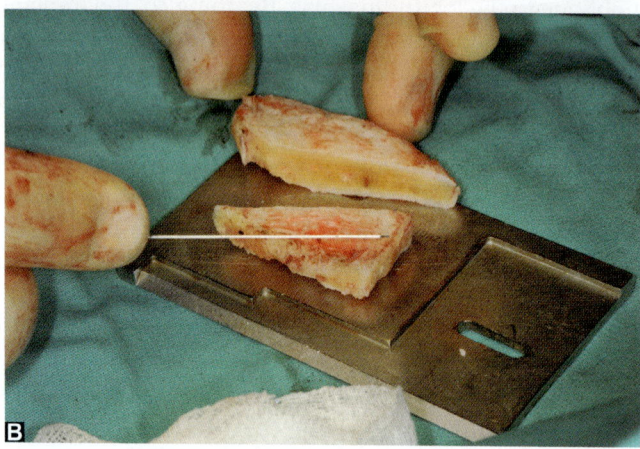

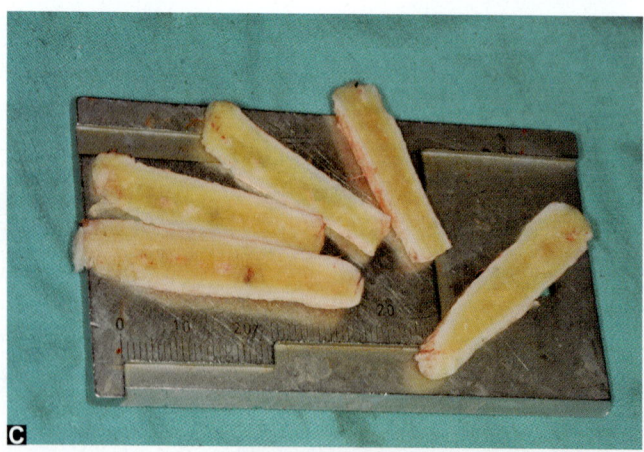

Figs 15.10A to C: (A) The eighth rib is used for the split technique; (B) The blade of a dermatome or microtome helps to make precise cuts obliquely; (C) Slices of different thickness and lengths can be obtained by this technique

II. Turbinate Surgery

In functional rhinoplasty, the inferior and the middle turbinates should be thoroughly examined. Anterior rhinoscopy is usually adequate for diagnosis in most of the cases when there is no septal deviation or mucosal swelling. Unfortunately, severely deviated septum prevents us to obtain a good view on the turbinates. Therefore, a reevaluation of the nasal passages should also be done during the operation. I would like to share some of my observations on the turbinates:

1. One-sided septal deviation very often causes contralateral inferior turbinate hypertrophy.
2. In C-type crooked noses, concha bullosa preventing the straightening of nasal septum is observed not infrequently.
3. In some cases, the tail of the inferior turbinate can be blocking the whole choana. Therefore, the posterior tail should also be evaluated as well. This is more often seen on the non-deviated side. Interestingly, in cases with one-sided severe septal deviation, the portion rear to the deviation can be hypertrophied as well.

A. Management of the Inferior Turbinate

There are many techniques used in the management of inferior turbinate hypertrophy:

1. Electrocautery
2. Radiofrequency ablation
3. Laser-assisted resection or ablation
4. Lateralization
5. Submucous resection
6. Turbinoplasty
7. Turbinectomy

1. *Electrocautery*: This technique can be applied both extramucosally or submucosally. Both techniques are more rarely used today. This is a fast and inexpensive method. It can be done during nasal surgery by using the electrocautery instrumentation ready on the operating table. Specially designed cautery tips can also be used, especially for submucosal applications. Submucosal application creates less complications such as crusting and synechia than extramucosal applications.
2. *Radiofrequency ablation*: This is a widely used mucosal-sparing method. It is easily applied under local anesthesia as an office procedure with some minor complications.[20,21] The needle probe is inserted into the turbinate in one or usually more points. The power and duration of the energy can be regulated in accordance with the experience of the surgeon with that particular gadget. If the inferior turbinate is decongested and smaller in size, balooning it with diluted local anesthetic usually facilitates application and prevents direct thermal exposure on the bone.
3. *Laser-assisted resection or ablation*: The most common lasers in use are the carbon dioxide and neodymium:yttrium-aluminum garnet.[22] This

was a popular application about a decade ago. It is currently more rarely used due to lower cost-effectiveness.

4. *Lateralization*: This is an often neglected technique which proved to be very beneficial in selected cases. An elevator can be used to lateralize the inferior turbinate to open the airway. It is possible to see the change in airway during surgery which usually stays.[23]

5. *Submucous resection*: In this technique, the entire inferior turbinate is injected with 1:1 diluted lidocaine and 1:100,000 adrenalin for additional anesthesia, hemostasis and hydraulic dissection. The anterior head of the inferior turbinate is vertically cut by no:11 blade. Mucosa is detached from the bony inferior turbinate on both lateral and medial aspects by using a Freer elevator. Then the hypertrophied turbinate bone is removed at the anterior portion or entirely.[24]

Another option is to use a microdebrider in debulking the submucosal soft tissue and/or bone.[25] Great attention should be reserved to prevent perforations of the mucosal flap. This is an elegant, but aggressive and expensive method. There is also a need for nasal packing.

6. *Turbinoplasty*: Apart from SMR, only the medial part of the mucosa is detached from the underlying bony part. By using a Heyman scissors, one full thickness horizontal cut throughout the inferior turbinate is done on the mucosa. Then, a similar second horizontal cut is done close to the connection point of the inferior turbinate preserving the medial mucosa and resecting the lateral side of the mucosa together with the bony turbinate and this composite piece is removed. The remaining medial mucosa is turned laterally to cover the remaining bony part of the turbinate. The nose is packed for 2–3 days.[26]

7. *Turbinectomy*: This technique involves partial or total removal of the enlarged inferior turbinate. This technique should be limited to cases with bony hypertrophy and tail hypertrophy blocking the whole choana.[24] It needs packing and crusting is a major problem during postoperative period. As microdebrider has become more favorable in reducing the bony hypertrophy with less postoperative discomfort, the use of this technique has become more limited in recent years. Besides, there are reports claiming that total or aggressive turbinectomy can lead to empty nose syndrome.[27]

In recent years, there is a trend of mucosal sparing techniques such as microdebrider-assisted inferior turbinoplasty and radiofrequency ablation.[28] Passali et al. reported the results of a 6-year randomized clinical study comparing turbinectomy, laser cautery, electrocautery, cryotherapy, SMR, and SMR with outfracture. They concluded that only SMR had given more physiologic results in terms of nasal patency, mucociliary clearance and local secretory IgA production.[29]

B. Management of the Middle Turbinate

When there is a concha bullosa, the most preferred technique is to remove the lateral lamella of it under endoscopic guidance.[30] An alternative method in selected cases can be reducing the volume by crushing it from sides by a long and large Takahashi forceps.[31]

III. Internal Valve

The internal valve area is surrounded by the caudal septum, caudal end of the upper lateral cartilages (ULCs), head of the inferior turbinate and the remaining tissues surrounding the pyriform aperture.[32]

The obstruction of the internal nasal valve can be due to mucocutaneous (swelling, adhesion, stricture), septal (deviation) and ULC (deflection, thickening) pathologies.[1]

Management of the Internal Nasal Valve

1. Spreader graft, flap

Spreader grafts are usually used to reconstruct the dorsal nasal roof, and restore the internal valves especially during reduction rhinoplasty.[33] These grafts should be carved from the septal cartilage when possible, but in case of shortage, conchal cartilage and costal cartilage can be used as well. They should be 20–25 mm in length, 3–4 mm in height and 2–3 mm in thickness.[33]

A viable alternative to the spreader grafts, spreader flaps, has been reported with successful results in certain cases.[34,35] In patients with a prominent hump, after the ULCs are separated from their junction with the septum and the bony-cartilaginous hump is removed, the ULCs are freed from the underlying mucoperichondrium, the surplus medial portion of the ULCs are folded inward and sutured to the lateral portion. The medial edges are then sutured to the dorsal edge of the nasal septum. This folding acts as a spreader and also widens the internal nasal valve (Figs 15.11A to C).

2. Upper lateral splay graft

Upper lateral splay graft is described to be used to obtain the natural "T" of the upper lateral and septal cartilages.[36] This graft is inserted in a pocket created just under the caudal half of the ULCs. The use of the conchal

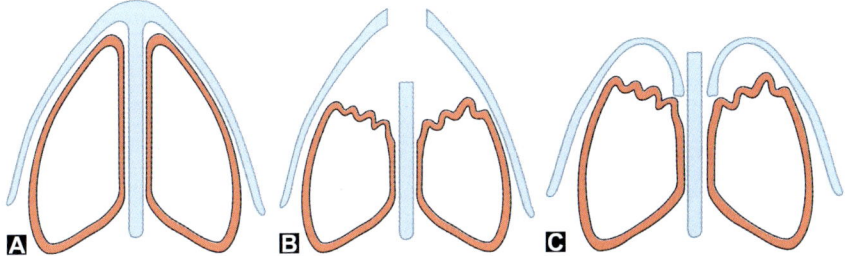

Figs 15.11A to C: (A) Cross-section of the nose at the middle vault; (B) The hump belonging to the dorsal segment is resected, but the upper lateral cartilages (ULCs) are saved; (C) ULCs are turned in, sutured on themselves and then to the septal cartilage as spreader flaps

cartilage is more desirable beacuse of its shape and its spring effect which can provide the necessary splay action.

3. Butterfly graft

Clark and Cook reported on the use of the ascending portion of the conchal bowl on the caudal half of the upper lateral cartilages to widen the internal nasal valve.[37] This graft is placed through either a closed or open approach. It is placed symmetrically over the nasal dorsum while the central "V-shaped" portion pointing caudally (Figs 15.12A to C). The only drawback of this graft is the additional supratip bulk from the profile and widened appearance from the frontal view.

4. Flaring sutures

Flaring sutures have been reported by Park to widen the nasal valve angle.[38] After a 4-0 PDS mattress suture placement from the caudal/lateral border of one ULC, across the nasal dorsum, and through the contralateral ULC, its tightening pulls the ULCs laterally opening the nasal valve angle. It has also been shown that these sutures could be more effective with the use of speader grafts.[39]

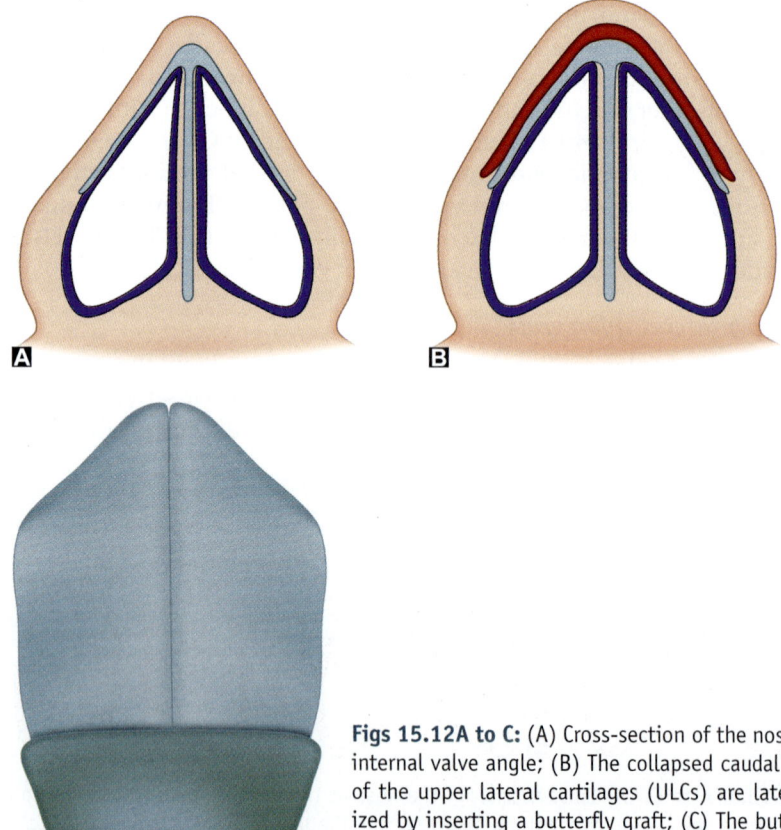

Figs 15.12A to C: (A) Cross-section of the nose at internal valve angle; (B) The collapsed caudal end of the upper lateral cartilages (ULCs) are lateralized by inserting a butterfly graft; (C) The butterfly graft is seen from above which is placed to the lower one-third of the ULCs

5. M-plasty

After the intercartilaginous incision, the caudal aspect of the ULC is freed from skin dorsally and from mucosa ventrally. A 2–3 mm of the caudal end of the ULC is resected horizontally, and then an additional medial triangle of the ULC can be removed submucosally after detaching from the septum. After the excess mucosa is trimmed, the incision is closed leaving an "M-shape" or linear line[32] (Figs 15.13A to I).

6. Suspension sutures

Suspension sutures are used to widen the nasal angle by suspending the caudal/lateral border of the ULC to a fixed point on the ipsilateral, medial infraorbital rim. It usually requires a small external incision above the point of fixation or can be done via a transconjunctival approach.[40-42]

IV. External Valve

The external valve is from the nasal entrance to the internal valve and it is the alar rim composed of lower lateral cartilages and nasal floor.[43]

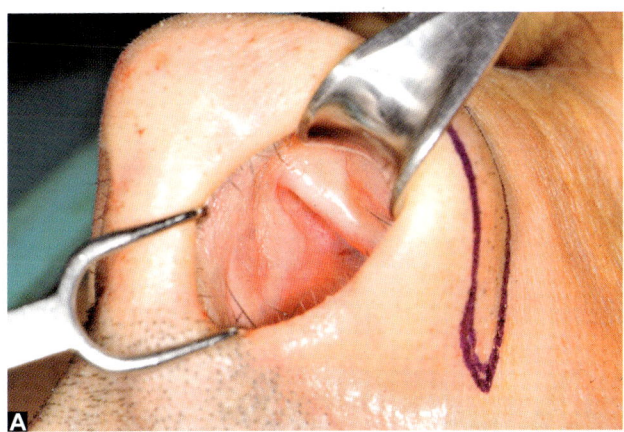

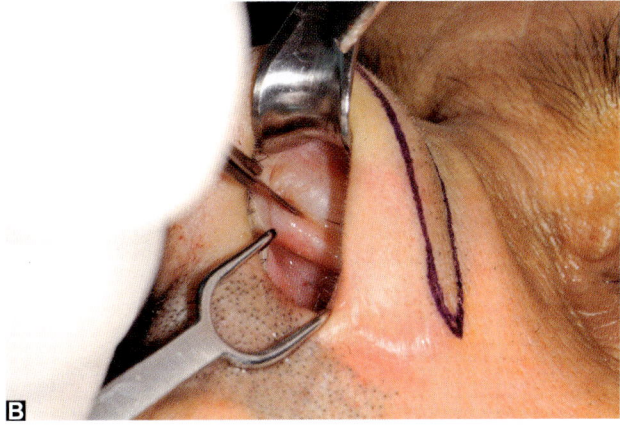

Figs 15.13A and B

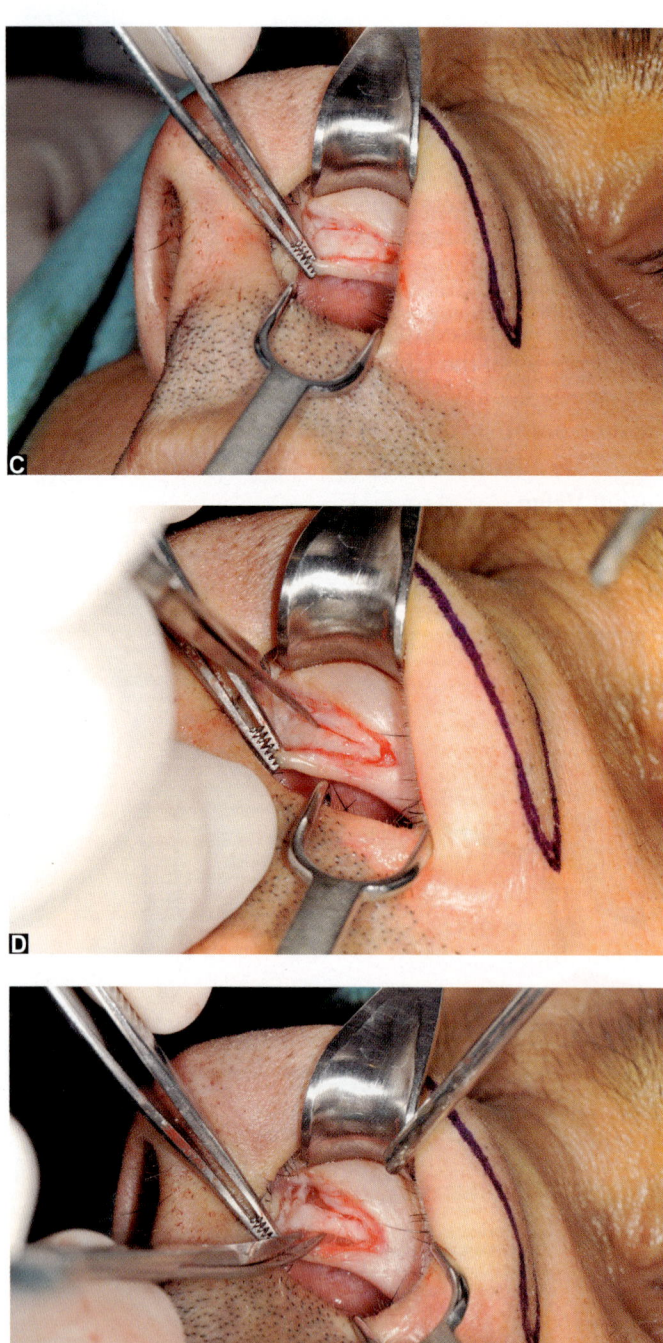

Figs 15.13C to E

Recent Advances in Otolaryngology – Head and Neck Surgery

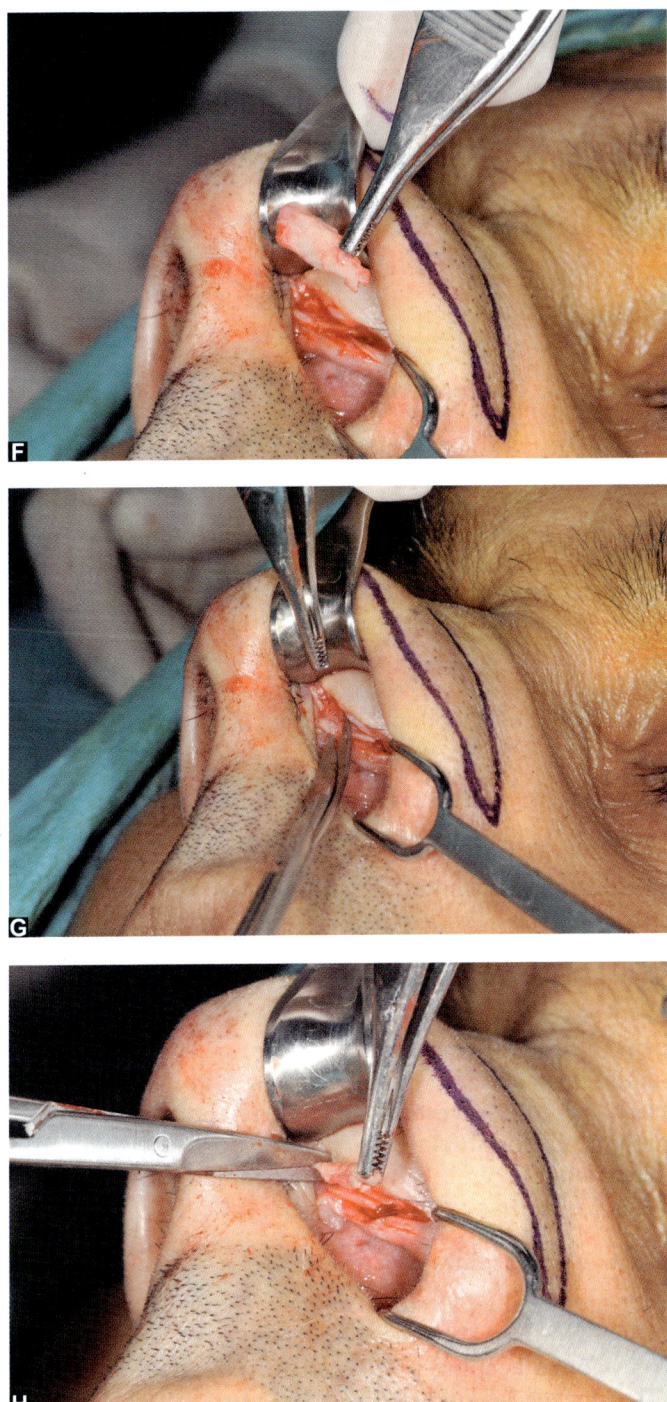

Figs 15.13F to H

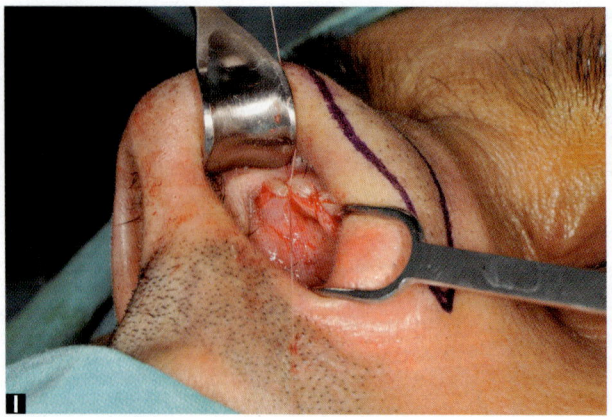

Fig. 15.13I

Figs 15.13A to I: Modified M-plasty. (A) The internal valve angle is narrow; (B) After local anesthetic injection, an intercartilaginous incision is performed; (C) The caudal portion of the ULC is exposed; (D to F) A 2–3 mm of cartilage strip is cut, detached from the underlying mucosa and then resected; (G) An additional triangle of cartilage is removed from the caudo-medial portion; (H) The surplus of mucosa is trimmed; (I) The incision is closed

Collapsing alar sidewalls, narrowed alar base and/or narrower nostrils can be the causes of obstruction at the level of the external nasal valve.[43]

Management of the External Valve Problems

1. Lateral crural dissection and repositioning

This method can be applied in two different ways.[44] The lateral crura can be inwardly concave with a pinched appearance. In this case, they are dissected free from the surrounding soft tissues, cut just lateral to the dome, reversed and sutured back to its bed again. Therefore, the concavity turns out to be a convexity (Figs 15.14A and B). A modification of this technique is to suture the resected lateral crura contralaterally.

In a situation where the lateral crura are cephalically oriented, they can be freed from the investing soft tissues and can be repositioned in more anatomically desirable beds.[44] The detached lateral crura can be supported by lateral crural strut grafts to guarantee a support and a better shape[45] (Figs 15.15A to C).

2. Lateral crural strut grafts

These grafts are usually placed via an open rhinoplasty approach. After a cephalic trim of the lateral crura is performed, the vestibular skin is undermined from above keeping it adhered to the lateral crus at the caudal border. The pocket is extended over the pyriform aperture. The linear axis of the pocket should be designed for maximum support of the lateral crura (Figs 15.16A and B). These grafts are usually obtained from the nasal septum, 3–4 mm in width and 15–25 mm in length. They are placed into

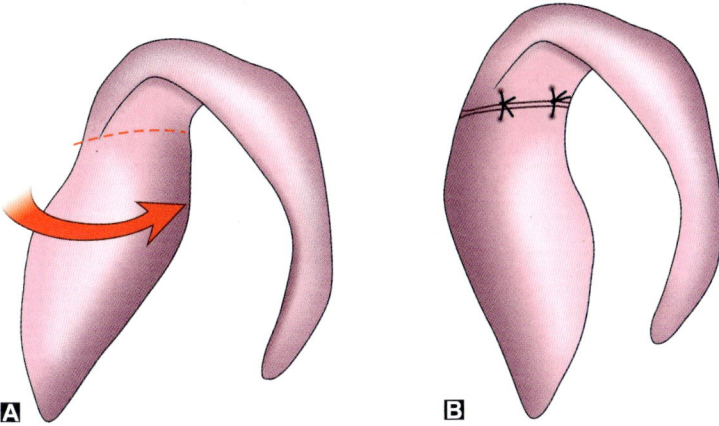

Figs 15.14A and B: (A) The lateral crus can be concave as a variant; (B) In order to open the external valve and obtain a more natural tip shape, the lateral crus can be dissected free of the underlying skin, divided vertically near the dome, flipped over and sutured to its bed again

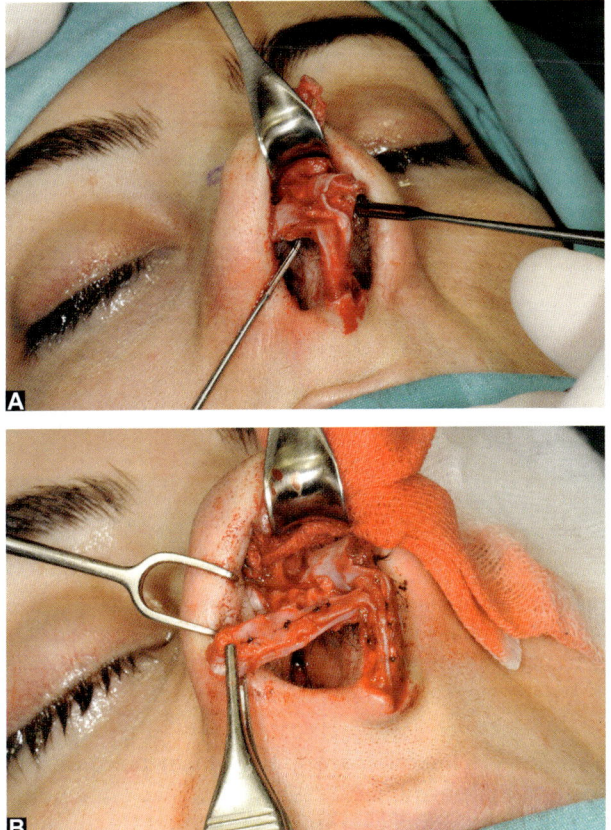

Figs 15.15A and B

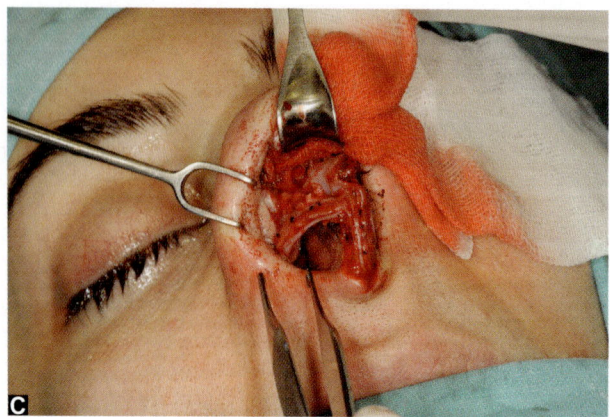

Fig. 15.15C

Figs 15.15A to C: (A) The cephalically oriented and buckled weak lateral crura are exposed; (B) Detached from the underlying soft tissues and supported by lateral crural strut grafts; (C) Then they are inserted in new pockets which enables them to turn to the direction of the lateral canthi

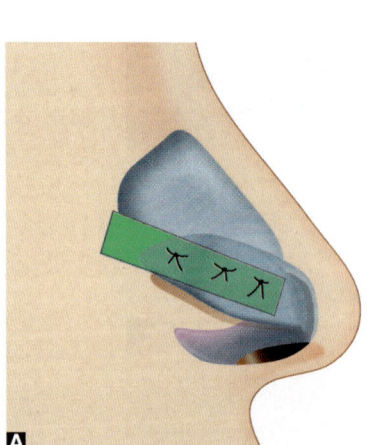

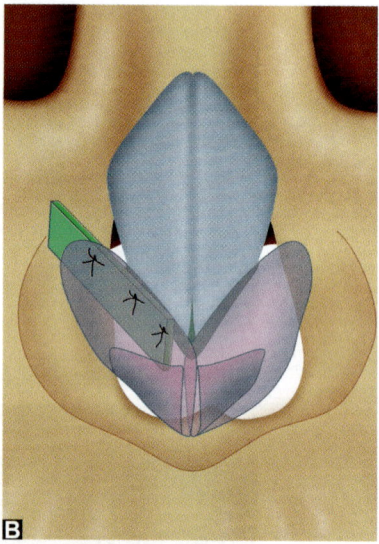

Figs 15.16A and B: Lateral crural strut grafts are very powerful grafts to support the lateral crura from the ventral surface. They have been shown to work well in cases of the boxy nasal tip, malpositioned lateral crura, alar rim retraction, alar rim collapse, and concave lateral crura

the pockets under the lateral crura and fixed in place by PDS mattress sutures. In case of malpositioned lateral crura, alar retraction, and severe cases of alar collapse, a longer strut going beyond the pyriform aperture is indicated. Gunter reported to use them for reshaping, repositioning, or reconstructing the lateral crura.[45]

3. Alar battens

Alar batten grafts are curvilinear cartilage grafts that are placed into a precise pocket at the point of maximal lateral wall collapse or supra-alar pinching.[46] The use of alar battens has been reported for the correction of both internal and external nasal valve collapse[47] (Figs 15.17A and B). These grafts can be obtained from the nasal septum, conchal cartilage and sometimes from the costal cartilage as well. They were described as 10–15 mm in length and 4–8 mm in width. It was also noted that larger grafts could be used in patients with severe collapse or thicker skin. My preference is usually to use larger grafts placed in a tight pocket whose tail usually exceeds the pyriform aperture. Regardless of the approach, I also prefer suturing them to the lateral crura for fixation. When these grafts are used for external valve which is usually the case in many occasions, they are usually placed on and under the lateral half or two thirds of the lateral crura. Porous polyethylene implants have been used as alar battens,[48] but sometimes with a rather high extrusion rate.[49]

4. Lateral crural turn-in flap

Tellioglu and Cimen used turn-in folding of the cephalic portion of the lateral crus to support the alar rim. They have operated 32 patients with this flap and followed them for a year. Four of these patients have undergone surgery for the treatment of a collapsed alar rim, and five more as a supportive measure against thick and sebaceous skin. Satisfactory results

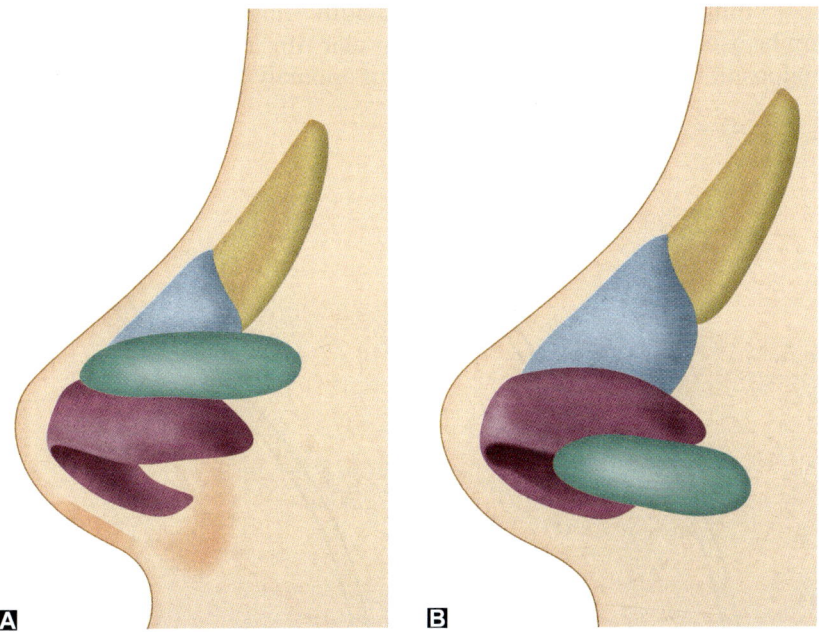

Figs 15.17A and B: (A) Alar batten grafts are curvilinear cartilage grafts that are placed into a precise pocket at the point of maximal lateral wall collapse or supra-alar pinching to correct both internal; (B) External nasal valve collapse

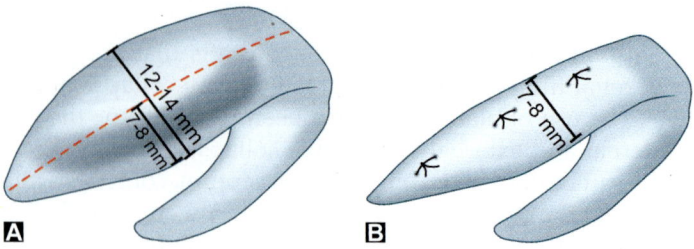

Figs 15.18A and B: Lateral crural turn-in flap is another method to reinforce the weak and deformed lateral crura. The cephalically trimmed piece of cartilage is folded inward to create a double layer of cartilage like a sandwich and sutured

have been obtained in all cases.[50] Murakami et al. have also reported the same technique to reinforce the alar cartilage after cephalic trimming.[51]

I did two modifications in this technique: (1) Instead of cutting and turning-in the medial two-thirds of the lateral crura, a partial linear cut was done along the horizontal axis of the lateral crus leaving a 7-mm caudal segment (Figs 15.18A and B); (2) The scroll area was not disturbed, i. e., the caudal part of the ULC stayed attached to the cephalic lateral half of the lateral crus (Figs 15.19A to C).

5. Alar rim grafts

Alar rim grafts are thin, soft cartilage grafts that measure approximately 12–15 mm in length and 2–3 mm in width[52] (Figs 15.20A and B). They can be used to support and/or contour alar rims namely in lateral crural malposition, alar retraction, alar contour anomaly and alar collapse.[53]

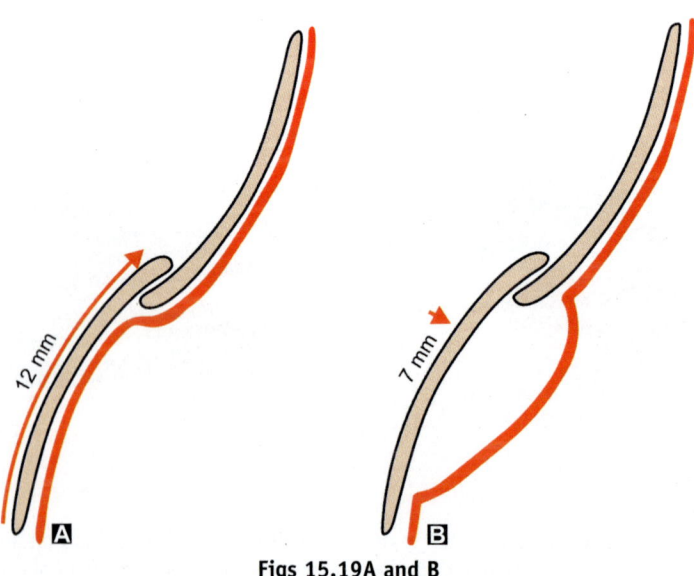

Figs 15.19A and B

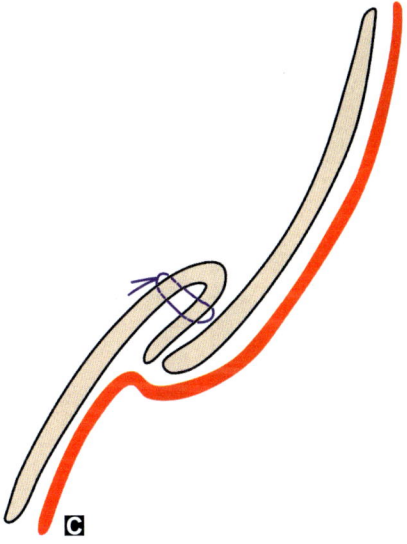

Figs 15.19C

Figs 15.19A to C: This sagittal slice shows the scroll area. While turning the partially cut lateral crus inward, the scroll is not disturbed, and the suture fixation prevents the collapse of the caudal part of the ULC

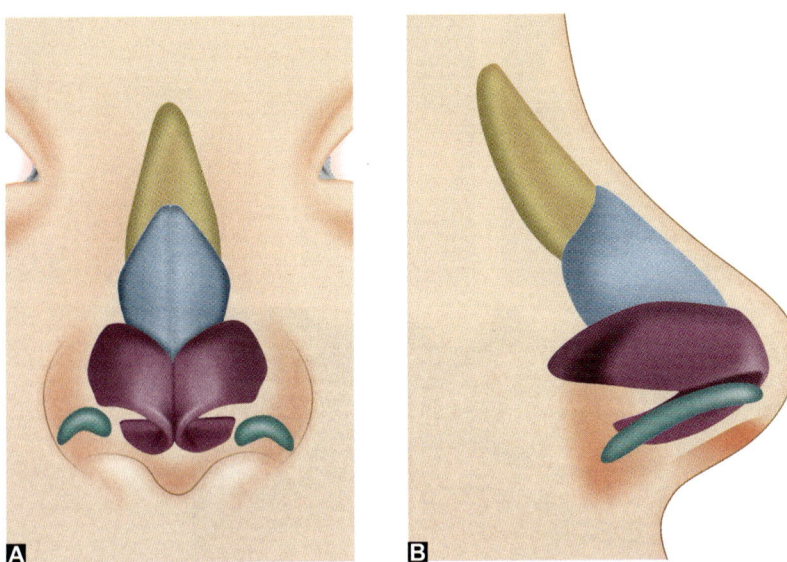

Figs 15.20A and B: Alar rim grafts can be used to support and/or contour alar rims in cases of lateral crural malposition, alar retraction, alar contour anomaly and alar collapse

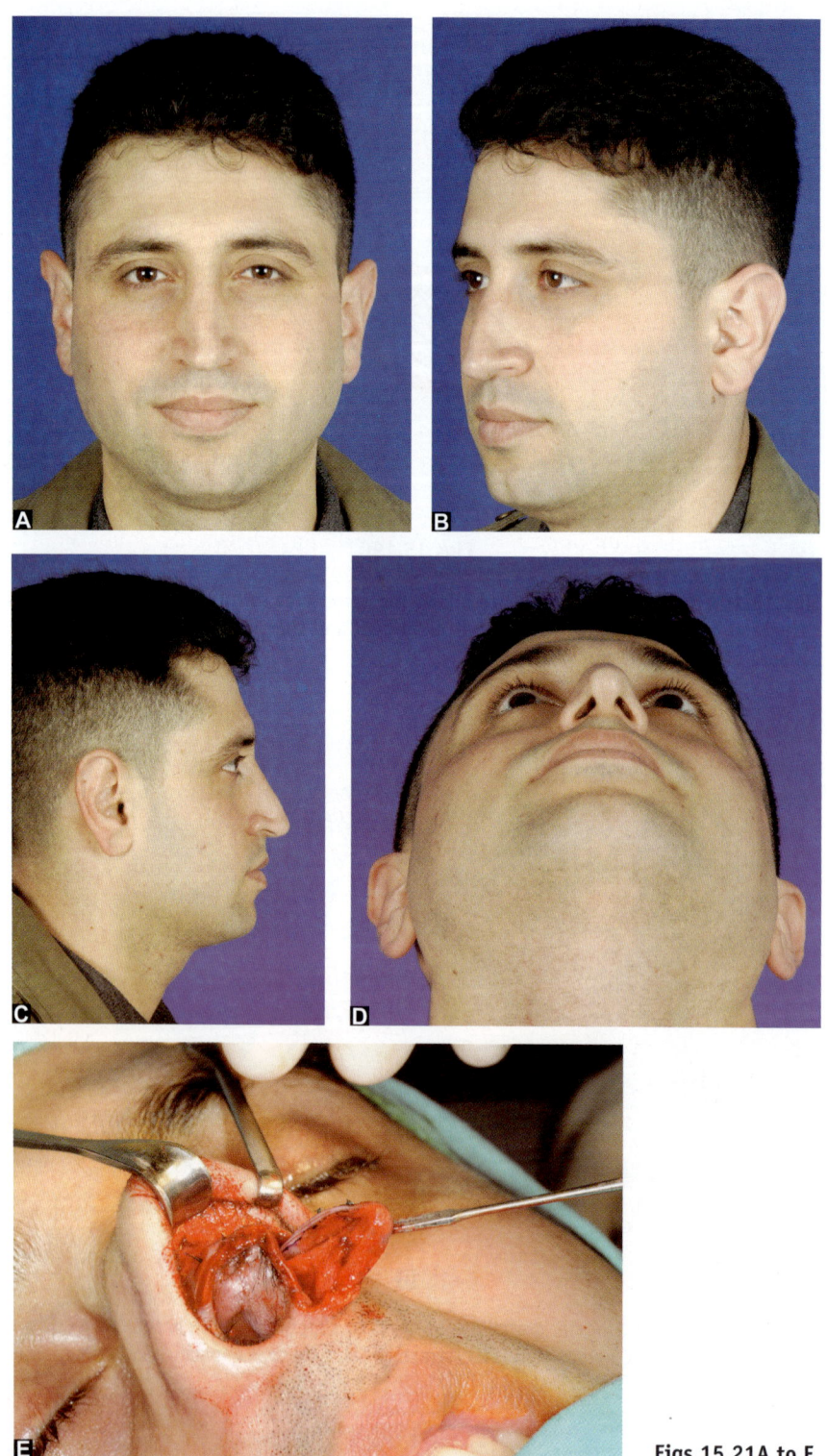

Figs 15.21A to E

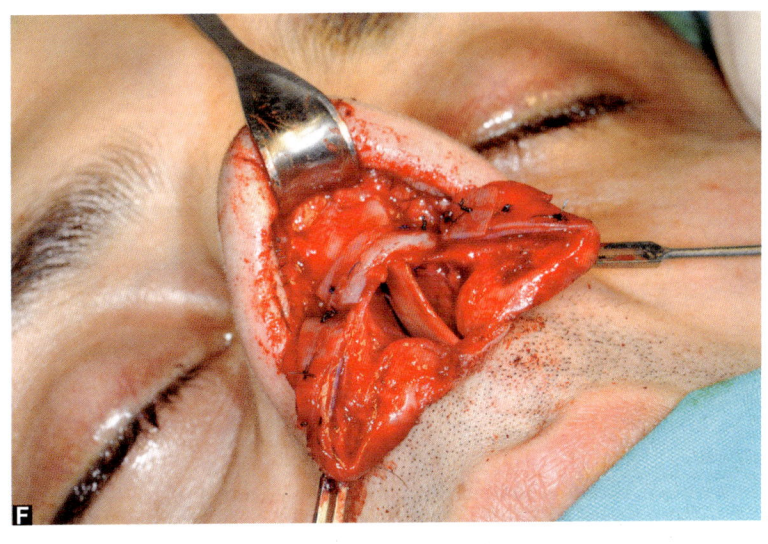

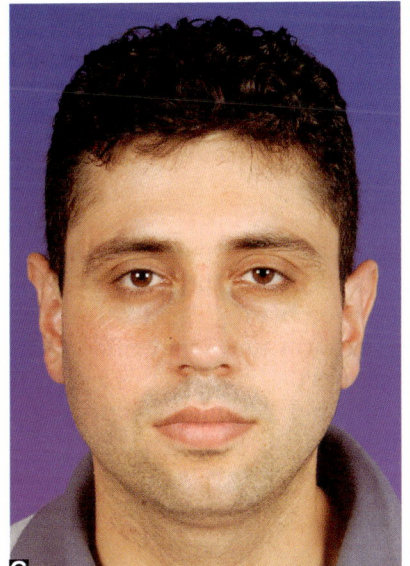

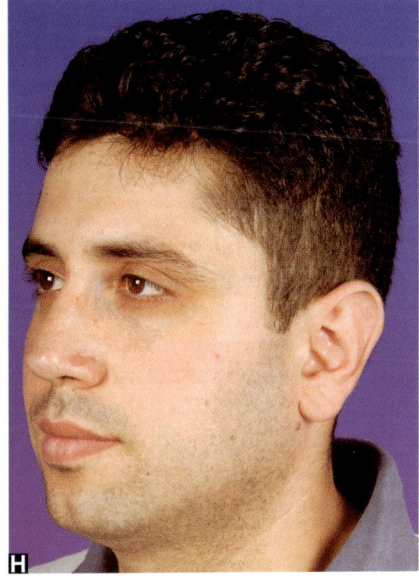

Figs 15.21F to H

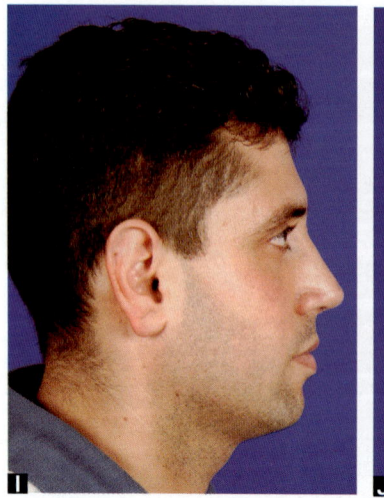
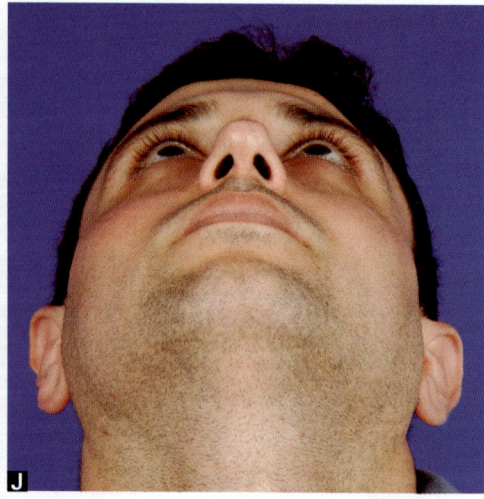

Figs 15.21I and J

Figs 15.21A to J: A 31-year-old male with nasal obstruction due to external and internal valve narrowing. In this particular case, butterfly graft, lateral crural turn-in flaps, alar battens, and alar rim grafts are all used. The patient is seen 1 year after surgery. He can breath better through his nose and he is also satisfied with the aesthetic outcome as well

CONCLUSION

The main focus on rhinoplasty should aim on adressing the four valves by using the techniques described above. In daily routine, the majority of the patients usually need a combination of these techniques (Figs 15.21 A to J). Therefore, a surgeon who is willing to perform functional rhinoplasty should have a wide spectrum of the techniques described in this article. It should not be forgotten that the main criteria in choosing the appropriate technique is the surgeon's own experience.

ACKNOWLEDGMENTS

No financial support has been taken from any institution. I would like to thank Yeliz Tuna, the medical photographer, and Merve Ulug, the medical illustrator, for their help.

REFERENCES

1. Kasperbauer JL, Kern EB. Nasal valve physiology. Implications in nasal surgery. Otolaryngol Clin North Am. 1987;20:699-719.
2. Guyuron B, Uzzo CD, Scull H. A practical classification of septonasal deviation and an effective guide to septal surgery. Plast Reconstr Surg. 1999;104:2202-9.
3. Mladina R, Cujić E, Subarić M, et al. Nasal septal deformities in ear, nose, and throat patients: an international study. Am J Otolaryngol. 2008;29:75-82.

4. Killian G. The submucous window resection of the nasal septum. Ann Otol Rhinol Laryngol. 1905;14:363-93.
5. Tzadik A, Gilbert SE, Sade J. Complications of submucous resections of the nasal septum. Arch Otorhinolaryngol. 1988;245:74-6.
6. Cottle MH, Loring RM, Fischer GC, et al. The 'maxilla-premaxilla' approach to extensive nasal septum surgery. Arch. Otolaryngol. 1958;68:301-13.
7. Giles WC, Gross CW, Abram AC, et al. Endoscopic septoplasty. Laryngoscope. 1994;104:1507-9.
8. Raynor EM. Powered Endoscopic Septoplasty for Septal Deviation and Isolated Spurs. Arch Facial Plast Surg. 2005;7:410-2.
9. Porter JP, Toriumi DM. Surgical techniques for management of the crooked nose. Aesthetic Plast Surg. 2002;26:18-31.
10. Wright WK. Principles of nasal septum reconstruction. Trans Am Acad Opthalmol Otolaryngol. 1969;73:252-5.
11. Pastorek NJ, Becker DG. Treating the Caudal Septal Deflection. Arch Facial Plast Surg. 2000;2:217-20.
12. Toriumi DM. Structural approach to primary rhinoplasty. Aesthet Surg J. 2002;22:72-84.
13. Foda HM. The caudal septum replacement graft. Arch Facial Plast Surg. 2008;10:152-7.
14. Toriumi DM. Subtotal reconstruction of the nasal septum: a preliminary report. Laryngoscope. 1994;104:906-13.
15. Rettinger G. Reconstruction of the pronounced saddle nose. Laryngorhinootologie. 1997;76:672-5.
16. Dyer WK 2nd, Yune ME. Structural grafting in rhinoplasty. Facial Plast Surg. 1997;13:269-77.
17. Tastan E. Presented at the 33th Annual Meeting of the European Academy of Facial Plastic Surgery, Antalya–Turkey, 1-4 September 2010.
18. Gubisch W. Extracorporeal Septoplasty for the Markedly Deviated Septum. Arch Facial Plast Surg. 2005;7:218-26.
19. Boenisch M, Nolst-Trenité GJ. Reconstruction of the Nasal Septum Using Polydioxanone Plate. Arch Facial Plast Surg. 2010;12:4-10.
20. Nease CJ, Krempl GA. Radiofrequency treatment of turbinate hypertrophy: a randomized, blinded, placebo-controlled clinical trial. Otolaryngol Head Neck Surg. 2004;130:291-9.
21. Back LJ, Liukko T, Sinkkonen ST, et al. Complication rates of radiofrequency surgery in the upper airways: a single institution experience. Acta Otolaryngol. 2009;19:1–5.
22. Janda P, Sroka R, Baumgartner R, et al. Laser treatment of hyperplastic inferior nasal turbinates: a review. Lasers Surg Med. 2001;28:404-13.
23. Buyuklu F, Cakmak O, Hizal E, et al. Outfracture of the inferior turbinate: a computed tomography study. Plast Reconstr Surg 2009 [Epub ahead of print].
24. Saunders WH. Surgery of the inferior nasal turbinates. Ann Otol Rhinol Laryngol. 1982;91:445-7.
25. Friedman M, Tanyeri H, Lim J, et al. A safe, alternative technique for inferior turbinate reduction. Laryngoscope. 1999;109:1834-7.

26. Mabry RL. Inferior turbinoplasty: Patient selection, technique, and long-term consequences. Otolaryngol Head Neck Surg. 1988;98:60-4.
27. Chhabra N, Houser SM. The diagnosis and management of empty nose syndrome. Otolaryngol Clin North Am. 2009;42:311-30.
28. Bhandarkar ND, Smith TL. Outcomes of surgery for inferior turbinate hypertrophy. Current Opinion in Otolaryngology and Head and Neck Surgery. 2010;18:49-53.
29. Passàli D, Passàli FM, Damiani V, et al. Treatment of inferior turbinate hypertrophy: a randomized clinical trial. Ann Otol Rhinol Laryngol. 2003;112:683-8.
30. Stammberger H. Functional Endoscopic Sinus Surgery. Philadelphia, PA: BC Decker; 1991. pp. 161-9.
31. Doğru H, Tüz M, Uygur K, et al. A new turbinoplasty technique for the management of concha bullosa: our short-term outcomes. Laryngoscope. 2001;111:172-4.
32. Kasperbauer JL, Kern EB. Nasal valve physiology. Implications in nasal surgery. Otolaryngol Clin North Am. 1987;20:699-719.
33. Sheen JH. Spreader graft: a method of reconstructing the roof of the middle nasal vault following rhinoplasty. Plast Reconstr Surg. 1984;73:230-9.
34. Byrd HS, Meade RA, Gonyon DL. Using the autospreader flap in primary rhinoplasty. Plast Reconstr Surg. 2007;119:1897-902.
35. Gruber RP, Park E, Newman J, et al. The spreader flap in primary rhinoplasty. Plast Reconstr Surg. 2007;119:1903-10.
36. Guyuron B, Michelow BJ, Engelbardt C. Upper lateral splay graft. Plast Reconstr Surg. 1998;102:2169-77.
37. Clark JM, Cook TA. The "butterfly" graft in functional secondary rhinoplasty. Laryngoscope. 2002;112:1917-25.
38. Park SS. The flaring suture to augment the repair of the dysfunctional nasal valve. Plast Reconstr Surg. 1998;101:1120-2.
39. Schlosser RJ, Park SS. Surgery for the dysfunctional nasal valve. Cadaveric analysis and clinical outcomes. Arch Facial Plast Surg. 1999;1:105-10.
40. Paniello RC. Nasal valve suspension: an effective treatment for nasal valve collapse. Arch Otolaryngol Head Neck Surg. 1996;122:1342-6.
41. Lee DS, Glasgold AI. Correction of nasal valve stenosis with lateral suture suspension. Arch Facial Plast Surg. 2001;3:237-40.
42. Rizvi SS, Gauthier MG. Lateralizing the collapsed nasal valve. Laryngoscope. 2003;113:2052-4.
43. Most SP. Analysis of outcomes after functional rhinoplasty using a disease-specific quality-of-life instrument. Arch Facial Plast Surg. 2006;8:306-9.
44. Tardy ME. Rhinoplasty: The Art and the Science, Vol II. Saunders; 1996.
45. Gunter JP, Friedman RM. Lateral crural strut graft: technique and clinical applications in rhinoplasty. Plast Reconstr Surg. 1997;99:943-52.
46. Tardy ME, Garner ET. Inspiratory nasal obstruction secondary to alar and nasal valve collapse: technique for repair using autologous cartilage. Operative Tech Otolaryngol Head Neck Surg. 1990;1:215-8.

47. Toriumi DM, Josen J, Weinberger M, et al. Use of alar batten grafts for correction of nasal valve collapse. Arch Otolaryngol Head Neck Surg. 1997;123:802-8.
48. Romo T, Sclafani A, Sabini P. Use of high-density polyethylene in revision rhinoplasty and in the platyrrhine nose. Aesthetic Plast Surg. 1998;22:211-21.
49. Ramakrishnan JB, Danner CJ, Yee SW. The use of porous polyethylene implants to correct nasal valve collapse. Otolaryngol Head Neck Surg. 2007;136:357-61.
50. Tellioglu AT, Cimen K. Turn-in folding of the cephalic portion of the lateral crus to support the alar rim in rhinoplasty. Aesthetic Plast Surg. 2007;31:306-10.
51. Murakami CS, Barrera JE, Most SP. Preserving structural integrity of the alar cartilage in aesthetic rhinoplasty using a cephalic turn-in flap. Arch Facial Plast Surg. 2009;11:126-8.
52. Toriumi DM, Checcone MA. New concepts in nasal tip contouring. Facial Plast Surg Clin North Am. 2009;17:55-90.
53. Boahene KD, Hilger PA. Alar rim grafting in rhinoplasty: indications, technique, and outcomes. Arch Facial Plast Surg. 2009;11:285-29.

Chapter

16

NASAL SEPTAL RECONSTRUCTION

Patrick C Angelos and Dean M Toriumi

INTRODUCTION

Nasal septal deformity is a significant contributor to nasal obstruction and is an extremely common problem encountered in functional nasal surgery as well as aesthetic rhinoplasty. It naturally follows that septal reconstruction or septoplasty are extremely frequent procedures performed in Otolaryngology for a diverse variety of septal deformities. As the complexity of the septal problem increases, in turn does the challenge of the reconstructive procedure.

Provided there is adequate preservation of the dorsal-caudal L-strut, mild septal deviation may be treated with traditional open and/or endoscopic septoplasty procedures that involve submucous resection techniques. In this technique, the non L-strut deviating portion of the septal cartilage is removed (Fig. 16.1). Since the introduction and incorpora-

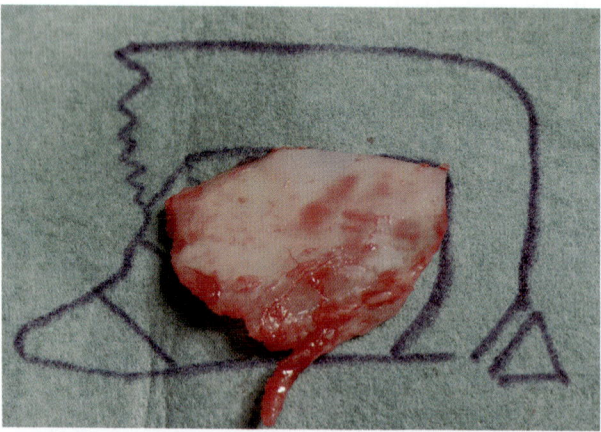

Fig. 16.1: Area typically removed during a traditional septoplasty. Note how extra cartilage is left along the ethmoid bone and near the nasal spine to insure adequate stability of the L-strut

tion of the nasal endoscope in paranasal sinus surgery, its benefits have carried over into septal surgery and many surgeons, especially in the case of concurrent sinus surgery, now perform endoscopic septoplasty.[1] While many patients are adequately treated with traditional septoplasty methods, more severe and complex deformities and revision cases may require advanced techniques of reconstruction beyond traditional methods. These procedures are typically executed via an external rhinoplasty approach with or without the use of the endoscope and may also include adjunctive procedures to address other areas of the nose including the nasal valves, dorsum, tip and alar base. A complete discussion of related procedures however is beyond the scope of this chapter, the purpose of which is to give an update on recent advances and techniques in nasal septal reconstruction.

A stable septal reconstruction will serve as a base for rebuilding the nasal framework in both functional and aesthetic rhinoplasty. Successful management of septal deviation or deficiency is challenging because it may be difficult to overcome the intrinsic memory of the cartilage and to some degree the overlying soft tissues. In addition to causing nasal obstruction, deviation of the dorsal septum can cause contour deformities in the middle third of the nose. Caudal septal deficiency may be due to congenital underdevelopment or to acquired factors such as prior septal procedure(s), cartilage destruction, or by trauma or infections. Loss of the caudal septal support leads to a weak, unstable tip that is easily displaced by the weight of the thick lobular skin and the constant pull of gravity.[2] As mentioned, deficiencies and deviation of the anterior and caudal septum may not be fully addressed with traditional septoplasty approaches, which provide limited access to the premaxilla and nasal spine.[3]

In the severely deviated nose, the underlying septal deformity can involve dorsal and caudal segments of the L-strut. After traditional submucous resection (SMR), the L-strut often remains deviated with weakened dorsal support (especially if overresected, crushed, scored, or incised). These efforts initially intended to straighten the septum, may lead to saddling, midvault collapse and recurrent deviation postoperatively.[4] Severe septal deviations have been categorized as either horizontal or vertical or a combination of both.[5] In each case, with the use of techniques described in this chapter, the reconstructive surgeon may have to overcome the limitations to more traditional septoplasty approaches.

This update is a review of more basic as well as advanced methods to septal reconstruction beyond traditional septoplasty techniques, especially as applied to caudal deviations. Traditional approaches to septoplasty may also include scoring of cartilage to release deviations as well as the "swinging door maneuver" in which trimming of the inferior septum allows it to swing back into the midline over the maxillary crest.[6] Minor modifications to the existing framework include septal splinting as well as cutting and suturing of the caudal L-strut.[6,7] A new and increasingly popular method to perform septal reconstruction involves the use of polydioxanone (PDS) resorbable plates (Mentor Worldwide).[8-10] Other techniques include placement of a columellar strut, the tongue in groove method, as well as more advanced techniques, such as caudal septal extension grafts. Extracorporeal septoplasty has been advocated as the ultimate reconstructive procedure for severe and complex nasal septal deformities.[5,11] This technique involves removal and replacement of the caudal septum with a caudal septal replacement graft (CSRG). Each technique serves as a tool in the armamentarium of the reconstructive surgeon to address the individual patient's particular problems. When appropriate, outcomes data are reviewed on the various techniques, as this data is becoming increasingly important not only as the basis for evidence based medicine, but also for physician grading, as well as for procedure reimbursement.

SEPTAL SUTURING AND SPLINTING TECHNIQUES

Septal incision and suturing techniques involve incising the most convex portion of the caudal septum and then reconnecting it with the cut ends of the caudal cartilage strut.[7] Performed endonasally, this approach is aimed to preserve the natural junction between the maxillary crest and the septal cartilage. In a series of 45 patients, Jang et al. describe their use of the technique via a hemitransfixion incision on the concave side of the deviating septal cartilage. Roughly two third of the patients underwent primary procedures and the remaining one third of cases were revisions. Their technique involves elevation of bilateral muco-perichondrial flaps, cutting the caudal strut with scissors at the most convex region (caudal-cephalic orientation). The excess portions of the strut are then overlapped and sutured together using 5-0 monofilament absorbable sutures. The degree of overlapping should be adjusted as not to adversely effect vertical height. If stability is questionable, a cartilaginous septal batten graft (harvested from the posterior, inferior non-L-strut portion of the septum) may be placed for further support, usually on the concave side. This batten must be very thin and carefully carved so it does not create excess bulk and block the nasal airway. This graft was used in just over half of the patients in the series and always in a unilateral manner.

Objective outcomes measures from this study on cutting and suturing techniques revealed decreased mean VAS (visual analog scale) scores for nasal obstruction, which were improved from 7.93–3.63, indicating that improvement in nasal obstruction was achieved at 6 months postoperatively ($P\_.001$).[7] Endoscopic examinations showed that 51% of patients had near complete correction of the septum and that 47% had improved but a little persisting caudal deviation and one patient had no change in caudal septal deviation. No significant difference was noted in the amount of VAS score improvement with or without concurrent inferior turbinate reduction. To assess the effect of the batten graft, they also compared the VAS score change between the groups and found that the batten graft showed an additionally beneficial effect on symptom improvement (with vs. without batten graft placement: 5.22 vs. 3.11, $P=.01$).

Since placement of a batten graft enhanced the effect of the cutting and suture technique significantly, it is not surprising that various techniques for septal splinting to support a weak L-strut have been described in the literature.[12] One of these techniques involves the placement of a "septal angle splinting graft" which is a modification of the septal crossbar graft. This is a structural graft that allows for anterior septal angle reconstruction during septorhinoplasty. It is touted to improve dorsal septal support and facilitate correction of the deviated nose.[4,13] Physically, the graft acts as a pillar supporting the cartilaginous dorsum. The original septal crossbar graft was described by Broccieri[13], as a spreader type crossbar graft in which a large 15-mm L-shaped caudal and dorsal strut is preserved. Incisions are placed along the L-strut and a cartilage graft is used to splint the bent dorsal septum towards the midline (Fig. 16.2). This graft may serve a dual purpose to straighten the dorsum as well as stent the internal nasal valve.

In a more recent update on surgical technique, Aziz et al. described their method of oblique placement of a septal crossbar graft for anterior septal angle reconstruction. In a prospective case series of nine patients, they reviewed their technique and as well as representative patient outcomes. An external rhinoplasty approach was used using standard dissection techniques for exposure. A generous graft of quadrangular cartilage is harvested preserving the L-shaped strut. A swinging door

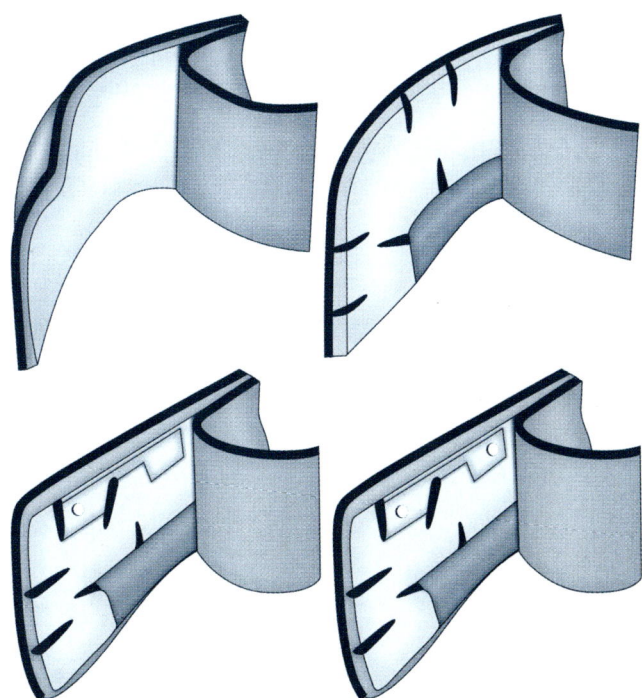

Fig. 16.2: Septal crossbar technique showing placement of septal cartilage along the deviated dorsal septum

maneuver is performed to reposition the subluxed septum and to secure it in the midline. Next, the harvested septal cartilage is fashioned into a graft approximately 20 mm (length) X 6 mm (height) X 2 mm (thickness) in size. This oblique septal crossbar graft is placed along the posterior third to half of the caudal strut to a point on the ipsilateral or contralateral side of the dorsal strut. The dorsal end may be adjusted and placed at various locations along the length of the dorsum, adjusting the lever arm (Figs 16.3A and B).

Advantages of this technique include additional structural integrity over SMR, preservation of the anterior septal angle and avoidance of extracorporeal septoplasty. It is limited by its additional bulk and potential for persistent nasal obstruction, widening and possible shadow effect of the tip lobule. The surgeon should be mindful of inherent weakness in the harvested cartilage graft, as the remaining septum may not always be suitable for this technique. Although this is a descriptive paper, other outcome based measures and long-term follow-up are needed to ensure lasting and sound improvement with this method.

POLYDIOXANONE PLATES

Drawing from previously used techniques in orbital floor repair, surgeons adapted the use of resorbable polydioxanone (PDS) to nasal septal reconstruction to help support cartilage fragments during healing.[8] PDS, a common suture material, is degraded by hydrolysis that is completely resorbed by the body. PDS plates are available in various sizes and thickness and they have been previously used in the restoration of bone discontinuities.[14]

Boenisch et al. evaluated the usefulness of resorbable PDS plate to support septal cartilage in external septoplasty, assessed its mechan-

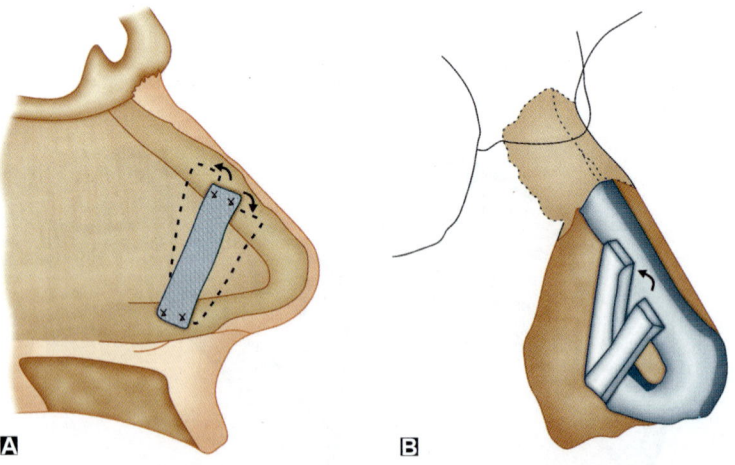

Figs 16.3A and B: Oblique septal crossbar graft. (A) Lateral; (B) Oblique views
Adapted from: Aziz ZS, Brenner MJ, Putman HC. Oblique septal crossbar graft for anterior septal angle reconstruction. Arch Facial Plast Surg. 2010;12:422-6

ical stability and described the surgical technique as well as the clinical experience in 396 patients since 1996.[8] The indication was typically post-traumatic severe septal deformity. This technique involves removal of the quadrangular cartilage and division into straight fragments, which are sutured to the plate and replaced as a free graft (Fig. 16.4). In this series, if inadequate cartilage was available, the missing cartilage was supplanted with auricular conchal cartilage. Functionally, all patients experienced varying degrees of improvement in nasal blockage. In a mean follow-up period of 12 months, maximum 10 years, straightening of the nasal septum was achieved in almost 90% of the patients, correlating with subjective improvements. To confirm this objectively, the authors performed rhinomanometry usually 2 months after surgery. The results showed remarkably improved nasal flow in 324 patients (81.8%). Eighteen patients (4.5 %) required revision surgery for persistent deviation or pollybeak deformity. There were no immediate postoperative complications reported and only three patients were reported to have long-term dorsal irregularities.

In a similar report, Tweedie et al. published their experience with perforated and unperforated forms of PDS plates in a retrospective review of 50 patients over a 4-year period.[10] The group used an external rhinoplasty approach and often employed extracorporeal techniques. If the septal cartilage was reconstructed *in situ* (corporeal approach), the PDS foil was inserted on the concave side of the deformity in a batten type fashion. If the cartilaginous septum was reconstructed extracorporeally, the fragments were laid out on a sheet of PDS foil and sutured into one large graft. Approximately half of the patients underwent septal reconstruction using perforated (first 26 patients) or unperforated (next 24 patients) plates. Three patients required minor revision surgery of the septum or tip. Four patients experienced moderate

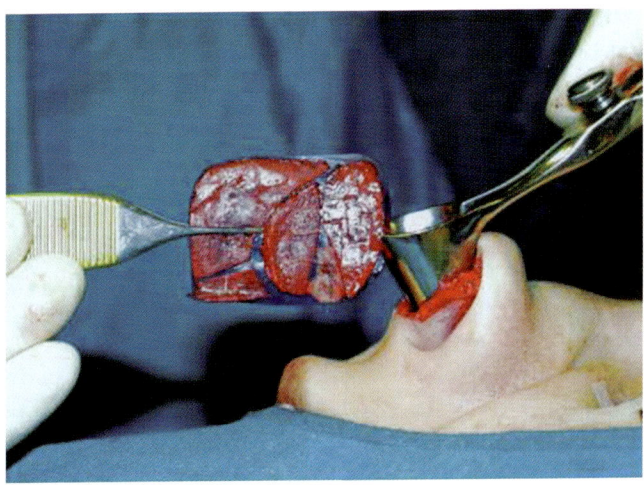

Fig. 16.4: Portions of septal cartilage sutured to a PDS plate

Adapted from: Boenisch M, Nolst Trenite GJ. Reconstruction of the nasal septum using polydioxanone plate. Arch Facial Plast Surg. 2010;12:4-10

saddling of the dorsum (all involved unperforated PDS foil) and underwent successful revision surgery using auricular cartilage grafts. No such complications were seen with the use of thin, 0.15-mm perforated foil. The authors warn against the use of unperforated PDS foil in this context.

In our experience with PDS plates, as yet to be published, we feel that they may be extremely useful in stabilizing an *in situ* or reconstructed L-strut without adding additional bulk to the construct. The most common application has been in primary septorhinoplasty, in which a septal angle splinting PDS plate is used to straighten a deviated dorsal/caudal L-strut. In this application, a triangular wedge of cartilage is removed at the inferior junction of the dorsal-caudal cartilaginous L-strut. Then the dorsal/posterior aspect of the PDS plate is sutured to one side of the dorsal septum and the anterior/caudal portion of the PDS plate is sutured to the opposite side of the septum (Figs 16.5A to F). For this indication, we only use 0.25-mm thickness PDS plate and frequently make a couple of holes in the plate using a 16-gauge needle. Typically, the PDS plate is sutured in place with using a 5-0 PDS suture. The major advantage of using the PDS plate in this capacity is that the PDS plate will resorb without leaving any bulk that can block the internal nasal valve.

TONGUE IN GROOVE

Deviation of the caudal aspect of the septum along with asymmetries of the medial crura are frequently addressed, but correction of deviations in these areas can be complex to achieve and difficult to maintain results over time. The tongue in groove technique, when used in combination with septoplasty and/or columellar modifying techniques, serves to aid in the maintenance of long-term correction of caudal septal deviations.

If the patient has a drooping tip due to a hanging columella and prominent caudal septum that would require trimming, the surgeon can set the

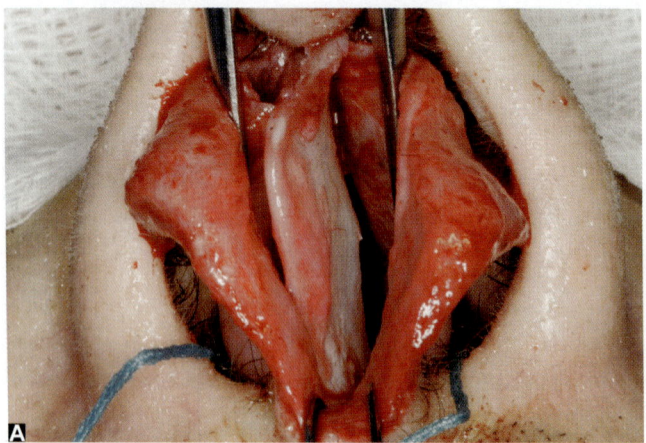

Fig. 16.5A

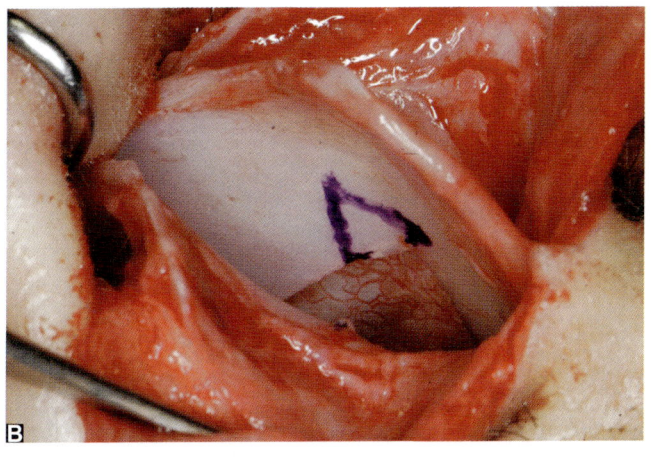

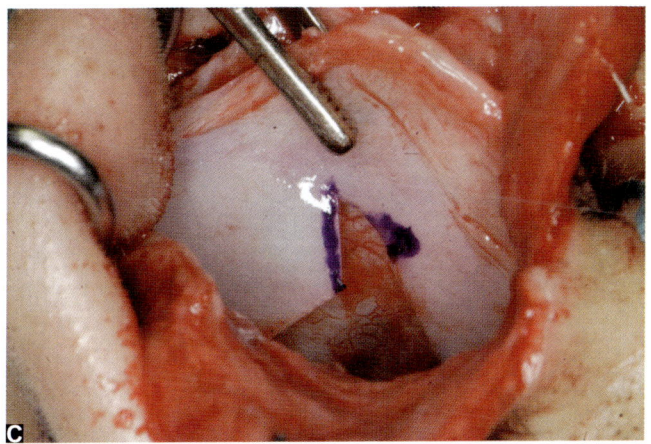

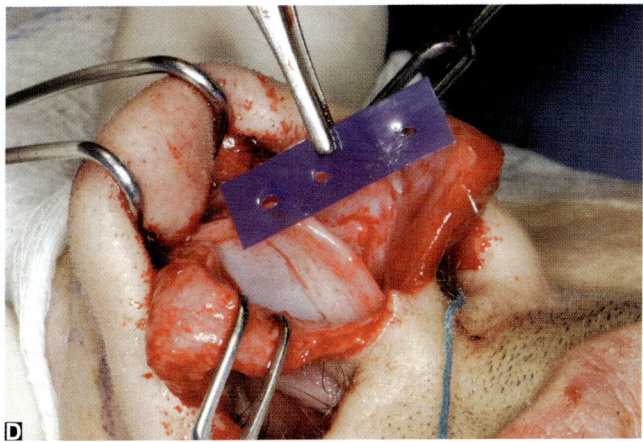

Figs 16.5B to D

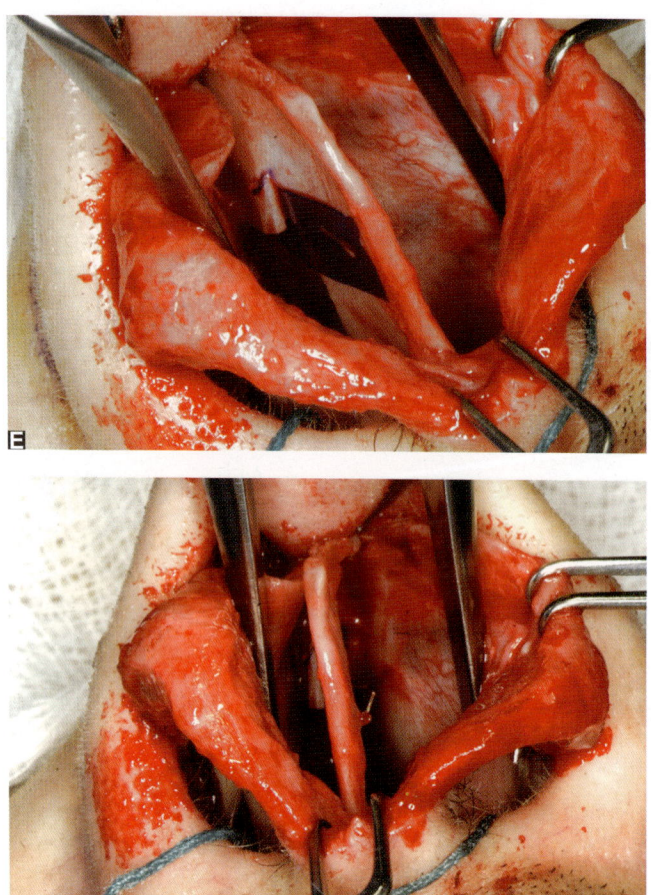

Figs 16.5E and F

Figs 16.5A to F: Use of the splinting septal angle PDS resorbable plate to straighten a deviated dorsal strut blocking the left internal nasal valve. (A) Note how the dorsal septum is deviating to the left; (B) A triangular segment of cartilage is removed from the inferior dorsal strut; (C) Cartilage segment is excised; (D) 0.25-mm PDS plate is perforated with a 16-gauge needle; (E) PDS plate is positioned to straighten the deviated dorsal strut; (F) Straight dorsal strut after placement of the PDS plate

medial crura back on the midline caudal septum "in a tongue in groove fashion" (Figs 16.6A to C). It is imperative that the caudal septum be in the midline to avoid asymmetries of the columella and nasal base. This method, described by Kridel et al. can be used instead of placing a columellar strut in selected patients.[15] Tongue in groove method was indicated to straighten a caudal septal deviation in almost half (94 of 200) of the patients in Kridel's study.

It is important to emphasize that this maneuver should only be used in patients who have a redundancy of caudal septal length that otherwise would require trimming. Patients with a hanging columella and short

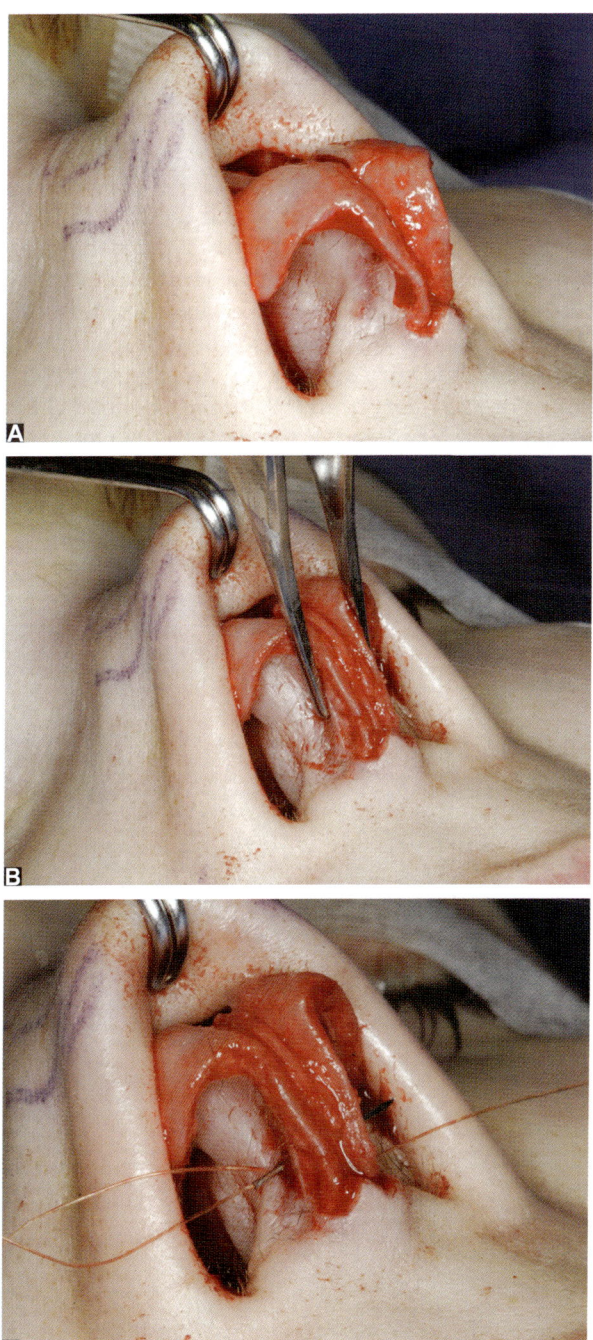

Figs 16.6A to C: Tongue in groove technique. (A) Hanging tip lobule; (B) Dissection between medial crura and movement of medial crura superiorly to suture to caudal septum; (C) Placing plain catgut on straight septal needle to fixate

Adapted from: Toriumi DM. New concepts in nasal tip contouring. Arch Facial Plast Surg. 2006;8:156-8

upper lip are ideal candidates because fixation of the medial crura to the caudal septum will usually lengthen the upper lip. Patients with a hanging columella due to a long caudal septum are ideal for this technique.[16]

COLUMELLAR STRUT

For minor caudal septal deviations in which the base of the nose is well supported by the medial crura along with a favorable alar-columellar relationship, a sutured-in-place columellar strut can effectively stabilize the base.[17] This graft is placed into a pocket dissected between the medial crura. If the base of the nose is severely deficient or if augmentation of the premaxilla is needed, the surgeon can use an extended columellar strut with or without a premaxillary graft.[16] With the extended columellar strut, it is best to fixate the inferior end of the graft to the nasal spine. This can be done by making a notch in the nasal spine and then fixating the inferior end of the extended columellar strut into the notch with some small splinting grafts to fixate to the nasal spine (Fig. 16.7). Another option is to flare the base of the strut, to cut a notch in the posteroinferior end of the

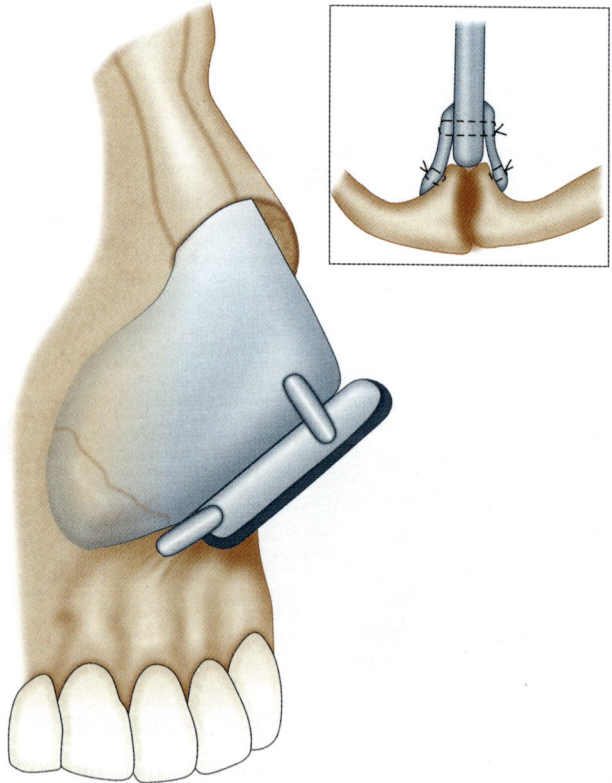

Fig. 16.7: Extended columellar strut sitting on nasal spine and stabilized using small splinting grafts

Adapted from: Toriumi DM. New concepts in nasal tip contouring. Arch Facial Plast Surg. 2006;8:156-85

graft so it may sit over the nasal spine. This will allow the caudal septum to integrate with the graft.

With reconstructive septal surgery, it may be necessary to alter tip projection, the alar-columellar relationship and/or the nasolabial angle. There are several reliable and versatile methods that can achieve these goals, which include using a caudal extension graft or CSRG. Which graft is used depends on each patient's specific anatomic deficiencies and surgical goals.[16]

CAUDAL SEPTAL EXTENSION GRAFT

If the caudal septum is deficient or if tip position must be altered or stabilized, a caudal septal extension graft may be placed to augment the caudal septum. This in turn can serve as a stable fixation point for the medial crura.[16,18] The caudal extension graft is a relatively straight segment of cartilage that slightly overlaps the existing caudal septum or is placed end-to-end with stabilization by splinting grafts on either side. When the graft is placed in an overlapping fashion, inherent deviations can be used to one's advantage to maintain a midline tip structure. Care must be taken to make sure the overlapping segment of the graft is not blocking the nasal airway. We rarely use the overlapping caudal extension graft and use almost exclusively an end to end orientation of the caudal septal extension graft. Splinting grafts and/or long extended spreader grafts that project caudally to the septum can also be used to stabilize the extension graft (Figs 16.8A and B).[19]

The shape and orientation of the caudal extension graft can be altered to provide different effects on tip position. If tip rotation is desired, the graft should be longer at its inferior margin. If nasal lengthening is needed, the graft should be longer superiorly to counter-rotate the tip and lengthen the nose.[16] Once the graft is in position, the medial crura can then be sutured to the caudal margin of the caudal extension graft with 5-0 PDS sutures. The PDS sutures are placed through the internal surface of the intermediate

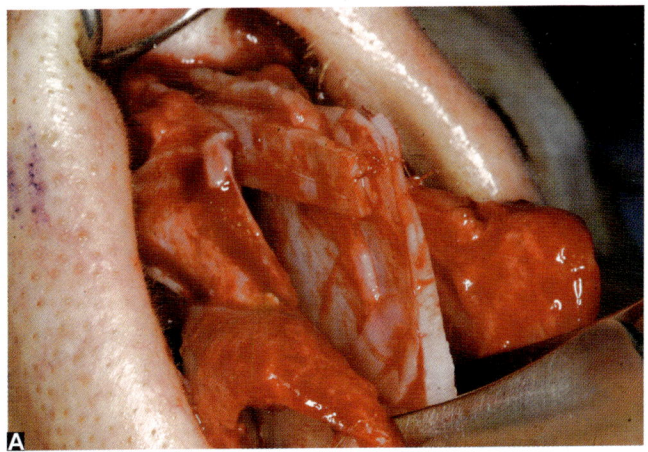

Fig. 16.8A

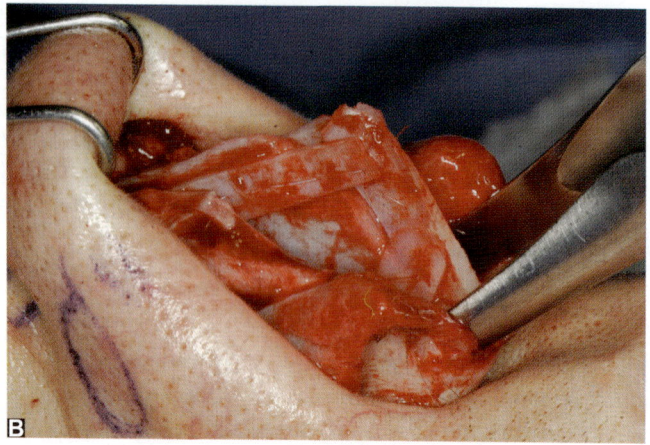

Fig. 16.8B

Figs 16.8A and B: Caudal septal extension graft stabilized using extended spreader grafts
Adapted from: Toriumi DM. New concepts in nasal tip contouring. Arch Facial Plast Surg. 2006;8:156-85

crura and then fixed to the caudal extension graft. If maximum support is needed, the caudal extension graft can be sutured inferiorly to the periosteum of the nasal spine or, as previously mentioned, it can be stabilized with splinting grafts or extended spreader grafts. The caudal margin of the caudal extension graft must be vertical and midline; otherwise, the tip will be deviated. The cephalic margin of the graft that overlaps the caudal septum should be trimmed or beveled so that it does not obstruct the airway. We frequently use 0.25-mm resorbable PDS plate to stabilize end to end caudal septal extension grafts (Figs 16.9A to E). Care must be taken to avoid using large pieces that could isolate the septal cartilage.

Patients undergoing placement of caudal extension grafts should be told that their nose will be stiffer after surgery with less tip compliance

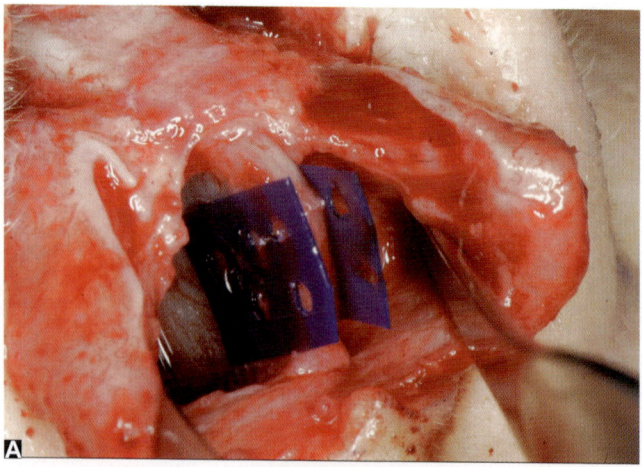

Fig. 16.9A

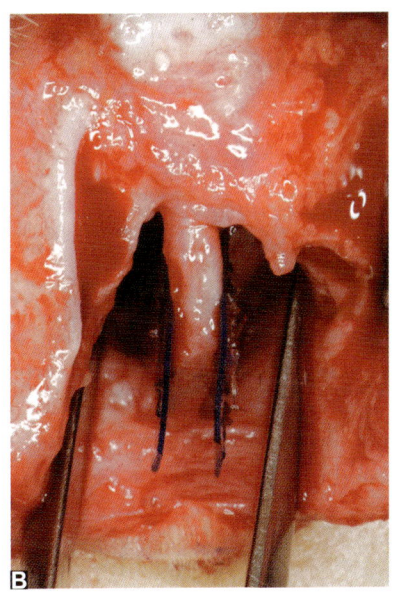

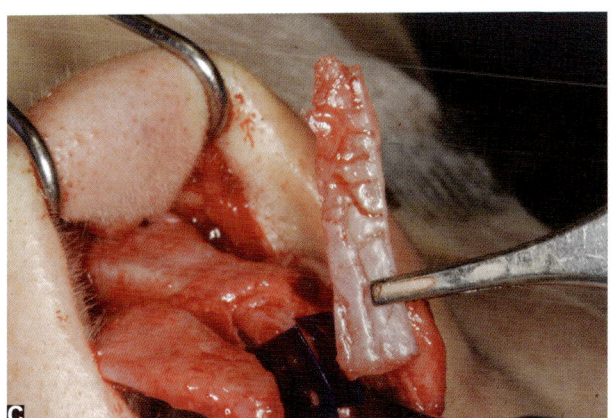

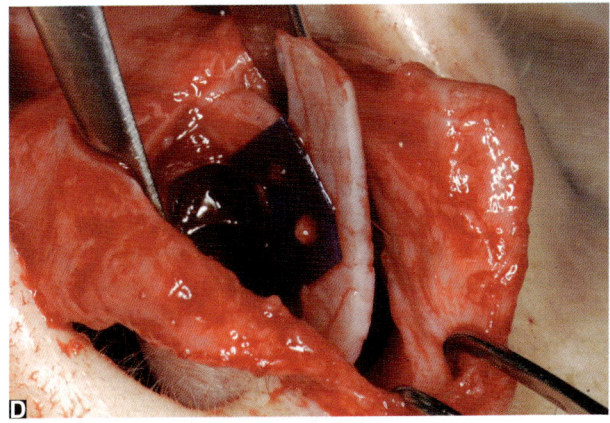

Fig. 16.9B to D

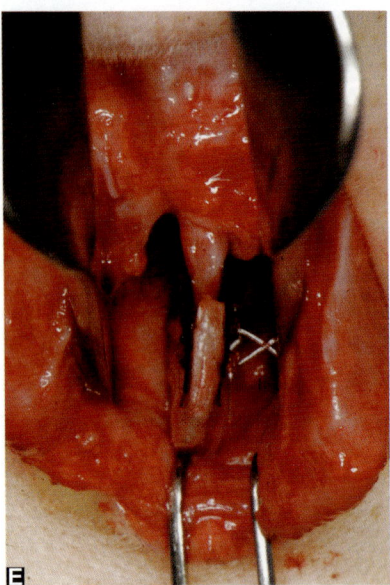

Fig. 16.9E

Figs 16.9A to E: Stabilization of caudal septal extension graft fixated using bilateral 0.25-mm PDS plates. (A) PDS plates sutured into position; (B) View from above; (C) Septal extension graft; (D) PDS plates fixating septal extension graft; (E) View from above showing septal extension graft placed end to end

and recoil. The use of caudal extension grafts requires special attention to the indication for placement, appropriately shaping of the graft with careful placement, stable fixation and setting proper tip position and alar-columellar relationship.

CAUDAL SEPTAL REPLACEMENT GRAFT

Almost a century ago, Metzenbaum emphasized the role of the caudal septum in supporting the nasal tip and described replacing the caudal septum versus submucous resection.[20] As these tenets for maintaining tip support hold true today, indications for total replacement of the caudal septum are severe deviations of the caudal septum as well as an unstable caudal septum. In 1994, Toriumi described a technique of subtotal septal reconstruction in which he would remove the damaged portion of the caudal and/or dorsal septum and then reconstructed it using septal cartilage harvested posteroinferiorly.[11] This graft is similar in concept to both the columellar strut as well as the caudal septal extension graft. The difference lies in the fact that, with this technique, the entire caudal aspect of the septum is removed and then replaced either with a straighter, more stable portion of posterior septal cartilage or autologous, typically costal cartilage graft. Replacing the severely deviated or unstable caudal septum can help to avoid the postoperative loss of tip projection which may result in a polybeak deformity, short nasal deformity, or an over-rotated nose.[16]

The caudal septal deficiency may also be associated with varying degrees of premaxillary deficiency due to an underdeveloped, previously resected, or damaged anterior nasal spine. In a series of 120 patients, Foda has described his experience with the CSRG.[2] A description of the technique includes restoring tip support using a CSRG along with premaxillary augmentation with Mersilene mesh (Ethicon Inc, Somerville, New Jersey). We do not recommend using Mersilene mesh in the nose and prefer to use autologous grafting materials such as septum, auricular cartilage or costal cartilage.

In an effort to measure the efficacy of a modified extracorporeal technique for anterior septal reconstruction, Most has reported his outcomes in a series of 12 patients.[5] In this prospective, observational study, pre and postoperative evaluation was performed using photographs and the Nasal Obstruction Symptoms Evaluation (NOSE) scale. The reported technique for anterior septal reconstruction is a modified extracorporeal technique, designed to preserve a dorsal remnant at the keystone area. This was performed via an external rhinoplasty approach along with a hemitransfixion incision of the left side. The dorsal strut that is preserved is at least 1.5 cm along its anteroposterior axis and the vertical height of the remnant is maximal at the keystone area, measuring at least 1 cm. It is critical to maintain the attachment of the dorsal septum to the nasal bones in order to maintain dorsal height and for support of the replacement graft. With this method, the replacement graft is placed on the concave side and acts as a spreader graft and serves to splint the dorsal remnant. The replacement graft is sutured between the dorsal remnant and the ipsilateral upper lateral cartilage with or without spreader graft(s) on the contralateral side. In analysis of the outcomes, no notching or saddling occurred over the average follow-up time of 5.4 months. Nasal obstruction was improved, with average NOSE scores decreased for patients who underwent anterior septal replacement, with or without turbinectomy (P<0.01).

In a retrospective clinical review, Andre et al. compared results of septal battens versus septal replacement using subjective self-evaluation and by postoperative clinical examination at follow-up.[21] While this study is limited by its subjective nature, the authors found no difference between patient self-reported evaluations, however there was a significant difference in postoperative septal position on clinical examination. They found that the septum was more often noted in the midline with the technique of septal replacement than in the septal batten group.

Specifically for reconstruction of a severe saddle deformity, we prefer to use a strong CSRG, extended spreader grafts secured to the preserved keystone are of septum, then using a separate dorsal onlay graft as needed. With this technique, a septal or costal cartilage replacement graft is placed into notch in nasal spine (or straddling the nasal spine), connected superiorly to extended spreader grafts which are stabilized to the dorsal septal remnant (Fig. 16.10). In most patients, we are able to correct septal deviations without resecting and reconstructing the caudal

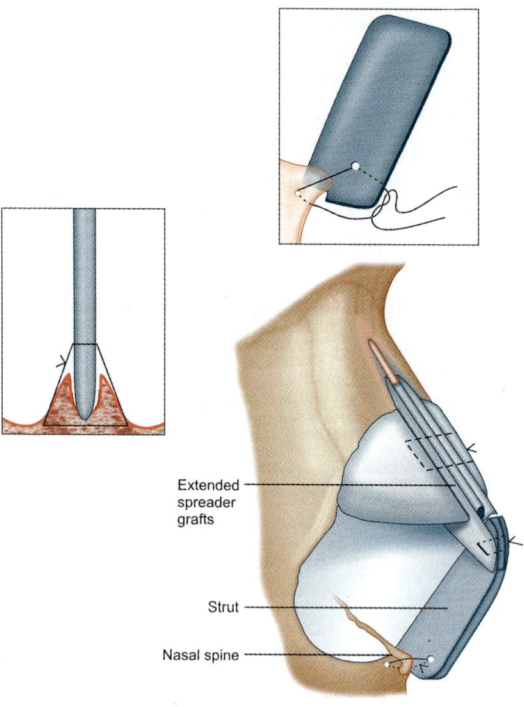

Extended spreader grafts

Strut

Nasal spine

Fig. 16.10: Caudal septal replacement graft fixed into notch in nasal spine and stabilized with bilateral extended spreader grafts

septum. Patients with deformities of the nasal base (deviated columella, asymmetric nostrils, deviated footplates) are more likely to need caudal septal replacement to provide proper correction of the deformity (Figs 16.11A to O).

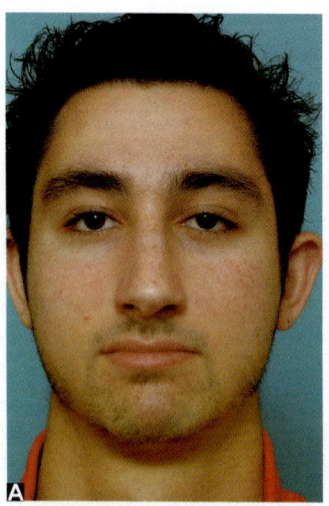

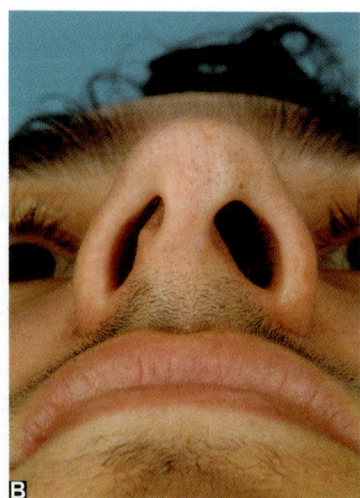

Figs 16.11A and B

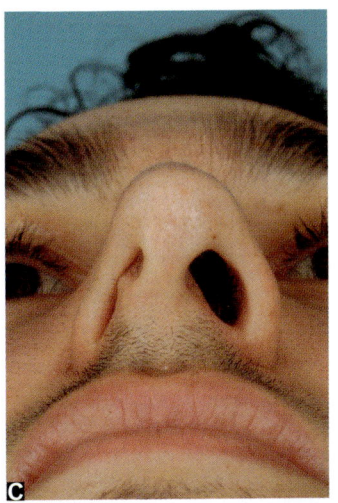

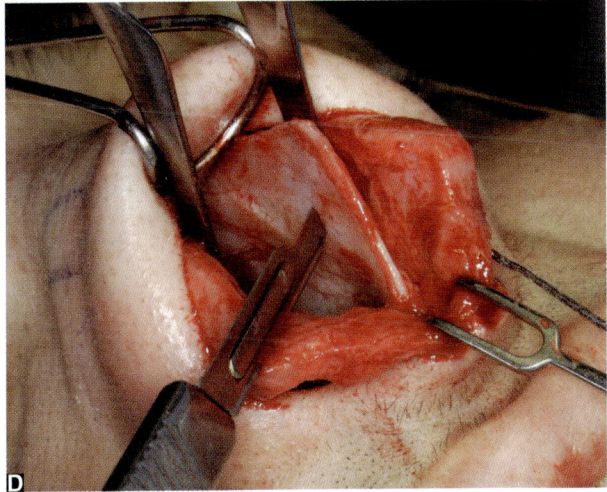

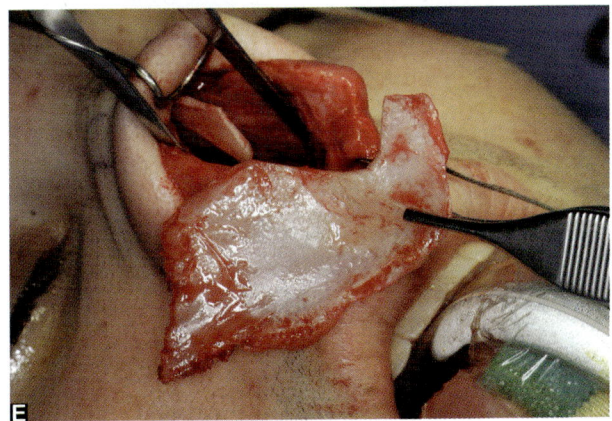

Figs 16.11C to E

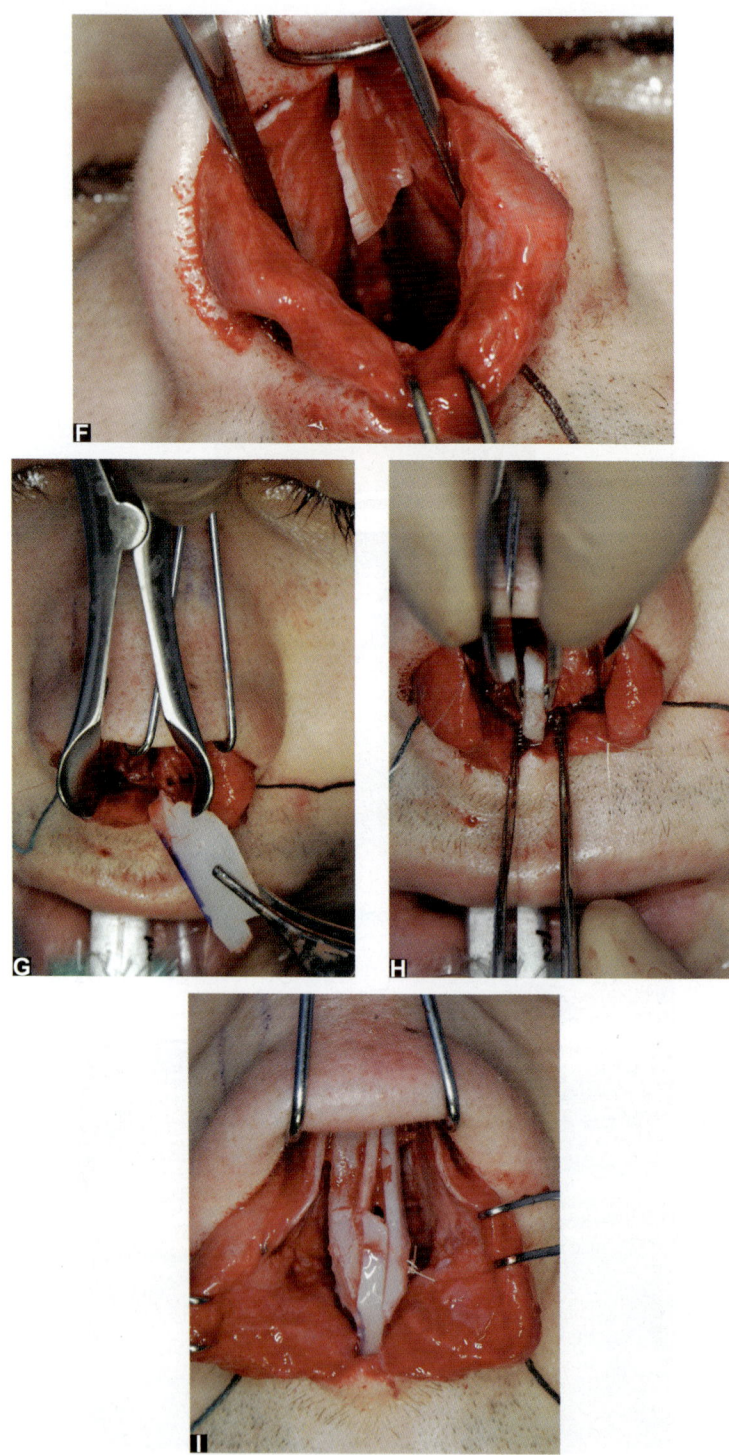

Figs 16.11F to I

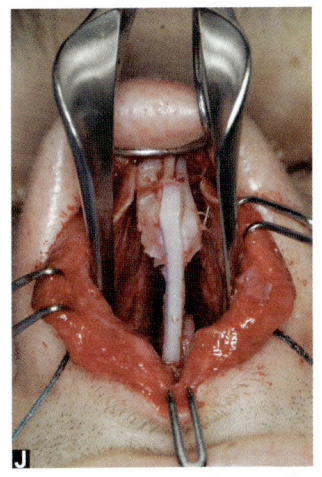

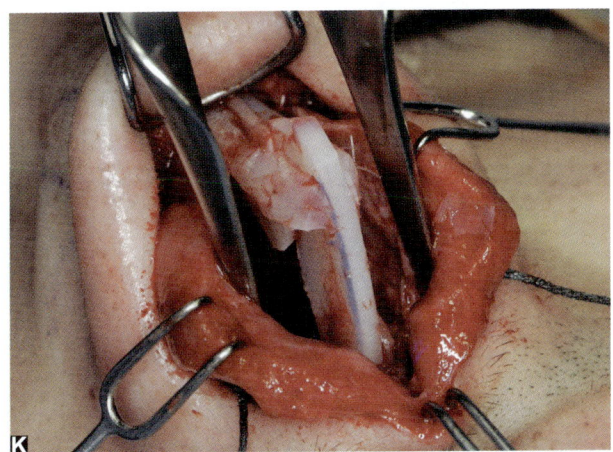

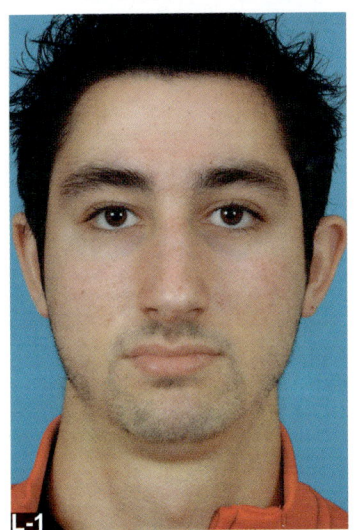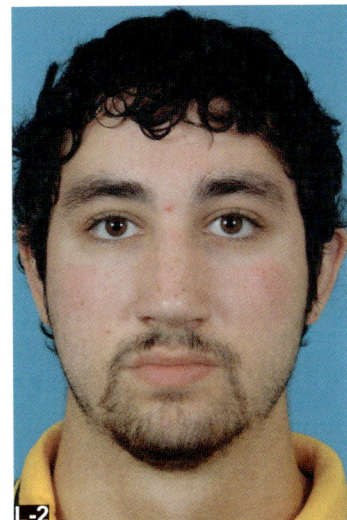

Figs 16.11J to L-2

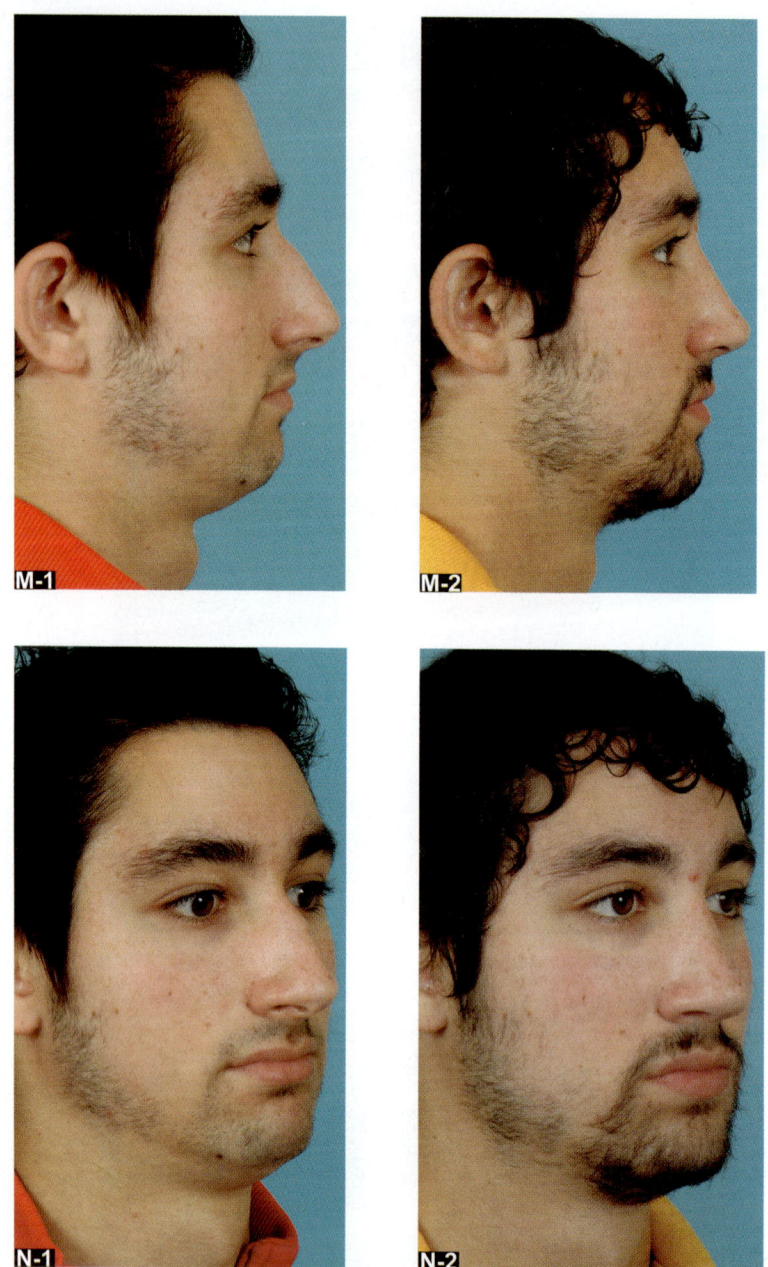

Figs 16.11M to N-2

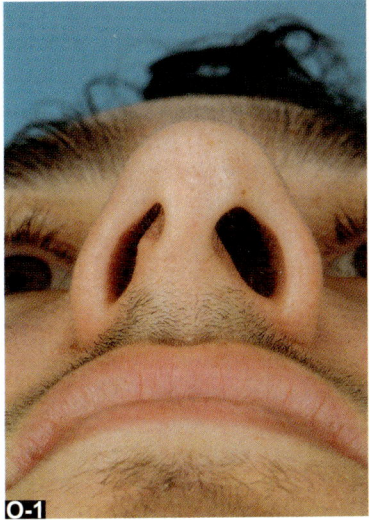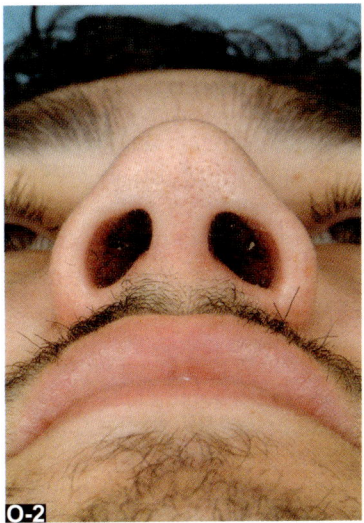

Figs 16.110-1 and 0-2

Figs 16.11A to 0: Patient presents with severe caudal septal deviation and severe asymmetries of nasal base. Patient has complete collapse of right nostril upon inspiration. (A) Preoperative frontal view showing asymmetries of nasal base; (B) Preoperative base view showing significant asymmetries of nostrils; (C) Preoperative inspiration base view shows complete collapse of right nostril; (D) Excising deviated segment of caudal septum. View also shows fracture of nasal septum; (E) Deviated caudal septum excised; (F) Dorsal septal strut remains attached to ethmoid bone at keystone area; (G) Caudal septal replacement graft with notch for attachment to nasal spine; (H) Placement of septal replacement graft into notch nasal spine; (I) Caudal septal replacement graft stabilized with bilateral extended spreader grafts; (J) Septal reconstruction as viewed from below. (K) Reconstructed septum from side view; (L1) Preoperative frontal view; (L2) One year postoperative frontal view; (M1) Preoperative right lateral view; (M2) One year postoperative right lateral view; (N1) Preoperative right oblique view; (N2) One year postoperative right oblique view; (01) Left: Preoperative base view; (02) One year postoperative base view

It is important to avoid potential complications of CSRG including dorsal irregularities, as well as notching and saddling. These can be avoided by ensuring the use of a straight and sturdy replacement graft. Our preferred grafting material for this technique is first posterior septal cartilage, followed by costal, then auricular conchal cartilage. In addition, inherent deviations of remnant septum may be corrected with the use of properly placed spreader or splinting grafts. Strict attention to detail is warranted over the dorsum to avoid dorsal irregularities, which may be camouflaged with soft tissue grafts, preferably of perichondrium. These irregularities may be more apparent in patients with thin skin.

COMMENTS

As reconstructive techniques continue to evolve, surgeons have a variety of options to treat deviations of the critical L-strut portion of the nasal septum. However, as we all know, every case is unique and requires recognition of the problem(s), an adequate plan to address the problem(s) and sound execution of the reconstructive technique. These advanced techniques in nasal septal reconstruction will serve as tools to correct a variety of severe septal deviations. It is clear that we need more prospective evaluations of advanced septal reconstruction techniques including validated outcomes measures. This evidence based approach will ultimately benefit patients as well as surgeons.

REFERENCES

1. Hwang PH, McLaughlin RB, Lanza, DC, et al. Endoscopic septoplasty: indications, technique, and results. Otolaryngol Head Neck Surg. 1999;120:678-82.
2. Foda HM. The caudal septum replacement graft. Arch Facial Plast Surg. 2008;10:152-7.
3. Kasperbauer JL, Facer GW, Kern. EB in Facial Plastic and Reconstructive Surgery. New York, NY: Thieme; 2009. pp. 649-61.
4. Aziz ZS, Brenner MJ, Putman HC. Oblique septal crossbar graft for anterior septal angle reconstruction. Arch Facial Plast Surg. 2010;12:422-6.
5. Most SP. Anterior septal reconstruction: outcomes after a modified extracorporeal septoplasty technique. Arch Facial Plast Surg. 2006;8:202-7.
6. Toriumi DM and Becker DG. Rhinoplasty Dissection Manual. Philadelphia, PA: Lippincott Williams & Wilkins; 1999.
7. Jang YJ, Yeo NK, Wang JH. Cutting and suture technique of the caudal septal cartilage for the management of caudal septal deviation. Arch Otolaryngol Head. Neck Surg. 2009;135:1256-60.
8. Boenisch M, Nolst Trenite GJ. Reconstruction of the nasal septum using polydioxanone plate. Arch Facial Plast Surg. 2010;12:4-10.
9. Gerlinger I, Karasz T, Somoqwari K, et al. Extracorporal septal reconstruction with polydioxanone foil. Clin Otolaryngol. 2007;32:465-70.
10. Tweedie DJ, Lo S, Rowe-Jones JM. Reconstruction of the nasal septum using perforated and unperforated polydioxanone foil. Arch Facial Plast Surg. 2010;12:106-13.
11. Toriumi DM. Subtotal reconstruction of the nasal septum: a preliminary report. Laryngoscope. 1994;104:906-13.
12. Foda HM. The crooked nose: correction of dorsal and caudal septal deviations. HNO. 2010;58:899-906.
13. Boccieri A, Pascali M. Septal crossbar graft for the correction of the crooked nose. Plast Reconstr Surg. 2003;111:629-38.
14. Iizuka T, Mikkonen P, Paukku, P, et al. Reconstruction of orbital floor with polydioxanone plate. Int J Oral Maxillofac Surg. 1991;20:83-7.
15. Kridel RW, Scott BA, Foda HM. The tongue-in-groove technique in septorhinoplasty. A 10-year experience. Arch Facial Plast Surg. 1999;1:246-56.
16. Toriumi DM. New concepts in nasal tip contouring. Arch Facial Plast Surg. 2006;8:156-85.
17. Johnson CMJ, T DM. Open Structure Rhinoplasty. Philadelphia, PA: WB Saunders; Co. 1989.

18. Toriumi DM. Structure approach in rhinoplasty. Facial Plast Surg Clin North Am. 2005;13:93-113.

19. Ha RY, Byrd HS. Septal extension grafts revisited: 6-year experience in controlling nasal tip projection and shape. Plast Reconstr Surg. 2003;112:1929-35.

20. Metzenbaum M. Replacement of the lower end of the dislocated septal cartilage versus submucous resection of the disloced end of the septal cartilage. Arch Otolaryngol Head Neck Surg. 1929;9:285-96.

21. Andre RF, Vuyk HD. Reconstruction of dorsal and/or caudal nasal septum deformities with septal battens or by septal replacement: an overview and comparison of techniques. Laryngoscope. 2006;116:1668-73.

Chapter

17

BALLOON SINUPLASTY IN THE TREATMENT OF SINUS DISEASE IN THE OPERATING ROOM

Iain F Hathorn and Amin R Javer

INTRODUCTION

Chronic rhinosinusitis (CRS) is a common condition affecting an estimated 13% of the US population.[1] This equates to 29 million people suffering with CRS in the US and 12.5 million visits to physician offices, hospital outpatient departments, and emergency departments per year.[1,2] CRS results in a considerable reduction in quality of life and also significant losses in productivity leading to large economic costs.[3] It has been estimated that in the US, CRS generates annual health-related costs of more than $5 billion.[4] Treatment is usually primarily medical, with surgery reserved for those cases unresponsive to conservative treatment or those with complications. Functional endoscopic sinus surgery (FESS) is the surgical approach of choice and provides very good outcomes for patients with CRS. It is minimally invasive surgery that is physiologically sound and allows more tissue preservation, reduced tissue trauma, lower complication rates and quicker recovery times than the previously utilized non-endoscopic techniques. Advances in FESS have resulted from the development of more refined instruments, increased surgical training and the application of navigation systems, initially used in neurosurgery. Balloon sinuplasty is a relatively new advance. It is a device that was first introduced in 2005 and developed from the success of balloon use in other specialties, utilizing Seldinger's technique to dilate the sinus ostia. The balloon compresses the surrounding mucosa and causes microfracture of the circumferential bone.[5,6] It has been argued that sinuplasty may enhance mucosal preservation, reduce local trauma, and restore the natural sinus drainage pathways resulting in effective relief of symptoms. Following its introduction, the technology received a lot of media attention and generated significant controversy within otolaryngology.[5] Despite continuing controversy regarding its application, many surgeons have been trained to use the device and large number of patients have had surgery using it. We will discuss the use of balloon sinuplasty in CRS with particular reference to its use in the operating room.

DEVICES

Balloon Sinuplasty

The first catheter-based system for dilation of the paranasal sinuses was introduced by Acclarent Inc. (Menlo Park, CA). This resulted from the work of California-based engineers adapting cardiac devices to perform sinus dilation. Having obtained US Food and Drug Administration (FDA) 510(k) approval in April 2005, the device was launched in September 2005 as 'Balloon Sinuplasty'. Traditional balloon devices were compliant and would conform to the anatomy on dilatation. However, this is a noncompliant device which when expanded displaces bone and tissue to open up the sinus drainage pathways. The majority of the literature relating to balloon catheter devices focus on the balloon sinuplasty system from Acclarent; this will be discussed in detail later (Fig. 17.1).

Technique

The patient is anesthetized using either general or local anesthesia. We are focusing on the use of balloon sinuplasty in the operating room and therefore, the majority of cases will use general anesthesia with a laryngeal mask airway or endotracheal tube. Initial access to the sinus ostia is gained with an appropriately angled guide-catheter that is placed in the nasal cavity pointing in the direction toward the target ostia under endoscopic visualization. A guide-wire is then introduced through the catheter and threaded toward the target sinus ostia (Figs 17.2 and 17.3). The correct placement of the guide-wire in the sinus can be confirmed using fluoroscopy or transillumination (Relieva Luma sinus illumination system; Acclarent) (Fig. 17.4). The guide-catheter can then be removed and the

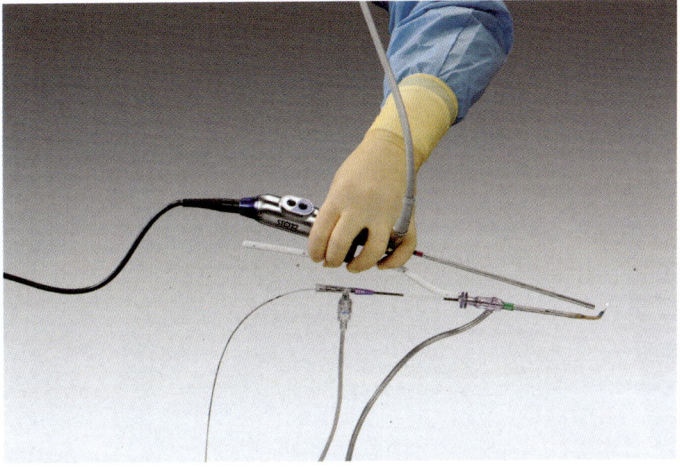

Fig. 17.1: Balloon Sinuplasty Integrated System
Source: Courtesy of Acclarent, Inc.

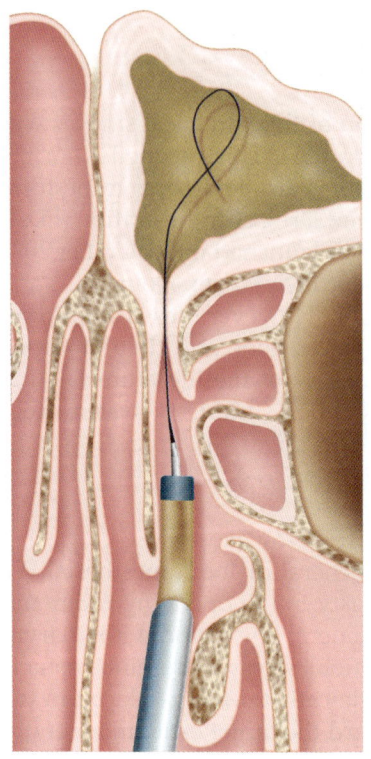

Fig. 17.2: Guide-wire passed through guide-catheter and into frontal sinus
Source: Courtesy of Acclarent, Inc.

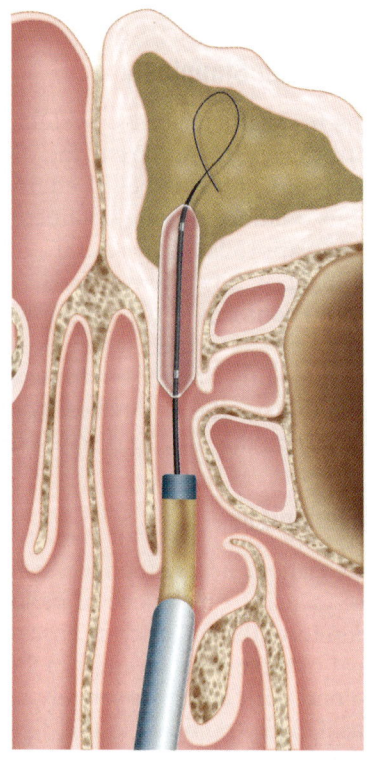

Fig. 17.3: The balloon catheter is passed over the guide-wire and into the sinus ostia and inflated
Source: Courtesy of Acclarent, Inc.

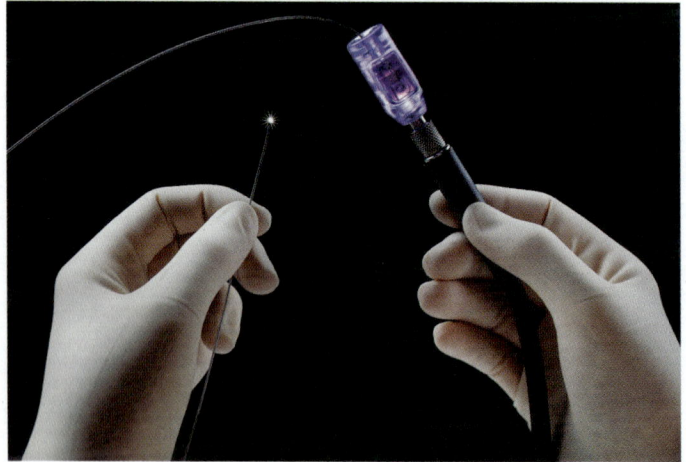

17.4: Relieva Luma sinus illumination system
Source: Courtesy of Acclarent, Inc.

balloon catheter is passed over the wire using the Seldinger technique into the sinus ostia. Following confirmation of correct placement, the balloon is inflated with saline achieving pressures of between 4 atm and 12 atm. The guide-catheter and balloons come in a range of angles and sizes for the various sinuses. Navigation can also be performed with calibrators. A standard inflation device is used (Fig. 17.5).[7,8]

In the majority of cases, the maxillary and sphenoid ostia require only a single inflation whereas the frontal recess, due to its longer outflow tract, may require repositioning and re-inflation of the balloon. Any other procedures that are indicated, such as septoplasty or turbinate surgery, should be performed following the dilatation so as to avoid bleeding and edema which may make passing the balloon catheter more problematic.

LacriCATH Device

The LacriCATH device (Quest Medical, Inc., Allen, TX) is used by ophthalmologists to dilate the lacrimal system to relieve nasolacrimal duct obstruction. They have been used off-label in the treatment of sinus ostia obstruction. The lacrimal duct balloons are soft and easily malleable into various angles. There is no guide-wire required and the balloon can be inflated up to

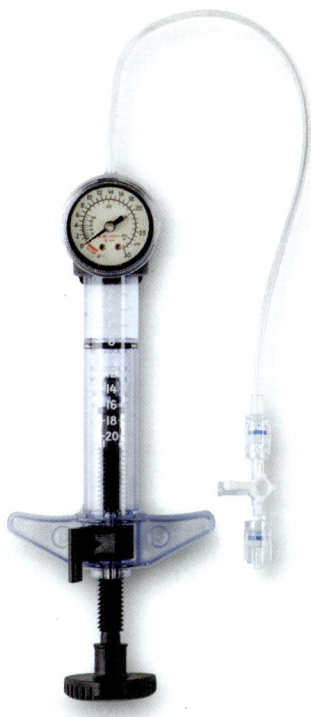

Fig. 17.5: Inflation device
Source: Courtesy of Acclarent, Inc.

8 atm with the ability to displace tissue and bone. A cadaveric study incorporating the LacriCATH device into FESS was performed without the use of fluoroscopy.[9,10] The frontal and sphenoid sinus dissection was successful using the balloon and standard surgical instruments. The maxillary sinus, however, was only successfully dilated in three of six sides due to difficulty passing the balloon into the sinus with an intact uncinate process. The conclusion was therefore that the lacrimal balloon could be incorporated into FESS as a composite or 'hybrid' approach. This approach obviated the requirement for fluoroscopy as catheter placement was facilitated by catheter guidance under endoscopic visualization. There was also a significant cost-saving compared to the Balloon Sinuplasty system, $300 versus $1,200.[9]

FinESS

The Functional Infundibular Endoscopic Sinus System, FinESS (Entellus Medical, Inc., Maple Grove, MN) cleared FDA approval in April 2008 and was launched in September 2008. This device uses a flexible endoscope (0.5 mm) and a dual-lumen cannula to locate the maxillary sinus ostia via the direct transantral route. A five or seven-millimeter balloon catheter can then be passed under direct endoscopic visualization into the ethmoid infundibulum and maxillary sinus ostium. The balloon is then inflated to 12 atm to dilate the outflow tract.[10,11] There are several advantages including no requirement for fluoroscopic guidance, minimal tissue trauma, and the procedure can be performed under local anesthetic making it an attractive option for office use. The prospective, multicenter Balloon Remodelling Antrostomy Therapy (BREATHE I) study evaluated the safety and feasibility of the device. Fifty-five of fifty-eight maxillary ostia were successfully dilated with 97% achieved under local anesthesia. CT scanning at 3 months confirmed ethmoid infundibulum and ostial patency in 95.8% and the Sinonasal Outcome Test (SNOT-20) improved at 6 months (from 2.9 to 0.8).[12] This gave some support to the use of the device in isolated maxillary sinus disease. However, the follow-up was short and it remains unclear whether it is applicable to a wider range of patients with CRS.

In 2010, Entellus launched XprESS, a dilation tool that can be used to treat the frontal, sphenoid and maxillary sinuses. It is a single, less invasive tool which can be used during functional endoscopic sinus surgery. It has a 2-mm atraumatic ball tip, similar to most sinus seekers, and also provides suction (Fig. 17.6). The XprESS, therefore, combines sinus seeker, balloon dilation and suction in a single tool which may provide improved efficiency in primary and revision FESS, as well as balloon only procedures. The tip of the device is malleable and can be reshaped for treatment of multiple sinuses and customized to the patients' anatomy.[13]

Ventera Sinus Dilation System

More recently, a new sinus dilation balloon and delivery instrument system has been introduced. The Ventera Sinus Dilation System (ENTrigue

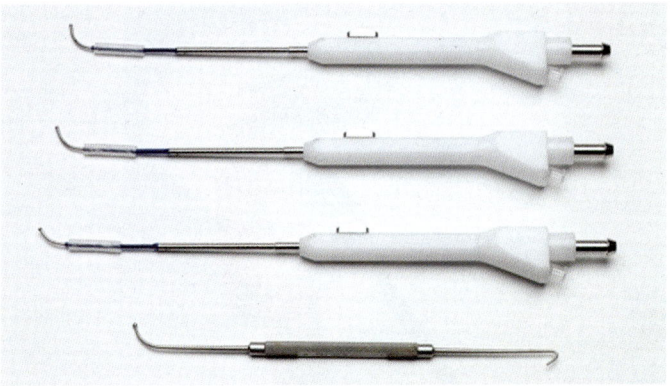

Fig. 17.6: The XprESS combines sinus seeker, balloon dilation, and suction in a single tool
Source: Courtesy of Entellus Medical, Inc.

Surgical, Inc., TX) consists of a disposable balloon and several reusable Articulating Delivery Instruments (Fig. 17.7). The sinus dilation balloon has a similar size (6 mm) and inflation pressures as other commercially available devices. The Articulating Delivery Instruments offer the advantage of allowing the surgeon to articulate the balloon into several positions to enable access into the desired sinus (Fig. 17.8). There is no guidewire or fluoroscopy required and the balloon is delivered using a handle portion similar to existing ENT instruments. This system is compatible with standard balloon inflation devices and is licensed in Canada but is not available for sale currently in the US.[14] This has the potential benefits of simplicity, improved handling, and is cost-effective due to the reusable delivery instruments with minimal disposables. It is being marketed as a useful addition to the instruments of a sinus surgeon but there is little clinical data available on its use and efficacy. Clinical trials are currently underway to evaluate this interesting system.

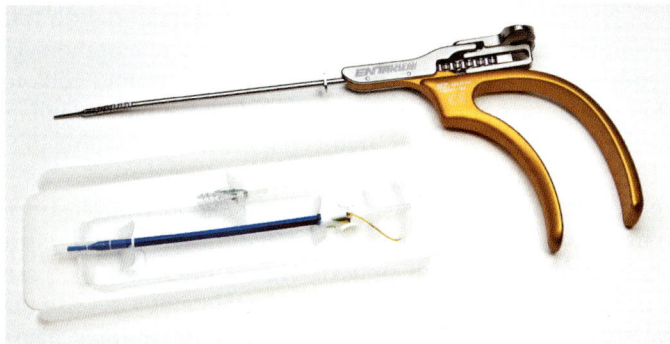

Fig. 17.7: The Ventera Sinus Dilation System consists of a disposable balloon and a reusable Articulating Delivery Instrument
Source: Courtesy of ENTrigue Surgical, Inc.

CHAPTER 17   Balloon Sinuplasty in the Treatment of Sinus Disease...   **339**

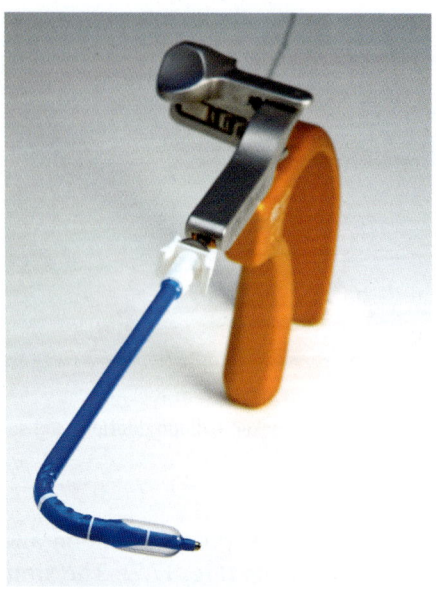

Fig. 17.8: The Articulating Delivery Instrument allows manipulation of the balloon to aid access to the desired sinus ostia

Source: Courtesy of ENTrigue Surgical, Inc.

Balloon-Only Versus Hybrid Procedure

The Balloon Sinuplasty device was initially marketed as an alternative to surgery for CRS patients and received a great deal of media attention. It is a misconception that these devices represent an alternative to surgery for all cases, but more accurately they can be classified as an instrument or tool that can be a useful addition to the surgeon's armamentarium in the treatment of patients with CRS.

In FESS, different techniques and instruments can be utilized to achieve the same end goal. In some cases, the balloon device is used as a 'stand-alone' device; however, their use in conjunction with traditional sinus instruments in a 'hybrid' fashion is much more common. This may involve endoscopic dissection of the obstructive ethmoid cells followed by dilation of the secondary sinuses (frontal, sphenoid, maxillary) ostia using the balloon device. Also, many patients will require FESS only, without balloon dilation.

There can be a patient perception that balloon sinuplasty does not involve cutting instrumentation or removal of tissue and therefore represents a nonsurgical treatment option. This is often not the case as the majority of patients with CRS will have ethmoid sinus disease that is not amenable solely to balloon dilatation. Many patients may also require additional surgery, such as nasal septal reconstruction or turbinate reduction. There is wide variability in how these devices are being used by individual surgeons. Some surgeons only use the balloon catheter in specific circumstances when they feel the technique provides definite advantages over other instruments. These indications may include 'high' obstruction in the frontal sinus not accessible by other instruments or repeated dilatation of recurrent stenosis of the frontal sinus. However, it appears that balloon sinuplasty is being used routinely by an increasing number of otolaryngologists.

Efficacy and Outcomes

Since its introduction in 2005, there have been many studies looking into the feasibility, safety and efficacy of the Balloon Sinuplasty system to treat CRS. The initial study used a cadaveric model to assess the feasibility and safety of the device.[6] All 31 ostia attempted were successfully dilated (11 frontal, 11 sphenoid and 9 maxillary). All were performed using fluoroscopic and endoscopic guidance. There was no orbital or skull base trauma noted on CT imaging. It was proposed following this study that Balloon Sinuplasty was feasible and may cause less mucosal trauma than the standard endoscopic techniques. The first human study was performed by Brown and Bolger involving 10 FESS patients.[15] Again, all planned sinus ostia were successfully dilated (10 maxillary, 5 sphenoid, 3 frontal) with no adverse events reported. Eight of the ten patients underwent a 'hybrid' procedure with concomitant ethmoidectomy. The maxillary sinus proved to be the most difficult to dilate and in approximately half of the cases, an uncinectomy was performed to confirm that the natural ostium was enlarged. The authors concluded that the device was easy to use and was well tolerated. However, there was a feeling by some otolaryngologists that the removal of normal tissue may be necessary for a long-term patency of the ostia and successful outcome.

It was following these initial studies that the controversy started. Acclarent Inc. increased their marketing campaign and there were several media reports emphasising the new technology, implying that Balloon Sinuplasty was a unique procedure and alternative to traditional FESS. This may have resulted in alteration of patient expectations and polarizing opinions. A period of controversy, debate, and confusion ensued with a variety of conflicting opinions and position statements generated by individuals and academic societies.[5,8,16-20] The emphasis of Balloon Sinuplasty then shifted to its role as a tool to be used in FESS, similar to the introduction of other instruments or technologies such as microdebriders, drills, or navigation systems.

The first multicenter trial was the Clinical Evaluation to Confirm Safety and Efficacy of Sinuplasty in the PaRanasal Sinuses (CLEAR) study.[21] This was a prospective, nonrandomised trial looking at 115 patients (358 sinuses) with CRS who had failed medical management and required FESS. Fifty-nine patients had a hybrid procedure while Fifty-six had sinuplasty alone. Six patients were unable to be cannulated and therefore excluded. At 24 weeks, the ostial patency rates were 91% for maxillary sinus, 82% for frontal sinus, and 61% for sphenoid sinus. However, large numbers of frontal and sphenoid sinus ostia could not be evaluated due to limited visualization during clinic endoscopy. The majority of these patients were not symptomatic. The overall patency of dilated ostia was 80.5%. The nonpatency rate was 1.6% with an 'indeterminate' rate of 17.9%. Of those that could be visualized, 98% were patent and 2% nonpatent. Patient symptom scores (SNOT-20) significantly improved from baseline in both balloon only and hybrid patient groups. In three sinuses (of three patients), a revision procedure was required, corresponding to a revision rate of 2.75%.

This cohort of patients was then followed up at 1 and 2 years.[22,23] Both studies demonstrated that significant improvements were maintained in Lund-Mackay CT scores and symptom scores (SNOT 20). At 1 year, ostial patency rates (assessed by a combination of CT and endoscopy) were 93% for maxillary sinus, 92% for frontal sinus and 86% for sphenoid sinus.[22] At 2 years, the same 65 patients (195 ballooned sinuses) were reevaluated. Again, the CT and symptom scores were significantly improved from baseline and stable compared to 6 months and 1 year in both hybrid and balloon only groups. Overall, 85% of patients reported an improvement of their symptoms, with 15% the same and 0% worse. Six patients required revision treatment, a revision rate of 9.2%.[23] These studies demonstrated that balloon sinuplasty is feasible and results in a significant improvement in symptoms that are maintained over a 2-year period.

However, many questions remain unanswered. The CLEAR and follow-up studies do not clearly define the patient population. The individual otolaryngologist at each site determined the diagnosis of CRS and appropriate medical and surgical management without defined criteria. The distribution of disease for this group of patients was not available and their low mean Lund-Mackay CT scores, suggesting mild disease, meant that it was unclear how applicable this study group was to the wider population of CRS patients.

The largest study on balloon sinuplasty is the retrospective review of balloon catheter use in sinus surgery in a multicenter registry of 1,036 patients across 27 otolaryngology practices.[24] The balloon catheters were used in 3,276 sinuses (maxillary, frontal, and sphenoid), an average of 3.2 sinuses per patient. Sinus symptoms improved in 95.2%, unchanged in 3.8%, and worse in 1.0% of patients. Revision surgery was required in 25 patients (2.4%). 73.8% of patients were free of infection in the follow-up period (average of 40.2 weeks) and overall postoperative sinus infections were less frequent and less severe than pre-surgery. This study did not define disease severity (CT/endoscopy) or their indications for surgery. Due to the lack of a comparator group in this and the CLEAR study, it is difficult to claim efficacy relative to FESS. Interestingly, if the results of the balloon only and hybrid groups (from CLEAR) are compared at 2 years, the hybrid group had higher preoperative SNOT-20 scores, suggesting more severe disease (2.42 vs. 2.14). The hybrid group improved to 0.64 at 2 years compared to 1.09 in the balloon-only group at the same point.[10,25]

This suggests that further comparative trials are necessary to better understand the role of sinuplasty in the management of CRS.

Friedman et al. compared FESS and balloon dilatation in a retrospective study of prospectively collected data.[26] The study included 70 patients (35 in each arm) and showed improvement in SNOT-20 scores in both groups at 3 months. The balloon group patients required less pain medication and reported higher satisfaction rates. However, this was a highly selective group of patients since patients with severe disease (Lund-Mackay ≥ 12) were excluded. In addition, the follow-up period was short (3 months) and the two groups were not randomised or matched, with the patients themselves selecting their treatment option.

■ Frontal Sinus

Frontal sinus disease continues to present a challenge to the sinus surgeon. There are many different surgical approaches to the frontal sinus and there is a higher failure rate in these patients. Surgeons can be nervous about dealing properly with the frontal recess due to the proximity of the skull base, anterior ethmoid artery, orbit and the unforgiving nature of this area. Failure can result from incomplete surgery, scar formation, mucosal stripping, edema and infection. The introduction of new angled-instrumentation, endoscopes and image guidance systems has resulted in more nonfellowship trained surgeons attempting to tackle this difficult area. In our experience, this has sometimes led to more destructive surgery with the use of powered instrumentation and drills often resulting in more complications related to osteogenesis and scarring of the frontal drainage pathway (Figs 17.9A and B). There is, therefore, a particular need

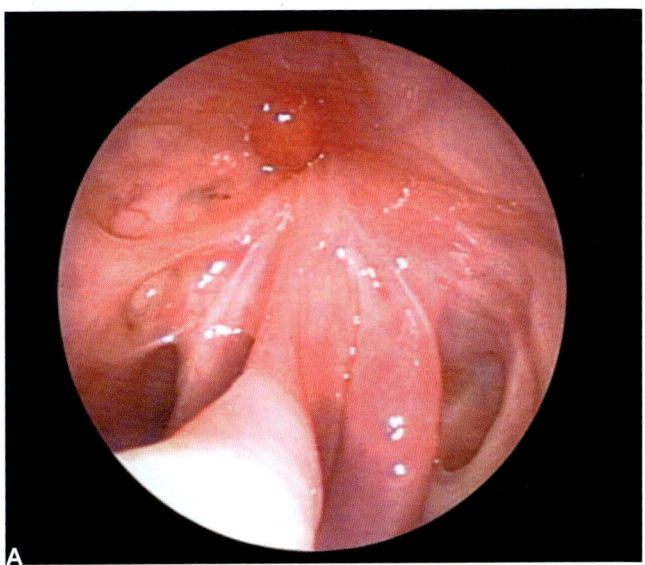

Fig. 17.9A

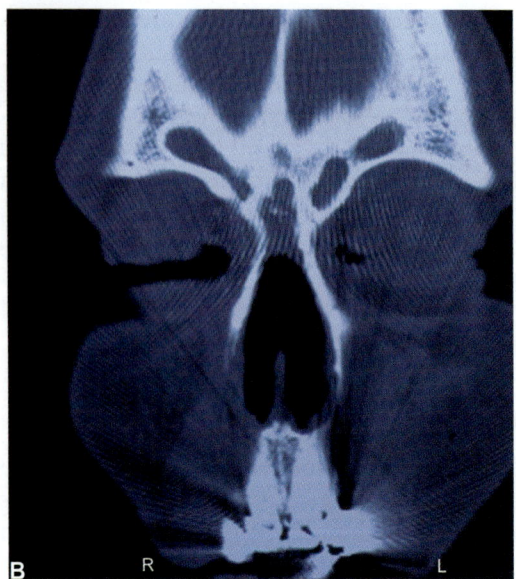

Fig. 17.9B

Figs 17.9A and B: Scarred nasal roof post-Lothrop procedure

and demand for a minimally invasive tool that can be used by the general otolaryngologist to work in the frontal recess while preserving mucosa (Figs 17.10 and 17.11). Catalano and Payne reviewed 20 patients who had undergone balloon dilatation of the frontal sinus outflow tract for

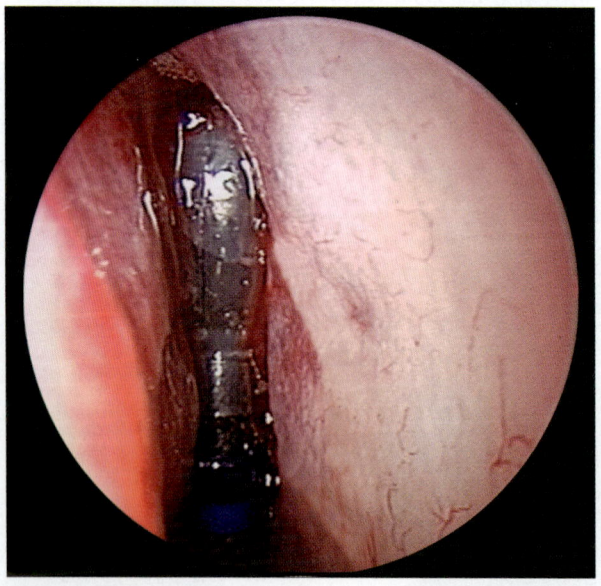

Fig. 17.10: Balloon inflated in the frontal recess
Source: Courtesy of Acclarent, Inc.

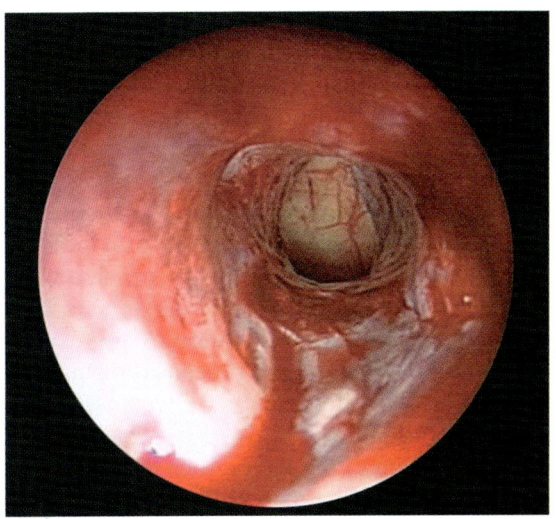

Fig. 17.11: Open frontal sinus ostia following balloon dialatation
Source: Courtesy of Acclarent, Inc.

chronic frontal sinusitis.[27] Improvements in imaging scores were noted in 48.3% of frontal sinuses with the best results seen in CRS patients without polyps (61.5%). These success rates are lower than those which have previously been reported for primary and secondary endoscopic frontal sinusotomy.[28-30] However, Plaza et al. have recently published the first randomised controlled clinical trial using balloon dilation of the frontal recess.[31] Thirty four patients were randomised into two treatment groups: hybrid versus FESS only (Draf 1 or 2a). Unlike many of the previous studies, there were well defined inclusion criteria. All patients met the criteria for CRS defined by the European Position Paper on Rhinosinusitis and Nasal Polyposis, and presented with nasal polyposis. They had total opacification of either frontal sinus (Lund-Mackay stage 2) and had failed an 8-week course of oral steroids, antibiotics and nasal saline irrigations. In all cases, polypectomy, uncinectomy, wide middle meatal maxillary antrostomy, and anterior ethmoidectomy were performed. Posterior ethmoidectomy and sphenoidotomy were performed as required dictated by the disease. Those patients allocated to the hybrid group had dilation of the frontal sinus outflow tract with a Relieva sinus catheter (Acclarent) under fluoroscopic control. The FESS group were treated with a Draf 1 or 2a procedure. 80.76% of frontal recesses were successfully dilated in the hybrid group and 91.7% in the FESS-only group. The lower success rate with the balloon was attributed to difficult frontal sinus anatomy and osteitis obstructing access. At 12 months following surgery, they demonstrated a statistically significant reduction in Lund-Mackay stage in both groups, related specifically to the frontal sinus and in general. The resolution of frontal sinus disease on CT was not significantly different between the two treatment arms, but seemed to be slightly more frequent following balloon dilation. The patency of the frontal recess seen by office endoscopy was statistically more frequent after balloon treatment (75% versus 63%), although, the treatment effect appears to be small. Visual analogue scales and Rhinosinusitis Disability Index Scores also decreased significantly in both groups, but no comparison was made between the two groups. Four patients required further surgery, one after balloon dilation (6.25%) and three after FESS only (18.75%).

No sample size calculation was performed to ensure adequate power to the study; instead, it was based purely on 'previous articles on sinuplasty'. There is, therefore, a risk that the group size was not adequate to detect a difference. However, the study was done independently from Acclarent and showed that balloon dilatation can be used successfully in cases of CRS with polyps as a hybrid procedure in the operating room. The authors found that the balloon catheter was useful in the treatment of the frontal sinus in patients with nasal polyposis as most of the frontal sinus opacification was due to mucous rather than polyps and therefore, tissue removal was not necessary in this area. It appears that careful patient selection and detailed assessment of the anatomy on CT imaging to assess feasibility of balloon use is necessary and important. This is supported by a recent study by Heimagartner et al. who looked into the etiology of failed access to the frontal sinus.[32] Out of 104 frontal sinuses operated on, dilation failed in 12 (12%). CT analysis was carried out on all of the patients with failed access and all cases revealed variations in the frontal recess anatomy (e.g. frontoethmoidal-cell, frontal-bulla-cell, agger nasi cell) or osteogenesis.

Use in Children

Functional endoscopic sinus surgery in children is far less common; however, the indications for surgery remain the same as in the adult population. When medical therapy fails in children, a minimally invasive device, such as the balloon catheter, with the ability to irrigate the sinuses would appear to be extremely useful. There are, however, very few studies looking at the use of balloon catheters in the pediatric population. The safety and feasibility of balloon sinuplasty in children as young as 4 years of age has been reported by Ramadan.[33] Successful cannulation was achieved in 91% of sinuses and no complications were noted. The average fluoroscopy exposure time was 18 seconds per sinus, with a range of 6–60 seconds per sinus. Adenoidectomy was also performed when indicated along with saline sinus irrigation. These patients were also included in a larger study looking at the quality of life of those treated with balloon sinuplasty with irrigation and adenoidectomy versus adenoidectomy alone. The results showed an improvement in symptoms after 12 months follow-up in 80% of the balloon group compared to 52% in the adenoidectomy alone group.[34] It is difficult to determine the impact of balloon dilation from these studies as maxillary sinus saline washes in addition to adenoidectomy have been shown to increase success rates versus adenoidectomy alone.[35] It is, therefore, unclear whether sinus dilation gives any additional benefit over irrigation alone in children also under-going adenoidectomy. It may be that patients with sphenoid or frontal disease, which are more difficult to irrigate, may be suitable for balloon dilation. However, it would be prudent to say that whilst studies have suggested safety of balloon catheter use in children, there is much more work required in this patient population before we can conclude whether it is effective, and if so, which patient groups would benefit most.

Complications

The placement of a balloon catheter into an enclosed space (sinus outflow tract) with subsequent inflation to a high atmospheric pressure results in the application of considerable direct force to the sinus ostia and surrounding tissue which could potentially lead to trauma and injury to adjacent structures. The original cadaveric study showed microfractures in the sinus ostial regions but there was no trauma noted to the orbit or skull base. In fact, the initial balloon catheter studies did not report any adverse events or complications.[15,21-23] The multicenter registry reports a total of eight complications, including six cases of minor bleeding requiring cautery or packing, and two CSF leaks.[24] The complications all occurred in the hybrid procedures and the rate of CSF leak in these cases was 0.3%. There were no reported complications in the balloon-only proce-dures. The Manufacturer and User Facility Device Experience (MAUDE) reported 18 incidents with Balloon Sinuplasty.[36] These included five CSF leaks, four orbital injuries, seven device malfunctions and two bleeding episodes requiring surgical intervention. Considering the number of balloon dilations performed, there seems to be a low number of reported complications. Overall, it appears to be a safe procedure. Another safety concern with the use of balloon catheters was the radiation dose during fluoroscopy to guide correct balloon placement. The main concern with fluoroscopy use is cataract formation and the development of malignan-cies if high or prolonged doses are used. A review of radiation expo-sure from fluoroscopy-guided balloon dilation of 108 sinuses noted low doses and fluoroscopy times.[37] An average dose of 4.2 mGy per eye was reported. This is much less than the 2 Gy acute dose or protracted expo-sure of 4 Gy for less than 3 months that might cause cataract formation.[38] The authors concluded that over 50,000 dilatations per year would need to be performed by a surgeon before reaching the occupational limit for the hand and 6,000 for the eyes, with fluoroscopy orientated in the poste-rior-anterior direction. Chandra estimated that the mean radiation dose to the lens per unit fluoroscopy time was 0.041 mGy/sec for the right eye, and 0.284 mGy/sec to the left eye by extrapolating data from fluoroscopi-cally guided balloon dacryocystoplasty.[39] If the threshold for lenticular opacity is estimated at 500 mGy, this would be attained in the left eye after approximately 29 minutes of fluoroscopy. The potentially higher dose of radiation received by the left eye is due to its proximity to the source during lateral projection. The total time of fluoroscopy will vary from case to case, depending on the number of sinuses requiring dilatation, the complexity of the anatomy and the experience and expertise of the surgeon. In Plaza's recent study, the mean duration of fluoroscopy was 3.2 minutes (range: 2.2–7.1 minutes), however, balloon dilation was only used for the frontal sinuses.[31] Therefore, radiation exposure should remain a concern for balloon catheter dilation. The need for fluoroscopy has been reduced due to the advent of lighted guide-wires, image-guided devices and newer-generation devices which are easier to use and place accurately in the correct position under endoscopic visualization. Friedmann and Wilson showed equivalent success rates in cannulation of the maxillary and frontal sinuses using fluoroscopy or transillumination-guided guide wire placement.[40] They found that transillumination was cheaper and resulted in shorter operating times. Transillumination cannot be used for the sphenoid sinus, however, the sphenoid ostium can be directly visualized without the need for either guidance technique. Transillumination of the frontal and maxillary sinuses seem to provide a real alternative to fluoroscopy and is useful in reducing radiation exposure associated with balloon sinuplasty procedures.

■ Cost

The majority of the balloon catheter systems on the market are single-use. However, a single balloon can be used to dilate multiple ostia during the same sitting. The cost of the Balloon Sinuplasty device (Acclarent, Menlo park, CA) is about $1200. The Ventera balloon is $325 and the reusable delivery instrument is $1500. Friedmann et al. found that the cost for primary procedures was similar between FESS and balloon dilation, whereas the cost for revision surgery using the balloon device was considerably less.[26] This was due to shorter revision surgery times with the balloon device and also shorter recovery and operating room time in patients undergoing surgery with local anesthesia. Thirty-one percent (all in the balloon dilation group) had surgery under local anesthetic. These savings would not be applicable for balloon use in 'hybrid' procedures as general anesthesia is usually required. A further study showed that using the Luma light reduced the cost by $454.00 or 37.5% compared to the use of fluoroscopy for guide-wire placement.[40] The operative time was also less using the Luma light. This further saving was not included in the cost comparison.

■ Future

The literature to date on balloon dilatation of the sinuses attests to the safety, feasibility and ability to achieve sinus ostia patency for up to 2 years. However, due to a lack of a comparative group in the majority of studies and poorly defined selection criteria, it still remains unclear if the current data can be applied to the general population with CRS. Also, many questions remain to be clearly answered; the main one being: are balloon dilation devices more effective than existing instruments used in FESS for the management of CRS? The recent Cochrane review on functional endoscopic balloon dilation of sinus ostia concluded that at present, there is no evidence to support its use above conventional surgical modalities in the management of CRS following failed medical management.[41] However, it would appear that balloon dilation devices have a useful role as a tool in the surgeon's armamentarium in the operating room. Certain anatomical variations lend themselves to balloon use such as high obstruction in the frontal sinus (e.g. Type III frontal cell) that can be difficult to access with traditional FESS instrumentation and may otherwise require a combined endoscopic and external approach. It has been suggested that the balloon catheter may be a safe and effective surgical option to treat immunocompromised and critically ill patients, acute rhinosinusitis, and revision cases.[42-44] Critically ill patients often have associated hematologic disorders such as thrombocytopenia, neutropenia and anemia. These patients would benefit from a noncutting minimally traumatic approach. This would be an additional role for the technology but again, further research is required before this becomes an accepted indication. The main indication for its use remains the same as for FESS, which is failed medical management for CRS. Since the majority of CRS patients have ethmoid disease and may also require adjunct procedures such as septoplasty or turbinate reduction, balloon catheter dilatation may not be effective by itself but could be useful as an adjunctive tool together with traditional FESS in the form of a hybrid procedure. The indications for its use are evolving and may expand to include patients with less severe disease than would have traditionally been considered for FESS. It has been suggested that patients with extensive mucosal disease and nasal polyposis are not generally candidates for balloon dilation alone due to the requirement for some tissue removal. However, Plaza et al. showed that the balloon sinuplasty device can play a role in the management of patients with nasal polyposis by incorporating its use into FESS.[31] The balloon dilation devices have increased the surgical options available to the sinus surgeon and provided an important and effective tool that can be very useful if used appropriately by the sinus surgeon. Further research is required to better define its indications and identify the patient groups that will benefit the most from this technology.

Futuristic dilatational devices that are currently being developed include slowly dilating stents that can be left *in situ* for prolonged and varying periods of time from 1 hour to 1 month; such devices would reduce the risk of trauma to surrounding tissue and would serve a dual purpose of dilating the ostia as well as providing a stent over a defined period of time. Exciting developments in the field of drug eluting stents may also be combined with such slow dilating stents creating a triple purpose dilatational device. Made to order balloon dilatational devices are also in the developmental phase; surgeons will be able to order the speed and pressure to which the balloon dilates and the drug that the surgeon wants to have eluting from the stent. The past decade popularized a strong trend toward larger openings and mucus membrane destruction of the frontal recess with drill-out procedures leaving behind a large number of patients with crippled and nonfunctional frontal sinuses. However, significant research and development continues in the field of balloon dilation surgery with the next decade likely providing a complete change in the surgical treatment of the frontal sinus from one of drilling and mucus membrane destruction to one of more physiologically sound mucous membrane preservation methodologies. In our opinion, a much-needed change is in the making and the pendulum may be swinging once again in the correct direction thanks to the development of these novel devices.

REFERENCES

1. Pleis JR, Ward BW, Lucas JW. Summary health statistics for U.S. adults: National Health Interview Survey, 2009. Vital Health Stat 10. 2010;(249);1-207.
2. Schappert SM, Rechtsteiner EA. Ambulatory medical care utilization estimates for 2007. Vital Health Stat 13. 2011;(169):1-38.
3. Fokkens W, Lund V, Mullol J, et al. European position paper on rhinosinusitis and nasal polyps 2007. Rhinol Suppl. 2007;(20):1–136.
4. Anand VK. Epidemiology and economic impact of rhinosinusitis. Ann Otol Rhinol Laryngol Suppl. 2004;193:3-5.
5. Vaughan WC. Review of balloon sinuplasty. Curr Opin Otolaryngol Head Neck Surg. 2008;16(1):2-9.
6. Bolger WE, Vaughan WC. Catheter-based dilation of the sinus ostia: initial safety and feasibility analysis in a cadaver model. Am J Rhinol. 2006;20(3):290-4.
7. Acclarent. Balloon Sinuplasty™ Technology. [online] Available from http:// www.acclarent.com/solutions/sinusitis-overview/balloon-sinuplasty/. [Accessed September, 2011].
8. Stewart AE, Vaughan WC. Balloon sinuplasty versus surgical management of chronic rhinosinusitis. Curr Allergy Asthma Rep. 2010;10(3):181-7.
9. Citardi MJ, Kanowitz SJ. A cadaveric model for balloon-assisted endoscopic paranasal sinus dissection without fluoroscopy. Am J Rhinol. 2007; 21(5):579-83.
10. Batra PS, Ryan MW, Sindwani R, et al. Balloon catheter technology in rhinology: Reviewing the evidence. Laryngoscope. 2011;121(1):226-32.
11. Entellus Medical, Inc. Take The Direct Approach. [online] Available from http:// www.entellusmedical.com/finess_overview.htm. [Accessed September, 2011].
12. Stankiewicz J, Tami T, Truitt T, et al. Transantral, endoscopically guided balloon dilatation of the ostiomeatal complex for chronic rhinosinusitis under local anesthesia. Am J Rhinol Allergy. 2009;23(3):321-7.
13. Entellus Medical, Inc. Treat Multiple Sinuses with a Single Multi-Functional Tool. [online] Available from http://www.entellusmedical.com/xpress_ overview.htm. [Accessed September, 2011].
14. ENTrigue Surgical, Inc. Ventera Sinus Dilation System. [online] Available from http://www.entriguesurgical.com/home/outside_US_products/ ventera. [Accessed September, 2011].

15. Brown CL, Bolger WE. Safety and feasibility of balloon catheter dilation of paranasal sinus ostia: a preliminary investigation. Ann Otol Rhinol Laryngol. 2006;115(4):293-9.

16. Lanza DC, Kennedy DW. Balloon sinuplasty: not ready for prime time. Ann Otol Rhinol Laryngol. 2006;115(10):789-90.

17. Bolger WE. Commentary: Misconceptions regarding balloon dilation of paranasal sinus ostia. Ann Otol Rhinol Laryngol. 2006;115:791-2.

18. Jones N. Commentary on safety and feasibility of balloon catheter dilation of paranasal sinus ostia: preliminary investigation. Ann Otol Rhinol Laryngol. 2006;115:300-1.

19. American Rhinologic Society (ARS). Revised Position Statement on Balloon Sinuplasty.[online] Available from http://www.american-rhinologic.org/position_balloon_sinuplasty. [Accessed May, 2007].

20. AAO-HNS. Revised position statement on dilation of sinuses. [online] Available from http://www.entnet.org/Practice/Balloon-Dilation.cfm. [Accessed March, 2007].

21. Bolger WE, Brown CL, Church CA, et al. Safety and outcomes of balloon catheter sinusotomy: a multicenter 24-week analysis in 115 patients. Otolaryngol Head Neck Surg. 2007;137(1):10-20.

22. Kuhn FA, Church CA, Goldberg AN, et al. Balloon catheter sinusotomy: one-year follow-up--outcomes and role in functional endoscopic sinus surgery. Otolaryngol Head Neck Surg. 2008;139(3 Suppl 3):S27-37.

23. Weiss RL, Church CA, Kuhn FA, et al. Long-term outcome analysis of balloon catheter sinusotomy: two-year follow-up. Otolaryngol Head Neck Surg. 2008;139(3 Suppl 3):S38-46.

24. Levine HL, Sertich AP 2nd, Hoisington DR, et al. Multicenter registry of balloon catheter sinusotomy outcomes for 1,036 Patients. Ann Otol Rhinol Laryngol. 2008;117(4):263-70.

25. Marple BF, Stringer SP, Batra PS, et al. Going to the next level: health care's evolving expectations for evidence. Otolaryngol Head Neck Surg. 2009;141(5):551-4.

26. Friedman M, Schalch P, Lin HC, et al. Functional endoscopic dilatation of the sinuses: patient satisfaction, postoperative pain, and cost. Am J Rhinol. 2008;22(2):204-9.

27. Catalano PJ, Payne SC. Balloon dilation of the frontal recess in patients with chronic frontal sinusitis and advanced sinus disease: an initial report. Ann Otol Rhinol Laryngol. 2009;118(2):107-12.

28. Chandra RK, Palmer JN, Tangsujarittham T, et al. Factors associated with failure of frontal sinusotomy in the early follow-up period. Otolaryngol Head Neck Surg. 2004;131(4):514-8.

29. Philpott CM, Thamboo A, Lai L, et al. Endoscopic frontal sinusotomy-preventing recurrence or a route to revision? Laryngoscope. 2010;120(8): 1682-6.

30. Chiu AG, Vaughan WC. Revision endoscopic frontal sinus surgery with surgical navigation. Otolaryngol Head Neck Surg. 2004;130(3):312-8.

31. Plaza G, Eisenberg G, Montojo J, et al. Balloon dilation of the frontal recess: a randomized clinical trial. Ann Otol Rhinol Laryngol. 2011;120(8):511-8.

32. Heimgartner S, Eckardt J, Simmen D, et al. Limitations of balloon sinuplasty in frontal sinus surgery. Eur Arch Otorhinolaryngol. 2011;268(10):1463-7.

33. Ramadan HH. Safety and feasibility of balloon sinuplasty for the treatment of chronic rhinosinusitis in children. Ann Otol Rhinol Laryngol. 2009;118(3):161-5.

34. Ramadan HH, Terrell AM. Balloon catheter sinuplasty and adenoidectomy in children with chronic rhinosinusitis. Ann Otol Rhinol Laryngol. 2010;119(9):578-82.

35. Ramadan HH, Cost JL. Outcome of adenoidectomy versus adenoidectomy with maxillary sinus wash for chronic rhinosinusitis in children. Laryngoscope. 2008;118(5):871-3.

36. US FDA. Manufacturer and user facility device experience (MAUDE) database. [online] Available from www.accessdata.fda.gov/scripts/cdrh/cfdocs/cfmaude/search.cfm. [Accessed August, 2011].

37. Church CA, Kuhn FA, Mikhail J, et al. Patient and surgeon radiation exposure in balloon catheter sinus ostial dilation. Otolaryngol Head Neck Surg. 2008;138(2):187-91.

38. Zammit-Maempel I, Chadwick CL, Willis SP. Radiation dose to the lens of eye and thyroid gland in paranasal sinus multislice CT. Br J Radiol. 2003;76(906):418-20.

39. Chandra RK. Estimate of radiation dose to the lens in balloon sinuplasty. Otolaryngol Head Neck Surg. 2007;137(6):953-5.

40. Friedman M, Wilson M. Illumination guided balloon sinuplasty. Laryngoscope. 2009;119(7):1399-402.

41. Ahmed J, Pal S, Hopkins C, et al. Functional endoscopic balloon dilation of sinus ostia for chronic rhinosinusitis. Cochrane Database Syst Rev. 2011;(7):CD008515.

42. Wittkopf ML, Becker SS, Duncavage JA, et al. Balloon sinuplasty for the surgical management of immunocompromised and critically ill patients with acute rhinosinusitis. Otolaryngol Head Neck Surg. 2009;140(4):596-8.

43. Hopkins C, Noon E, Roberts D. Balloon sinuplasty in acute frontal sinusitis. Rhinology. 2009;47(4):375-8.

44. Wycherly BJ, Manes RP, Mikula SK. Initial clinical experience with balloon dilation in revision frontal sinus surgery. Ann Otol Rhinol Laryngol. 2010;119(7):468-71.

Index

Page numbers followed by *f* refer to figure and *t* refer to table